HANDBOOK OF CONTEMPORARY CHINESE PULSE DIAGNOSIS

HANDBOOK OF
Contemporary Chinese
Pulse Diagnosis

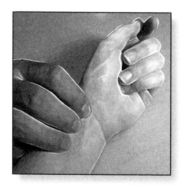

EDITED BY
Leon Hammer, M.D. & Karen Bilton, L.Ac.

EASTLAND PRESS ▶ SEATTLE

Published by Eastland Press, Inc.
P.O. Box 99749
Seattle, WA 98139, USA
www.eastlandpress.com

Library of Congress Control Number: 2012933267
ISBN: 978-0-939616-76-3

2   4   6   8   10   9   7   5   3

Cover design by Gary Niemeier
Book design by Gary Niemeier

Table of Contents

Human life depends on the pulse. The ten pulse types parallel the types of song. Therefore, healing requires knowing the pulses, and then knowing what song to use as a remedy.

Laying on of hand confers wisdom. Thus, Moses laid his hand on Joshua to give him wisdom. The Torah says, 'Joshua, son of Nun, was full of the spirit of wisdom because Moses had laid his hands upon . . . him.' Joshua thus became a man 'who has wind-spirit in him.' This meant that he knew how to determine each person's wind-spirit, which is manifested in that person's pulse.

—The Stories of Rabbi Nachman of Breslov

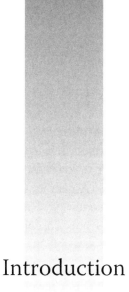

Introduction

This handbook summarizes the key elements of *Chinese Pulse Diagnosis: A Contemporary Approach* in a portable edition. It is the result of the very hard work, by many people, of extracting the essentials from each area of this subject. The names of these contributors are associated with individual chapters. To each of them I am eternally grateful, especially Karen Bilton, L.Ac., for her overall editing and with whom I collaborated throughout. In addition to Karen, other contributors include Oliver Nash, Jamin Nichols, Ross Rosen, Hamilton Rotte, and Brandt Stickley.

Particular recognition is accorded Wen-Huai (Richard) Chang, CMD, DDS, of Taiwan, who was responsible for an exhaustive comparative review of *Chinese Pulse Diagnosis: A Contemporary Approach* and this handbook, and for the very valuable corrections and suggestions that were incorporated into this book.

My deepest regard, respect, and gratitude is extended to Eastland Press and to John O'Connor, who conceived the idea for this handbook. I would also like to thank Chris Flanagan and Kira Isacoff for their perceptive and precise editing.

I am likewise indebted to others who did not directly contribute to the handbook but whose work over the years has deepened and enlarged our view of this subject. Among them are Sybill Huessen and Scott Tower in Europe, Elizebeth Pelzner, Brian La Forgia, and Celia Dermont in California, Helen Miller in the midwest, Lsisha Canner in Florida, Robee Fian and Phyllis Bloom in New York.

I wish to express my special appreciation to my longest continuous student and associate, Robert Heffron, M.D., who, with Marie Dauenheimer, contributed the graphic representations of the principal pulse qualities in this book. I am also grateful to Bruce Wang for his drawings that illustrate the positions of the fingers in taking the pulse.

I wish once more to thank Karen Bilton for her singular research on the reliability of this pulse system, the subject of her doctoral thesis[1] at the University of Technology in Sydney, Australia, which establishes the inter and intra rater reliability of the pulse system.

Where there is a difference in content between *Chinese Pulse Diagnosis: A Contemporary Approach* and this handbook, the handbook should be accepted as more correct due to new information or simply past regrettable error. For example, in Ch. 3 and throughout the handbook I have corrected a long-standing error with regard to intensity and amplitude in which I have used the term 'intensity' when the term should have been 'amplitude'. Similarly, we have replaced the term 'intensity' and substituted 'width' where the breadth of the pulse is involved (Ch. 10).

I wish to note in passing that in either book when the term 'heat from excess' is used, my meaning is 'excess heat', and when the term 'heat from deficiency' is used, I mean 'deficient heat'. 'Heat from' describes etiology whereas my intention is to indicate a condition. With this volume I have also begun to eliminate some of the special terms such as 'Heart large' that were introduced by my teacher, Dr. John Shen, for which Chinese conditions have long been introduced and which were never clinically informative. These terms, however, are defined in the glossary at the back.

In *Currents of Tradition in Chinese Medicine 1626–2006*, Volker Scheid traces Dr. Shen's lineage back hundreds of years to some of the most illustrious Chinese physicians of the Ding lineage and the Menghe current. Shen's photo and a brief biography are included in that text, and reference is made to *Chinese Pulse Diagnosis: A Contemporary Approach* in the bibliography and endnotes.[2] While Dr. Shen, over the years, often mentioned his study and apprenticeship with the Ding family's College of Chinese Medicine in Shanghai, he never elaborated on the extensive degree to which he borrowed from this tradition, as shown, for example, in the writings of Ding Gan-Ren (see Ch. 2).

The pulse diagnosis system presented in this book has been taught around the world as Contemporary Chinese Pulse Diagnosis, or the Shen-Hammer pulse system. A list of individuals who have been trained and certified as qualified instructors in this system can be found at the website of Dragon Rises Seminars, *www.dragonrises.org*.

---

1. Karen Bilton, "Investigating the Reliability of Contemporary Chinese Pulse Diagnosis." *Australian Journal of Acupuncture and Chinese Medicine;* Volume 5, Issue 1, 2010.

2. Volker Scheid, *Currents of Tradition in Chinese Medicine 1626–2006* (Seattle: Eastland Press, 2007): 393-94, 481, 494.

Mistakes are made and corrected as quickly as they are recognized. They constitute a small percentage of the total volume of information that I have shaped from my apprenticeships and clinical experience. Those who see the gold in the raw ore of this information and help me separate one from the other know that, at my age, no one has time for the perfection that, if accepted, will be their burden to bear.

A full list of pulse qualities, together with brief descriptions of their associated sensations and interpretations as we currently understand them, will be posted at the Resources tab of the Eastland Press website:

www.eastlandpress.com/resources/

Finally, my work here and elsewhere must be seen as work in progress in which I am constantly learning and passing on information. Findings in this pulse system are often early signs of disharmony not yet detectable by biomedical methodology. The emergence of the Choppy quality, once rare and now common, as a sign of the escalating environmental chemical and inhalant toxicity, and the Leather-Hard quality as a sign of the massive increase in electromagnetic fields, are examples of the changes that Chinese medicine and pulse diagnosis must make to reflect the changes that occur in society. Despite its long lineage, it is for this reason that this method of pulse diagnosis is called 'contemporary'.

— Leon Hammer, M.D.

1

Preliminary Reflections

Oliver Nash, L.Ac., M.B.Ac.C.

In our experience, the method of pulse diagnosis set forth in this book, which we call Contemporary Chinese Pulse Diagnosis, is unsurpassed in obtaining the greatest amount of physical and psychological information about an individual. We call it *contemporary* because it recognizes that pulse diagnosis must continue to develop over time. During the past century, at the hands of master pulse diagnostician Dr. John Shen and his apprentice Dr. Leon Hammer, it has evolved to better reflect our modern lifestyles. It is our intention to keep this system contemporary in our ever-changing world through its continuing development and refinement by generations of practitioners to come.

TRADITION AND REVISION

This system of pulse diagnosis draws on the classical traditions of Chinese medicine (Table 2-1), for which we have the greatest respect. However, we remain mindful of the fact that centuries of development within the oral traditions of Chinese medicine have seen this system evolve considerably.

For example, the severe, acute medical disorders mentioned by the ancients that were characteristic of preindustrial agricultural societies—things such as malarial disorder and internal cold obstruction—are rarely seen today by most practitioners in the West; our screened houses and central-heating systems lessen our exposure to the natural world. Instead, practitioners are more often confronted with chronic disease largely due to a variety of stresses: emotional, physical, chemical. Furthermore, today most acute symptoms are treated with modern biomedical modalities. As our work has evolved from treating mainly acute to mainly chronic phases of disharmony, the interpretation of pulse qualities such as Tense, Tight, and Wiry has also changed.

Despite the importance we place upon the classical traditions of Chinese medicine, it is dangerous to base treatments on interpretations of the pulse that are inconsistent with contemporary living conditions. If we interpret a Tight pulse to indicate acute cold stagnation when in fact there is chronic yin-deficient heat, we are obviously working against the patient's best interest. The classification and interpretation of pulse qualities in this book are, we believe, more in keeping with current clinical experience and allow for a more logical and rational treatment program.

Not only has the interpretation of some pulse qualities evolved, so too has the clarity of the nomenclature. An example of this can be seen in Wang Shu-He's description of the Choppy pulse quality. In his influential third-century text *The Pulse Classic (Mai Jing)*, Wang describes the Choppy pulse as "fine and slow, coming and going with difficulty and scattered or with interruption, but has the ability to recover." [1] Commentators on the pulse have repeated this description verbatim for nearly two millennia, [2] yet the terminology is confusing. In his attempt to describe the sensation of the Choppy quality, Wang is using terms that are themselves distinct pulse qualities, each of which has markedly different significance from that of the Choppy quality itself. While these other qualities—fine, slow, scattered, interrupted—may on occasion coexist simultaneously with the Choppy quality, they do not have the same meaning. Instead, they may signify one of its etiologies or represent a related yet distinct condition. [3]

Wang associated the Choppy quality with blood stasis or stagnation, but the use of a pulse quality such as "slow" to describe its sensation is misleading. The Slow quality often signifies Heart qi deficiency and impaired circulation. Since qi moves the blood, it would be correct to say that qi deficiency is one cause of blood stagnation. However, it does not follow that the Slow quality (revealing qi deficiency) is therefore necessarily a sign of blood stagnation, any more than the Choppy quality (revealing blood stagnation) is necessarily a sign of qi deficiency. Obviously, to treat a patient with qi deficiency for nonexistent blood stagnation could be very harmful to his health.

We have attempted here to clarify often confusing traditional terminology, particularly with regard to descriptions of pulse quality sensations, and for some qualities we have presented what we consider to be more clinically relevant interpretations.

TERMINOLOGY

Only the pulse qualities, the special complementary pulse positions, and the names of the organs in the traditional medical system are capitalized in this book. Terms unique to Dr. Shen, such as 'qi wild' and 'Heart nervous', enclosed by single quotation marks, are briefly defined in the glossary.

The term *principal position* refers primarily to the six major traditional individual positions: the distal, middle, and proximal positions of the radial pulses on both wrists. The term *complementary position* is used to refer to certain parts of the anatomy and physiology that are represented on the pulse, located proximally, distally, medially, laterally, or between the distal, middle, and proximal principal positions.

The term *level* refers to the three burners: upper, middle and lower. The term *depth* refers to the vertical layers—qi, blood, and organ—from the top of the pulse, just below the surface of the skin, to the bottom, above the bone. The term *function* refers to the natural function of an organism or one part of the organism. *Yin organ* refers to a solid organ and *yang organ* to a hollow one.

CLASSIFICATION AND NOMENCLATURE

GENERAL COMMENTS

Table 1-1 provides a comparison of the most widely used English terms for the principal pulse qualities and reveals the current confusion among the differing nomenclatures in Chinese medical terminology. This book offers a uniform nomenclature based on sensations easily recognized by those familiar with the English language.

Many of the qualities described in this book do not appear in Table 1-1. One reason for this is that some of our sensory descriptions and interpretations differ from those of the texts referenced in the table, another is that we have simply identified more qualities than are listed in those texts. Each quality (sensation) delineated by Contemporary Chinese Pulse Diagnosis (CCPD) has been confirmed by many practitioners over many years.

CLASSIFICATION BY SENSATION OR BY CONDITION

Pulse classification should be organized on the basis of the experience of the clinician, who first accesses the pulse through his sense of touch before making mental associations with those sensations. The nomenclature used in this book is therefore organized according to these sensations. For example, we perceive Tight before we diagnose yin-deficient heat, although with experience these two processes become nearly synonymous.

One example of how our descriptions differ from those used elsewhere is seen with the Wide quality. In traditional texts this quality is referred to as 'big' or 'large', yet descriptions of the physical sensation associated with the quality emphasize its width; Wu Shui-Wan, for example, notes that it is "twice as wide as a normal pulse."[4] As neither 'big' nor 'large' clearly conveys the principal identifying sensation of width, we use the term Wide as a more accurate label for

Table 1-1 Comparison of pulse terminology in English

Chinese	The Pulse Classic Wang Shu-He, trans. Yang Shou-Zhong	The Web That Has No Weaver Ted Kaptchuk	Practical Diagnosis in Traditional Chinese Medicine, Deng Tietao, trans. Marnae Ergil	Pulse Diagnosis Li Shi-Zhen, trans. Hoe Ku Huynh
Fú 浮	Floating	Floating	Floating	Floating
Chén 沉	Deep	Sinking	Deep	Deep
Chí 遲	Slow	Slow	Slow	Slow
Shùo 數	Rapid	Rapid	Rapid	Rapid
Xū 虛	Vacuous	Empty	Vacuous	Empty
Shí 實	Replete	Full	Replete	Full
Huá 滑	Slippery	Slippery	Slippery	Slippery
Sè 澀	Choppy	Choppy	Rough	Choppy
Cháng 長	---	Long	Long	Long
Duǎn 短	---	Short	Short	Short
Hóng 洪	Surging	Flooding	Surging	Flooding
Dà 大	---	Big	Large	Big
Wēi 微	Faint	Minute	Faint	Minute
Jǐn 緊	Tight	Tight	Tight	Tight
Huǎn 緩	Moderate	Moderate	Moderate	Leisurely
Xián 弦	Bowstring	Wiry	String-like	Wiry
Kōu 芤	Scallion-stalk	Hollow	Scallion stalk	Hollow
Gé 革	Drumskin	Leather	Drumskin	Leather
Láo 牢	---	Confined	Confined	Firm
Rú 濡	Soft (?)	Soggy	Soggy	Soft
Ruǎn 軟	---	---	---	---
Ruò 弱	Weak	Frail	Weak	Weak
Sàn 散	Dissipated	Scattered	Scattered	Scattered
Xì 細	Fine	Thin	Fine	Fine
Xiǎo 小	---	---	Small	---
Fú 伏	Hidden	Hidden	Hidden	Hidden
Dòng 動	Stirring	Moving (Spinning Bean)	Stirring	Moving
Cù 促	Skipping	Hurried	Skipping	Hasty
Jié 結	Bound	Knotted	Bound	Knotted
Dài 代	Interrupted	Intermittent	Regularly Intermittent	Intermittent
Jí 急	---	---	Racing	---

Chinese	*The Essentials of Chinese Diagnostics* Manfred Porkert	*The Chinese Pulse Diagnosis* Wu Shui-Wan	*Acupuncture: The Ancient Art of Chinese Healing* Felix Mann	C.S. Cheung & Jenny Belluomini
Fǔ 浮	Superficial	Floating	Floating	Floating
Chén 沉	Submerged	Deep	Sunken (Deep)	Sinking
Chí 遲	Slowed down	Slow	Slow	Slow
Shùo 數	Accelerated	Rapid	Rapid	Rapid
Xū 虛	Exhausted (Depleted)	Empty	Empty	Deficient
Shí 實	Replete	Full	Full	Excess
Huá 滑	Slippery	Slippery	Slippery	Slippery
Sè 澀	Grating	Choppy	Choppy (Rough)	Difficult
Cháng 長	Long	Long	Long	Long
Duǎn 短	Brief	Short	Short	Short
Hóng 洪	Flooding	Overflowing	Overflowing	Tidal
Dà 大	Large	Big	---	Large
Wēi 微	Evanescent	Minute	Minute	Diminutive
Jǐn 緊	Tense	Tight	Tight	Tight
Huǎn 緩	Languid	Slowed-down	Slowed-down	Leisurely (Relaxed)
Xián 弦	Stringy	Wiry	Bowstring	Bowstring
Kōu 芤	Onion stalk	Hollow	Hollow	Leek stalk
Gé 革	Tympanic	Leather	Leather	Leather
Láo 牢	Fixed	Firm	Firm (Hard)	Prison
Rú 濡	Frail	Weak-Floating	Weak-Floating	Soft
Ruǎn 軟	Soft	---	---	---
Ruò 弱	Infirm	Weak	Weak	Weak
Sàn 散	Dispersed	Scattered	Scattered	Scattered
Xì 細	Minute	Fine	Fine	Small
Xiǎo 小	Small	---	---	Small
Fú 伏	Recondite	---	Hidden (Buried)	Hidden
Dòng 動	Mobile	Moving	Moving	Agitated
Cù 促	Agitated	Hasty	Hasty	Accelerated
Jié 結	Adherent	Knotted	Knotted	Nodular
Dài 代	Intermittent	Intermittent	Intermittent	Replacement
Jí 急	Racing	---	Fast (Hurried)	Rushing (Swift)

this pulse quality. In fact, we use Wide and Thin to describe the two extremes of sensation palpated within the general category of width.

Most sources list between nineteen and twenty-eight pulse qualities. Table 5-2 (Ch. 5) summarizes our classification of pulse qualities, categorized according to sensation, and organized according to clinical experience. (Also in Ch. 5, Table 5-3 classifies the pulse qualities according to their associated conditions.) At first glance, our system, which describes many more qualities, seems more complicated than others. Actually it is simpler because it corresponds to what one feels at one's fingertips, especially in relationship to the presenting clinical condition. In our experience, students absorb these distinctions with less difficulty than anticipated and with a growing and lasting appreciation of their clinical application. The subtleties of this system may seem initially intimidating, but the rewards—even for the novice—are quickly apparent to those who persist.

CONTEMPORARY CHINESE PULSE DIAGNOSIS IN THE CONTEXT OF MODERN PRACTICE

TIME REQUIREMENTS

The consideration of the cost effectiveness of the time required for obtaining an accurate reading of the pulse is a question that arises in busy clinical settings. During teaching seminars and initial patient visits we require approximately thirty to forty-five minutes for pulse taking, and about five to ten minutes during subsequent visits. Dr. Shen required less than five minutes, and some students use as little as ten minutes. How much time is necessary seems to depend on the individual's pace. It is certainly cost effective once one has achieved a certain level of competence because of the amount, accuracy, and quality of diagnostic information one receives so quickly.

SIGNIFICANCE

Students of many different schools of acupuncture theory and practice have found this method of pulse diagnosis to be compatible with, and useful in, their own practices. All the information found on the pulse is real and deserving of attention, however some findings are more relevant to the current complaint than others. By combining the pulse with others signs and symptoms and by using one's own experience, the clinician will be able to determine which of the findings are most significant.

The pulse contains layers of information about rate, rhythm, organs, substances, body systems and areas, pathology, activity (heat and cold) and function. The practitioner can avoid feeling overwhelmed by all this information by viewing the pulse assessment as a current snapshot of the process of disease from birth to death.

This system is organized so that the most accessible information can be applied by the beginner, even before he has the experience to read the deeper subtleties of the pulse. A beginner should be able to gain information about the body's basic substances (qi, blood, yin, yang, and essence) and activity (heat and cold) that will aid him in prescribing the proper treatment.

POTENTIAL FOR PULSE DIAGNOSIS

No single diagnostic technique can provide us with the whole truth about the state of an individual's health, yet to an experienced practitioner the pulse can deliver a tremendous amount of information. It can reveal information about a patient's past: constitution, course of life, previous illnesses, emotional states, and lifestyle habits such as work, exercise, nutrition, drugs, and sex; and also about his present lifestyle and habits, overall body condition, the state of the interrelationships among the various organ systems, and the status of the body's fundamental substances.

Additionally, the pulse can provide information about past or present trauma (physical or emotional), the mental state and behavioral style of the patient, and the stage of disease. It is also a useful tool for assessing the course of treatment, even when the change is subtle. Because it reveals information about the past and present, pulse diagnosis can be used to predict possible future disharmonies, thus enabling the practice of preventive medicine (see Ch. 16).

The key to the potential of pulse diagnosis is the Normal pulse described in this book. It includes characteristics such as rate, rhythm, stability, waveforms, volume, depth, width, buoyancy, shape, and position. Small deviations from the sensations that define the Normal pulse are easily detectable, often long before symptoms appear, rendering this system a very sophisticated tool in the prevention of disease.

As times have changed, new diseases and new problems associated with modern civilization have begun to appear in pulse diagnosis. The Choppy quality, once uncommon, is now prevalent due to an escalation in environmental toxicity (in water, food, and air). Previously, the Leather quality was rarely felt except in irradiated cancer patients, but is now commonly found due to our increased exposure to electromagnetic fields (wifi, cell phone radiation, etc.).

Hopefully, with the information provided in this book and the skills developed in pulse seminars, practitioners will be even better equipped to explore new worlds and serve future generations.

LIMITATIONS OF PULSE DIAGNOSIS

Pulse diagnosis is an individually developed art form, a type of meditation, a simultaneous connection between one's deepest parts and those of another human being. It can be influenced by many transient events: emotions, acute illness, activity, a full bladder, diet, medication, imminent or concurrent menstrual flow, biorhythms, the season, and even the time of day. It can also be influenced (fleetingly) by the practitioner's energy. Nevertheless, with experience, a practitioner can distinguish these transient influences from the more enduring and authentic pulse qualities.

Pulse qualities can also be dependent on the condition of the body, the terrain at the time a problem first appeared, the intensity of the event, its location in the body, and the length of time that has elapsed since its appearance. A trauma that occurred at a time when the body was weak will be revealed by a different quality than one where the trauma occurred when the body was strong. For example, a trauma to the chest might create an Inflated quality in a strong person and a Flat quality in a weaker person in the upper burner positions.

The meanings of the qualities themselves can also differ depending on where on the pulse they appear and whether they are found in combination with other qualities (either at the same location or elsewhere on the pulse). The Slippery quality found at the left middle organ depth can indicate a Liver infection; if found at the blood depth, it may be a sign of blood toxicity or excess viscosity (elevated blood lipids); if found at the qi depth, it indicates differing conditions depending upon whether the rate is Slow or Rapid; and if found over the entire pulse, it can signal pregnancy or Heart qi deficiency.

THE PULSE AND OTHER METHODS OF DIAGNOSIS

Pulse diagnosis is not intended to be used alone but is designed to be integrated with other diagnostic tools: listening, looking, questioning, and forms of palpation other than pulse-taking. Sometimes there is a disparity between the pulse and other diagnostic sources of information. If this happens, the pulse is generally more accurate when interpreted by an experienced practitioner, unless the other diagnostic signs are more in agreement with the symptoms. In the latter case, diagnosis should lean more in the direction of the symptoms. An example of this disparity might be when the pulse indicates an internal deficient cold disorder, but the symptoms and tongue signs overwhelmingly suggest the diagnosis of a hot disorder.

Cold and hot disorders can coexist and our management decision may be to treat both, with an emphasis on the one that shows the most severe signs and symptoms. Also, in certain situations false cold or heat may be present. In either case the pulse can often be used to clarify the information gleaned from other methods of diagnosis.

Ultimately, the pulse can be the most important diagnostic tool available to a practitioner of Chinese medicine, if one is willing to focus, practice, search, and be patient.

THE PRACTITIONER

Within Chinese medicine, a practitioner's sensory awareness, intelligence, intuition, experience, and common sense become diagnostic instruments, providing a window to the inner world of another human being. They do, however, often reveal seemingly unrelated and sometimes disparate information, and this can also be the case with pulse diagnosis. As Amber observes, taking the pulse "may call for some mechanical skill, but the interpretation of its story is an art".[5]

The western scientific model neither encourages nor develops the ability to seek relationships between seemingly unrelated pieces of information and blend them into a unified picture of the whole person.[6] For example, modern allopathic physicians are not trained to seek the relationship between a hemorrhoid and angina, yet these may be two expressions of a single systemic process such as blood stagnation. It is the ability to make these connections that enables a practitioner of Chinese medicine to utilize the pulse as an aid in the art of diagnosis.

Pulse diagnosis relies on the sense of touch, but of the senses we possess, some will develop more than others. Every individual is different, and while practitioners should make use of their innate gifts, they should not be restricted by them. If someone finds his sense of touch to be less than satisfactory, it should not become a source of frustration or of feelings of inadequacy. Developing competency in pulse diagnosis can instead provide an opportunity to expand one's abilities in this lifetime.

When using this book it is perhaps important to remember that there is a fine line between the wisdom that results from thousands of years of experience, and simple dogma. Knowledge is not a rigid framework within which to become trapped; it is an ever-expanding tool that can be inspired by one's own intuition and experience.

REFLECTION

The diversity of diagnostic modalities in Chinese medicine is great. However, it would be fair to say that, over the long period of time that Chinese medicine has been practiced, the pulse has been considered to be the most revealing mode of assessing the general and specific condition of a patient. If studied and applied in gradual increments, it will provide ever-increasing joy and the most profound satisfaction to the practitioner of Chinese medicine.

Practitioners who require unity[7] and a deep personal connection to their work through both their senses and their intelligence, and for whom impersonal detachment is anathema, will be drawn to and gratified by the practice of Chinese medicine and its premier diagnostic treasure, pulse diagnosis.

2

Pulse Positions through History

Oliver Nash, L.Ac., M.B.Ac.C.

HISTORICAL CONSIDERATIONS

From the time of the *Yellow Emperor's Inner Classic (Huang Di Nei Jing)* two thousand years ago up to the present day there have been a variety of opinions regarding the significance of the six positions of the pulse. As shown in Table 2-1, the main differences have been, first, whether the pulse has two or three depths, and second, the precise location on the radial artery of each of the organ systems and body areas.

At the dawn of the twenty-first century, we find two prevailing schools of pulse diagnosis. One, predominant in Europe and parts of America, favors the two-depth system and the Wang Shu-He interpretation; the other, predominant in China, employs three depths and is based on the perspective of the renowned Li Shi-Zhen.

WANG SHU-HE

Through his book *The Pulse Classic (Mai Jing)*,[1] written in the third century, Wang Shu-He has had a profound influence on the practice of pulse diagnosis. In Wang's system, each of the six pulse positions is associated with a particular phase (element), and each has two depths. The deeper depth at each position represents the yin (solid) organ associated with that particular phase, and the more superficial depth represents its paired yang (hollow) organ.

Li Shi-Zhen

The author of the sixteenth-century work *Lakeside Pulse Studies (Bin Hu Mai Xue)*, Li Shi-Zhen has had an equally profound influence on pulse diagnosis. The system described in his text relates each of the six positions to one of the five solid yin organs. Each position has three depths: the most superficial reveals the qi aspect of the associated organ, the middle depth reveals the blood aspect, and the deepest represents the yin-substance aspect.

Classic of Difficulties (Nan Jing)

In this important text there are lively debates about several methods of pulse diagnosis, including one that involves five beans of pressure versus another with nine beans of pressure, neither widely practiced today, as well as arguments in support of Wang Shu-He's methodology.

Ding Gan-Ren and the Menghe Lineage

In his youth, John Shen was a student at the Shanghai Technical College of Chinese Medicine, a school that was established in 1916 by physician-scholar Ding Gan-Ren. Ding was part of a famous medical lineage, reaching back to the early 17th century, known as the "Menghe current," which was named for the town in eastern Jiangsu province where it originated. This current of medical thought, centered around a handful of families and their social networks, produced some of the most influential physicians of the 19th and 20th centuries. Among other things, they were famed for their skills in pulse diagnosis.

Ding Gan-Ren himself published a book entitled *Summary of Pulse Study*.[2] In the Foreword to that book, Ding noted that he was integrating the styles of Li Shi-Zhen, Chen Xiu-Yuan, and Jiang Zhi-Zhen. The former two are authors of well-known works on pulse diagnosis. The latter is claimed to be the author of a secret manual passed down in the Fei family. Another physician of the Menghe current, Ma Guan-Qun, also wrote a book on pulse diagnosis in which he mentions a physician named Jiang Zi-Yang as influencing his own style and it is possible that this influence was passed on to the other physicians in this lineage. It would therefore be fair to assume that John Shen himself is part of the Menghe lineage, and it is this tradition of pulse diagnosis that was passed on to him at the Shanghai Technical College of Chinese Medicine, and that he subsequently developed and taught when he immigrated to the United States.[3]

In our time, when interpreting a single position on the pulse, history tells us that we have a choice: either the entire position represents the qi, blood, and yin-substance aspects of a yin organ, as held by Li Shi-Zhen, Dr. Shen, and the *Yellow Emperor's Inner Classic*, or it represents the yin (solid) and yang (hollow) paired organs of a phase, as described by Wang Shu-He.

Other perfectly valid systems of pulse diagnosis completely ignore or partially combine the part played by the radial pulse with other pulses in other locations,

Table 2-1 Historical correlations among pulse positions and organs

	Nei Jing c. 100 BC	*Nan Jing* c. 200 AD	*The Pulse Classic* Wang Shu-He Late 2nd century	*Pulse Diagnosis* Li Shi-Zhen 1564	*Collected Treatises* Zhang Jie-Bin 1624	John H.F. Shen* Late 20th century
LEFT WRIST POSITION						
Distal						
Superficial:	Sternum	Arm *tai yang*	Small Intestine	—	Pericardium	**
Deep:	Heart	Arm *shao yin*	Heart	Heart	Heart	Heart/Pericardium
Middle						
Superficial:	Diaphragm	Leg *shao yang*	Gallbladder	—	Gallbladder	**
Deep:	Liver	Leg *jue yin*	Liver	Liver	Liver	Liver/Gallbladder
Proximal						
Superficial:	Abdomen	Leg *tai yang*	Bladder	—	Bladder/Lg. Int.	**
Deep:	Kidney	Leg *shao yin*	Kidney	Kidney (Life Gate)	Kidney	Kidney/Lg. Intestine
RIGHT WRIST POSITION						
Distal						
Superficial:	Chest	Arm *yang ming*	Large Intestine	—	Sternum	**
Deep:	Lungs	Arm *tai yin*	Lungs	Lungs	Lungs	Lungs
Middle						
Superficial:	Spleen	Leg *yang ming*	Stomach	—	Stomach	**
Deep:	Stomach	Leg *tai yin*	Spleen	Spleen	Spleen	Stomach/Spleen
Proximal						
Superficial:	Abdomen	(Text unclear)	Triple Burner	—	T.Burner/Sm.Int.	**
Deep:	Kidney	(Text unclear)	Kidney (Life Gate)	Kidney (Life Gate)	Kidney	Bladder/Sm.Intestine

* This selection does not include the complementary pulse positions in the Shen system.

** In the Shen system the superficial depth is associated with qi, the middle depth with blood, and the deep depth with the parenchyma of the yin organs.

Fig. 2-1 Pulse positions according to Hammer, based on the Shen model. Arrows indicate the direction in which the finger should be rolled to assess the given pulse.

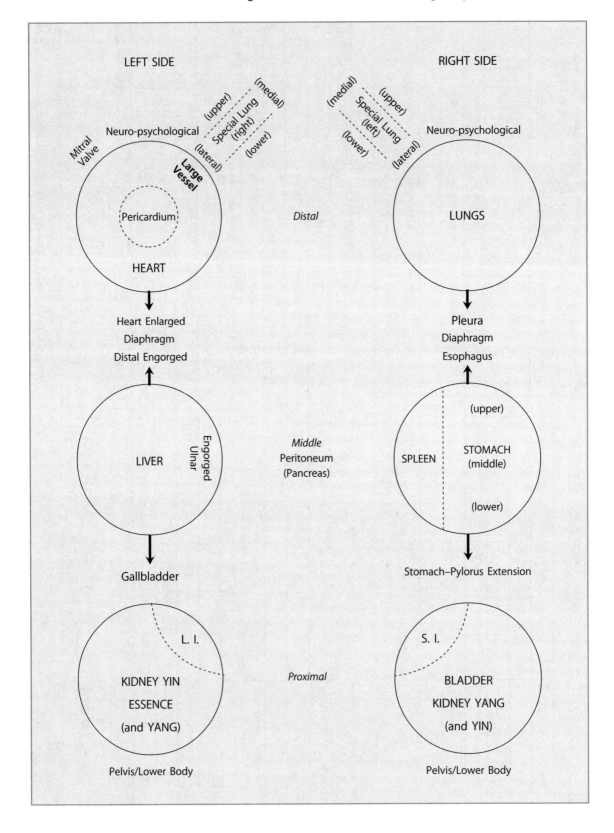

Fig. 2-2 Pulse positions according to Shen. Asterisks denote pulse positions differentiated by quality.

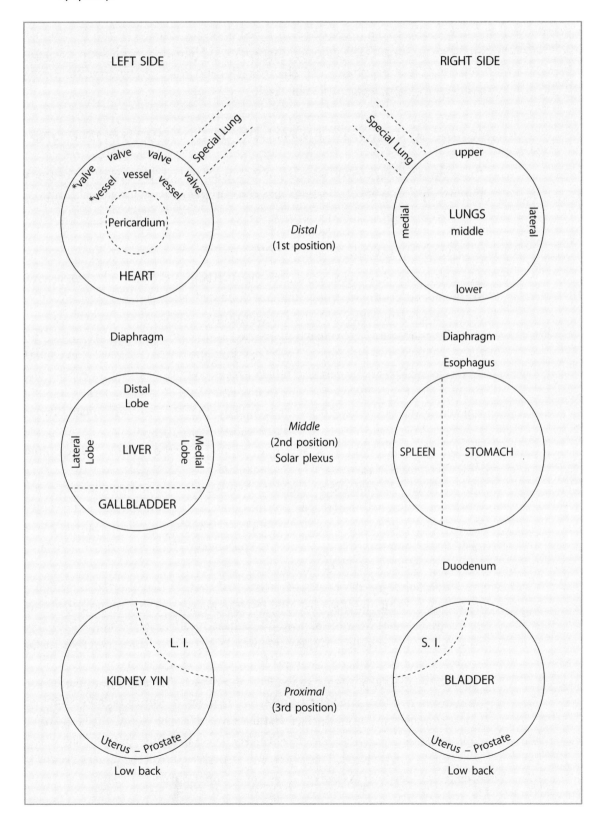

such as the carotid artery and the pedal pulses. As an organism, the body broadcasts information about itself in many ways. That we can hear these messages at all is far more important than arguing over the best way to listen to them.

The pulse system in this book is based upon the interpretations of Dr. Shen and leans toward an emphasis on the work of Li Shi-Zhen, with some concepts reflecting the interpretations of Zhang Jie-Bin and others drawn from the *Yellow Emperor's Inner Classic* (see Table 2-1).

PRINCIPAL AND COMPLEMENTARY INDIVIDUAL POSITIONS

Based on Dr. Shen's work, we present two general types of individual positions: the principal individual positions and the complementary individual positions (Figs. 2-1 & 2-2).

PRINCIPAL POSITIONS

The principal positions correspond to the six traditional ones, with three at each wrist, and with some variations that are discussed in Ch. 4. Each position represents a major yin organ, with two exceptions: the right middle position, which partially represents the Stomach (more excess qualities), and the proximal positions, which represent different aspects of the same organ (Kidney yin and yang). The proximal positions can also reflect excess conditions in the Intestines and Bladder (see Ch.4). Except for the distal positions that have two depths, superficial and deep, each pulse position has nine depths: qi, blood, organ (subdivided into organ-qi, organ-blood, and organ-substance), Firm, Hidden, Floating and Cotton. The last four of these depths are named after the specific pulse qualities with which each is associated. The Firm and Hidden depths are close to the bone and are rarely encountered except in extreme conditions, and the Floating depth is just under the surface of the skin. While it usually appears over the entire pulse, the Floating quality has been felt at only the right distal position (Lungs) in the early stage of an invasion by an external pathogen. The Cotton depth is located between the skin and the qi depth.

When palpating the positions, it is worth noting that there is a tendency for qualities in the middle positions (middle burner) to expand into the other positions, especially the distal positions. Anatomically, the abdominal area represented by the middle positions is much less confined than the chest (distal positions) and somewhat less confined than the pelvis (proximal positions). Thus the qi in the middle burner is more prone to expand. The tendency of the middle positions to overflow is also partly due to the expansive nature of gases contained in the Stomach, and from the fact that the Liver stores blood. As the blood often contains some degree of heat, it will likely cause the pulse position associated with the Liver to expand. This is why it is necessary to roll the fingers distally in order to properly access the qualities in the upper burner (see Ch. 4).

The right middle position primarily reflects the state of the Spleen, especially in conditions of deficiency. It also represents the Stomach in conditions of excess, such as excessive heat and damp-heat, and in stagnation of qi, food, and phlegm.

Of the proximal positions, traditionally the right is said to reflect Kidney yang and the left to reflect Kidney yin. Clinically, the proximal positions (singularly or together) may depict Kidney yin deficiencies, Kidney yang deficiencies, or both. The most likely scenario is that the left proximal position would reveal the hard qualities (such as Tight or Wiry) that relate to Kidney yin-essence deficiency. However, when this position is Feeble or Absent, it is also a sign of Kidney yang deficiency.

There will be Robust Pounding and Flooding Excess at the right proximal position when there is active pathology in the Bladder or Small Intestine. Active pathology in the Large Intestine may be marked by similar robust qualities at the left proximal position.

When both Kidney yin and Kidney yang deficiency are present simultaneously, the pulse qualities in either the left or right proximal position can reveal both these deficiencies, and will do so by changing back and forth from Tight to Feeble. However, when yin and yang deficiency are approximately equal, the yin deficient qualities of Tight and Wiry will tend to override the yang deficient qualities of Feeble or Absent at either or both proximal positions.

COMPLEMENTARY POSITIONS

Within this pulse system there are twenty-one complementary positions that represent either the yang (hollow) organs or parts or areas of the body. These positions, some of which are bilateral, include the Neuro-psychological, Pericardium, Mitral Valve, Large Vessels, Heart Enlarged, Diaphragm, Special Lung, Pleura, Liver Engorgements (distal and ulnar), Large Intestine, Esophagus, Gallbladder, Spleen, Stomach-Pylorus Extension and Small Intestine. Pathology in the pancreas/peritioneum and duodeneum is indicated by a combination of findings in the other complementary positions and the Pelvis/Lower Body (which includes the pelvis, low back, lower extremities, ovaries, fallopian tubes, uterus, and prostate).

The complementary positions have only two relevant aspects, superficial and deep. Qualities in the complementary positions sometimes have different interpretations than when found in the principal positions; for example, a Tight quality at the Large Intestine position usually indicates an overactive, irritable, or inflamed intestine, rather than yin deficiency (see discussion of complementary positions in Chs. 4 and 12).

Rolling the Fingers on the Pulse

The complementary positions are located either medial or lateral to, between, or distal or proximal to the six principal positions, and are accessed by rolling the fingers. It is important to accurately learn the rolling technique; Dr. Shen used it as an essential aspect of pulse diagnosis. Fig. 2-2 shows his system of pulse location, in which the fingers are rolled within the position up and down and sideways.[4]

This technique was mentioned in the translation of George Soulié de Morant's book,[5] indicating that although this technique has recently been neglected in China, it was known and practiced up to the start of the twentieth century. Its practice is also implied in the *Classic of Difficulties (Nan Jing)*.[6] Both Wang Shu-He[7] and Deng Tietao make references to it, the latter in a text that refers to Zhen Jia-Shu's "lifting, seeking, pressing and pushing."[8]

Contemporary Chinese Pulse Diagnosis

Dr. Shen taught that certain positions would show no qualities if they were normal. This is so for the Large Vessel position (where it is clearly best if there are no perceptible qualities), Mitral Valve, Diaphragm, Liver Engorged, and Spleen positions. Conversely, an Absent quality at the Special Lung position could be a sign of danger.

According to Dr. Shen, in order to be considered normal the other complementary positions should have the same quality as the principal positions. Although we have found this to be true for the Stomach-Pylorus Extension, we feel that the Gallbladder, Pelvis/Lower Body, and Intestine positions should be judged independently of the principal positions with which they are associated.

3

Basic Axioms and Other Considerations

Ross Rosen, L.Ac.

THE PULSE AND CHINESE PHYSIOLOGY

COMBINATIONS OF PULSE QUALITIES THAT SEEM PARADOXICAL

Often apparently paradoxical qualities can be presented at the same position and depth of the pulse. For example, a Hollow quality at the blood depth, which may signify blood deficiency or hemorrhage, can be felt as the finger pressure is increased from the qi to the organ depth. Simultaneously, a Wide quality, which may signify the presence of blood heat, can be felt as the finger pressure is released from the organ up to the qi depth.

Therefore, we have two entirely different sensations at the same blood depth, depending on whether we are applying or releasing pressure. Being aware that the pulse can convey multiple messages helps us to be flexible about our preconceived notions and to see things as they are, rather than as we think they should be.

PARADOX AS A SIGN OF ILLNESS

When the pulse qualities and the disease correspond—such as a Robust and Pounding pulse seen in an acute disease, and a Reduced one in a chronic disease—the prognosis is better than when they are incompatible or paradoxical.[1] Examples of paradoxical presentations include the presence of a very high temperature and a very low pulse rate, or a very low temperature and very high pulse rate, which are signs of serious physiological chaos ('qi wild').

PULSE QUALITIES AS PREDICTORS OF PATHOLOGY

The pulse accesses a physiology and pathology at a more subtle level than the threshold for perceptible symptoms can be assessed by the diagnostic tools of modern biomedicine. This time lag between the two exists until the pulse signs associated with impending death appear, when the signs and the underlying reality are finally unified. Because the signs obtained from the pulse are several steps ahead of the organism's outward manifestations of disease, it is an instrument for prediction and prevention (see Ch. 16 for a more thorough explanation of this topic).

POSITIVE AND NEGATIVE SIGNS: A LIFE RECORD

The pulse record is a statement of a person's condition along the continuum from birth to death. It highlights our weaknesses, but it also tells us of our strengths. Intact proximal positions (the lower burner) tell us that we have root, ground on which to stand and heal. Intact middle positions (the middle burner) tell us that we can restore and cleanse ourselves. Intact distal positions (the upper burner) tell us that we can reach out to the world with awareness of our creative being, and with the strength to both communicate and protect this being, and to maintain mental and emotional stability despite the "slings and arrows of outrageous fortune" with which we are constantly bombarded.

Even with signs of Heart disharmony, a Normal rhythm tells us that there is strength to recover. Normal complementary positions inform us that the pathology found in their associated principal positions is not as serious as first thought and that the chances for restoration of health are good.

Above all, remember this: an accurate pulse record is a precise and faithful catalog of a person's physiology and pathology at a given moment in life. It is the road to early diagnosis and prevention, the true reality of who we are, and a better guide than any other diagnostic parameter for therapeutic management.

RELATIONSHIP BETWEEN HARD AND PLIABLE QUALITIES IN ACUTE AND CHRONIC CONDITIONS

Often the pulse quality of an acute condition supersedes the quality of a chronic condition. For example, the Deep, Feeble, Absent, or Reduced qualities associated with Kidney deficiency can be overshadowed by the Tight, Rapid, Flooding Excess, Robust Pounding, or Slippery qualities seen in acute infections such as fulminating colitis, cystitis, or prostatitis.

In general, the yin gives the body substance and suppleness and the yang gives it expansiveness and force. When yin becomes deficient, the pulse becomes Hard. When yang (qi) is deficient, the pulse becomes Yielding. When these two conditions exist simultaneously in the same position, the harder qualities can override the more yielding and pliable (softer) qualities or may even switch back and forth, reflecting both conditions. It is important to remember that the condition whose pulse quality has been displaced still exists.

OBFUSCATION

Patients who do not wish to reveal themselves can, for a limited period of time, withdraw qualities, continually change them, and change qualities from side to side, among other confusing maneuvers. What seems to the organism as the overriding concern—concealing itself—can briefly override all other messages revealed through the pulse. The cited article illustrates this in detail.[2]

THE PULSE AND WESTERN PHYSIOLOGY

Over the years, many biophysiological theories of Chinese medicine and the pulse have arisen, though none has yet stood the test of time. It is our impression that such efforts to bridge the gap between the two physiological models by explaining one in terms of the other misses the essential point that they are complementary but conceptually and operationally different, and that each can fill the other's gaps.[3] Like Einstein's analogy of reality as a watch that can be observed but never opened, a model of reality must not be confused with the truth: its only value is its usefulness, not its appeal.

LARGE SEGMENT AND SMALL SEGMENT PULSE SIGNS

LARGE SEGMENTS

The large segments of the pulse include rhythm, stability, and rate as well as uniform qualities that are found over the entire pulse, at one or another of the three burners, or on one side of the wrist. The large segments also include the qi, blood, and organ depths of the entire pulse. Although it is important to study the individual positions and qualities, it is the larger aspects of the pulse that are the keys to successful diagnosis. It is here that a condition first manifests and where its effect on the entire organism can best be assessed (see Ch. 14).

Rhythm, stability, and rate are aspects that take precedence over other qualities or combinations of qualities in terms of diagnosis and treatment. Deviations from the norm among these parameters are generally the most critical in determining the seriousness of disharmony and the sequence of treatment. Frequently, when the rhythm, instability, and rate of the pulse are brought into order and balance, the other qualities and signs will themselves change.

Rhythm

Rhythm is the most significant measure of Heart and circulatory function and must be addressed first. Instability in the emperor (Heart) is tantamount to chaos in the empire and anarchy among its ministers and subjects. Irregularity of rhythm is considered in terms of whether it occurs at rest or during movement, whether or not the rate can be perceived, whether the changes in rate are small or large, and whether its irregularity is constant or occasional (see Ch. 6).

Rate

Classically, the rate of the pulse has been correlated with conditions of heat or cold such that a uniformly Rapid pulse is interpreted to mean a condition of heat or hyperactivity and a uniformly Slow pulse to indicate a condition of cold and hypoactivity. However, clinical experience suggests that rate is most frequently associated with the Heart and with circulation. Thus deviations from the norm are more often the result of either a shock to the Heart in utero, at birth, emotional shock during life, and/or some alteration in the circulation of blood and qi due to factors outside of, but ultimately affecting, the Heart. When there is severe deficiency, it is important to remember that the pulse can sometimes be temporarily very Rapid—especially upon exertion—due to the instability of qi, particularly the qi of the Heart (see Ch. 7).

Stability

By stability we mean the capacity of an organism to return easily to equilibrium after stress, and its capacity to maintain operational parameters within optimally functional limits over time. Apart from the regularity of the pulse, stability is associated with the steadiness of the amplitude, qualities, and rate of the pulse as well as with the balance of yin and yang and among the pulse positions (see Ch. 6).

Separation of Yin and Yang

One should consider the differences between pulse qualities in which yin and yang are in contact and those in which they are not—associated with the more serious variety of deficiency. The qualities associated with each can occur over the entire pulse or in just one position.

The Feeble quality occurs in a situation where there is still contact between yin and yang; it is a sign of significant deficiency. By contrast, the Empty quality occurs when yin and yang are out of contact, and if found in one position, is a sign of extreme dysfunction in its associated organ. When the Empty quality is found over the entire pulse, yin and yang are out of contact in the organism as a whole, referred to as 'qi wild'. If yin and yang are separated in one organ, this can eventually destabilize the entire system and thereby lead to a 'qi wild' state throughout the organism.

The 'separation of yin and yang' is a process that begins in utero and grows, usually gradually with the wear and tear of daily life, until the final complete separation at death (see Ch. 6).

Changes in Qualities

A Change in Qualities is an advanced sign that yin and yang are separating. If the qualities are changing in one position, it is a sign of extreme dysfunction in the organ represented by that position. If qualities are changing in many positions, it constitutes the serious imbalance of 'qi wild' (see Ch. 6).

Changes in Amplitude

Amplitude is the height to which the pulse is generated from the organ to the qi depth or beyond, and is a measure of the yang force (i.e., basal metabolic functional heat). High amplitude reflects a strong yang force while low amplitude is a mark of diminished yang force. Consistent, ongoing Changes in Amplitude over the entire pulse are indicative of either circulatory or Heart problems. In just one position it is most often a mild to moderate sign of the separation of yin and yang, or less often, a transition in the energy of that organ or area from better to worse or vice versa. Changes in Amplitude over the entire pulse may be found at the first impression stage: if constant, it reflects blood circulation and Heart function; if inconsistent, it reflects qi circulation (usually Liver qi stagnation) (see Ch. 6).

Changes in Width

The change on the pulse back and forth from Thin to Wide is found much less frequently than the Change in Amplitude. The blood is the repository of excess heat and toxins as retained pathogens that the blood is attempting to discharge. The 'change in width' is a measure of that activity.

Fig. 3-1 Normal pulse wave

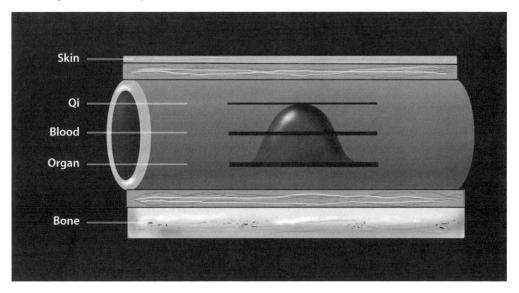

Wave Form

The wave associated with a Normal pulse is a sine wave or bell curve, as illustrated in Fig. 3-1. Deviations from this norm are indications of pathology that are discussed more fully in Chs. 4, 8, and 13.

SMALL SEGMENTS

Every depth at the principal positions reflects the integrity of its associated organs. The organ depth is the repository of information about the qi, blood, and yin-substance of the yin-solid organ; the qi depth tells us about the organ's contribution to the total true qi, and the blood depth about its contribution to the total blood of the organism. When the qi and blood depths are inaccessible at a particular individual position, the yin organ is no longer making a full contribution to the total function, but instead is retaining the qi and blood for its own survival.

QUANTITY VS. QUALITY

Many systems of pulse diagnosis note only a *quantity* of impulse at each position, such as 'two plus' or 'two minus' for a moderately strong or weak pulsation, and give little regard to the *qualities*, such as Tense or Feeble. This can be very misleading as the quantitative measure of the pulse conveys none of the subtlety that has made the pulse the foundation of Chinese medical diagnosis since antiquity. Preserving this subtlety by studying and recording the shades of quality is the focus of this book.

Furthermore, there is a sometimes misguided association of excess pulse qualities with 'strong' conditions. For example, the Reduced Pounding quality may be interpreted only as excess because of the Pounding quality, overlooking its more subtle Reduced aspect, which reflects an attempt to compensate for deficiency and continue function. Likewise, the hard qualities of Tight and Wiry—seemingly signs of excess or strength—are actually signs of yin and yin-essence deficiency. Treatment management based on such misinterpretations can be detrimental to the healing process.

Jiang Jing seems to support this view:

> Students of pulse diagnosis often make rudimentary mistakes by considering a strong pulse as an indication of a strong organ. ...
> More often than not, a strong pulse should be looked at more closely to discover what big changes are taking place in the organ.[4]

Often the nature of the quality inherently depicts and encompasses the quantity, for example, the Flooding-Excess or Full-Overflowing qualities that are by definition expressions of overabundant quantity, and the Absent or Empty qualities that are likewise statements of deficient quantity. For many qualities, such as Robust Pounding or Changing Amplitude, we can indicate the degree with a numbering system, from one to five, with one as the least and five the most.

CONDITIONS AND CIRCUMSTANCES THAT AFFECT PULSE QUALITIES AND THEIR INTERPRETATION

Environment and Etiology

Environmental and cultural considerations have played a considerable role in the form and substance of Chinese medicine. In preindustrial societies, excess conditions of cold, heat, wind, and dampness causing blockage of circulation of qi and blood were common. Although rare today, excess from these pathogenic influences must be considered if there are signs supporting its presence, such as a very Rapid rate, high temperature, acute pain, and a Robust Pounding and Flooding Excess pulse wave. New pathologies of the industrial-digital age such as toxicity and radiation have replaced older ones.[5]

Age at Onset of Qi Deficiency

The causes of qi deficiency are usually a combination of factors including constitutional deficiency, an impoverished environment, overwork, exercise beyond one's capacity, drug abuse, premature or excessive sex, or toxicity and radiation. Ignoring constitutional deficiency for the moment, the earlier in life that these factors play a major role, the more likely one encounters pulse qualities indicating energetic chaos and severe deficiency in later life.

Age and the Interpretation of Qualities

It generally takes more than half a lifetime to develop the pulse qualities associated with deficiency. Should qualities such as Feeble-Absent (qi deficiency) or Tight (yin deficiency) occur in a young person, one must seek another explanation than those associated with the normal wear and tear of the aging process. An adolescent with a Feeble-Absent pulse quality, in the absence of extreme deprivation, probably has a constitutional deficit. A young person with a very Tight generalized pulse quality is more likely to be in general pain than to be suffering from yin deficiency.

Furthermore, children's pulses should be considered differently from those of adults, where the same degree of chaos may instead reflect their immaturity and state of constant change, rather than a serious disease. Each case must always be considered on an individual basis, as we have seen some cases when this chaos in children was an indicator of serious illness.

GENDER

A Thin pulse quality in a man represents a greater degree of deficiency and a more serious condition than when it is found in a woman. A Wide pulse in a woman represents more excess heat than the same pulse in a man.

BODY CONDITION

The diagnostic significance of a pulse quality can be affected by other factors. Two important ones are body condition (terrain) and stress, discussed next, and lifestyle, which follows later.

VULNERABILITY: TERRAIN AND STRESS

All things being equal, disharmony will occur first and foremost in the most deficient organ. For example, if a person does heavy physical work after eating, the Inflated quality can appear in either the Stomach or the Intestines position, whichever organ is most deficient. Likewise, if a person is angry and the Lung is more deficient than the Liver, the Lung will be affected first, even though the Liver is commonly associated with anger.

This vulnerability of organ systems depends on three variables. The first is constitution, which Dr. Shen defined as having three aspects: heredity, pregnancy, and delivery. The second is body condition or terrain, more specifically determined over time by the interplay between the initial terrain and the stressful experiences in infancy and childhood between birth and adulthood. The third variable is called life, and refers to stressful adult habits and lifestyles, such as work, sex, drugs, exercise, and nutrition.

If one performs within one's capabilities and listens to the messages that presage overuse, one can stay free of disease. If instead, one works beyond one's innate energies (terrain), illness is inevitable. All of life is a variation of this relationship between extraneous stresses and the terrain of the body.

FOUNDATION[6]

The foundation for all human functions is composed of Kidney qi, yin, yang, and essence. Kidney yin and yang are derived from essence. Kidney qi is the combined functional aspects of Kidney yin-essence and yang-essence. Supported by stored Kidney essence, Kidney qi represents the foundation on which rests, and out of which is expressed, the functions of all organ systems throughout life. Please refer to the source text for a more detailed account of the systems that are dependent on Kidney function.

Abuse of the Foundation

The Kidney organ is profoundly affected by constitutional and congenital factors. As the foundation for all the other organ systems, Kidney qi, yin, yang, and essence are quickly exhausted in a life marked by abuse, often manifested by a Deep pulse quality in the proximal positions.

Proximal Pulses and the Foundation

It is our clinical impression that deficiencies of Kidney essence, yin, and yang can all be found at either or both the left and right proximal positions, and that the differentiation depends on the qualities found there: Kidney yin deficiency is seen as a Tight quality, Kidney yang deficiency as a Feeble-Absent quality, and Kidney essence deficiency as a Wiry and increasing Leather-Hard quality. Yin deficiency tends to show up first on the left, and qi-yang deficiency on the right, proximal position. When both occur simultaneously, the left might be Tight and the right Feeble, or they may both reflect Change in Qualities, from Tight to Feeble.

The Feeble-Absent quality in all but the aged is usually associated with a constitutional etiology and the Tight quality with an etiology that has occurred later in life—usually a result of over-thinking and overworking of the 'nervous system'[7] (see Ch. 15). The Wiry quality is associated with the extreme phase of yin-essence deficiency, as a sign of pancreatic dysfunction (diabetes) and/or circulatory issues (hypertension), or of severe pain in the lower burner.

Emotions and the Foundation

The propensity toward depression is rooted in Kidney energy deficiencies. Depressions that begin early in life and are independent of circumstance (endogenous depressions) are rooted in constitution, intrauterine exigencies, and very early-life misfortune. This and other aspects of emotional life and Kidney energies are discussed in Ch. 15.

History

History refers to specific life events, including in utero and at birth. For example, a Flat pulse in the left distal position may result from a birth delivery complication of the umbilical cord having been wound around the neck after the head was outside the mother's body, which will often also present with Feeble-Absent proximal positions.

There are many other causes of a Flat distal pulse including emotional trauma ('Heart closed'), physical trauma, or shock. The real etiologic event becomes significant in terms of intervention and can be determined by reviewing the history and through other diagnostic signs and symptoms in conjunction with the pulse.

Organ Systems and Body Areas

As a rule, pathologies in areas or regions of the body, such as the chest or pelvis, are distinguishable when the same quality appears bilaterally at the same position, bilaterally between the distal and middle positions (diaphragm), or laterally between all positions (musculoskeletal disorders). See Ch. 14 for further discussion.

POSITION, SENSATION, AND SIMILARITY

The sensations of the pulse qualities are generally consistent but some qualities will *feel* somewhat differently at different positions. A Tight pulse at the Pericardium position feels more like a sharp point sticking the finger compared to the longer, more string-like Tight sensation at the left middle and proximal positions.

Qualities with a similar sensation (e.g., Rough) are sometimes difficult to distinguish. The Vibration (buzzing) and Choppy (grating) qualities are both Rough sensations that have completely different interpretations. The Spreading, 'separating', and Pounding from below qualities can cause the wave to move in two directions (Pseudo-Slippery) and all are frequently confused with the Slippery sensation that moves in only one direction. (See the source text for detailed descriptions of each of these). All of the above can be easily distinguished with a little instruction.

POSITION AND INTERPRETATION

Interpretation of the qualities is generally consistent, but the same quality sometimes has a different *meaning* from position to position. A Slippery quality at the organ depth of the left middle position can mean infection; in the Mitral Valve complementary position it can indicate regurgitation of blood from a mitral valve prolapse; in the left distal position it represents phlegm 'misting' the Heart; in the right middle position or SPEP it can reflect Spleen dampness or stagnant food; over the entire pulse at all depths, pregnancy, parasites, or elevated lipids; and at the blood depth, it can reflect turbulence in the blood vessels. (See the source text for further elaboration regarding different meanings based on position.)

IMMEDIATE OBSCURING FACTORS

The Robust Pounding, very Rapid, Interrupted, and Intermittent qualities, as well as medications—both stimulating and calming substances—aerobic exercise, physical and emotional trauma, or heavy lifting can temporarily obscure the real pulse. Overeating will also temporarily obscure the real pulse, but to a much less significant degree than these other factors. The obvious solution is to first attend to the etiology of these obscuring signs.

RECREATIONAL SUBSTANCES (DRUGS)

LSD, marijuana, and heroin are cooling and associated with an Empty quality at the left middle position. The stimulants cocaine and amphetamines cause Tense, Robust Pounding, and Flooding Excess qualities first at the left middle position and then in the left distal position, finally becoming Tight-Wiry in both middle and distal positions. (The source text has further descriptions of specific drugs, their effects on the organs, and related pulse qualities.)

ORIGIN OF DISHARMONY

Serious (often Chronic) Conditions

At one time, when excess conditions predominated, a useful and very general guide to tracing the etiology of a serious and/or chronic disharmony was that the organ that had a Feeble-Absent quality, or the pulse position that reflected the greatest chaos ('qi wild'), is where the problem had ended; while the organ that had a hard (Taut, Tense, Tight, or Wiry) pulse quality is where the problem presently resided and is beginning. However in our time, when deficiency predominates, the qi deficient qualities of Feeble-Absent, Reduced Substance, Diffuse, Deep, and 'qi wild' are appearing in very young people at the onset. The old rule no longer holds, and the deficient qualities are found where the problem began.

Mild (often Acute) Conditions

Mild, often acute patterns show a different pulse picture. The position associated with the origin of the acute problem usually presents with a more Tense, Rapid, Tight, Robust Pounding, or Flooding Excess quality than the other positions. Floating qualities are found over the entire pulse with early stages of external pathogenic factors, less often at one position such as the right distal position (Lungs).

FOCUS OF INTERPRETATION

When searching for the organ system suffering the greatest functional distress the focus is on the positions that show the greatest chaos with Changes in Amplitude, and Changes in Qualities, or those that show Empty qualities.

OVERLAPPING PATHOLOGIES AND QUALITIES

Pulse qualities associated with disease progressions moving toward qi and blood deficiency, such as Diminished, Thin, or Feeble qualities, may appear at the same time as those reflecting yin deficiency, such as Tight and Wiry. As already noted, often the harder sensations will seem to override the more pliable qualities. When, through therapy, we relieve the Kidney yin deficiency and the Tight quality disappears, we may be surprised to find a Feeble quality at the proximal positions, requiring that we then treat the deficient Kidney qi. More often, the qualities will change back and forth from Feeble-Absent to Tight, informing us of the simultaneous presence of both conditions.

ACUTE

In terms of treatment, acute conditions usually take precedence over chronic ones unless the latter present an immediate threat to life. When an acute sign appears, ongoing treatment for chronic conditions should be reduced or interrupted temporarily until the acute condition is resolved. However, the sudden worsening of a chronic deficiency would take precedence over an acute disorder.

Among acute signs there is a hierarchy as well. A Leather-Hollow quality (especially if Rapid) represents imminent bleeding and is an immediate threat to life and takes precedence over all other qualities. Other pulse qualities that signify serious acute states—Flooding-Excess, Leather-Hollow, Very Tight Hollow Full-Overflowing and Tight (pain)—are the Bean (Spinning); abrupt overwhelming Smooth Vibration (sudden extreme worry); abrupt appearance of very strong Rough Vibration over the entire pulse (Heart shock); very Slow (40 beats/min) (hypothermia); very Rapid (febrile states or Heart shock); suddenly very Rapid with very low fever; suddenly very Slow with very high fever; and suddenly Interrupted Hollow and rate unquantifiable (acute serious heart failure).

CHRONIC

With chronic illness, the seriousness of its pulse qualities is based on the degree of chaos, deficiency, or stagnation that each quality represents, so that an Empty quality ('separation of yin and yang') is a more serious sign than a Deep or Feeble-Absent quality. The organs showing the greatest chaos or deficiency are likely to be most reliably identified with the etiology of a chronic disease process.

In treating chronic illness, several conditions exist that often must be dealt with simultaneously. For example, although the Muffled quality at the left distal position (depression) is not as serious as the Interrupted quality, it may be necessary to overcome the qi stagnation that the former represents concurrently, before completely regulating the rhythm, if the symptoms associated with the Muffled quality dominate the clinical picture.

A Muffled quality (4-5) in the Pelvis/Lower Body position could also take precedence over an Empty quality over the entire pulse—generally a serious sign—if one suspects malignancy in the pelvis.

FENG SHUI AND SOCIAL FACTORS

It is our impression that certain pulse qualities appear more frequently in some parts of the earth than others, for example, the 'qi wild' in the earthquake-prone San Francisco Bay area, and the Slippery Neuro-Psychological pulses in several areas of western North Carolina, with no explanation other than that practitioners report a high degree of ear infections in the population and that the toxicity levels around Asheville are said to be the highest in the nation. This *feng shui* connection warrants much further scrutiny and observation since the data is very limited and precludes any assumptions.

THE SERIOUSNESS OF DISHARMONY

CONSISTENCY AND RESPONSE TO TREATMENT AND REST

Generally, qualities that appear consistently are signs of a greater disharmony than those that appear occasionally. A condition that responds to a moderate period (1-2 weeks) of absolute rest, or that changes after a short period of treatment, is a qi (functional) disease rather than an organic disease, that is, a 'disease' defined by allopathic medicine. In Dr. Shen's view, healing is an "up and down process" like the motion of the ocean waves, with the "up" waves gradually predominating.

STAGNATION

The qualities most often associated with the term qi stagnation are the Taut and Tense pulse qualities. These qualities occur when the moving qi of the body and/or mind, irresistible forces, are opposed by an immovable object, such as repression. These represent two opposing and usually strong forces within an area or organ, for example, Liver qi stagnation, where the qi wants to move and spread but is opposed and restrained, usually by repressive emotional forces.

Other pulse qualities reflecting qi stagnation include:

- **Inflated:** a sign of qi or heat trapped in an area or organ when it was robust
- **Flat:** a sign of qi unable to enter an area where it is deficient
- **Cotton:** a sign of superficial qi stagnation reflecting suppression, resignation, or physical trauma
- **Muffled or Dead:** revealing the presence of potential, imminent, or present tumor formation or other life-threatening disease
- **Bean (Spinning):** a sign of severe fright and intense pain
- **Firm, Hidden Excess qualities:** associated with severe internal cold
- **Short Excess:** involves qi, blood, or food stagnation between yin organs

RESTORATION OF EQUILIBRIUM AND QUALITIES ASSOCIATED WITH STAGES OF DISHARMONY

Each pulse quality is a sign of the body's attempt to restore equilibrium, or of its failure to do so. A Rapid rate or Reduced Pounding pulse may reflect the organism's attempted compensation for a state of overwork beyond one's energetic capability; the Empty pulse signifies that its compensatory restorative measures are failing.

The early stages of chronic disease are due to interference with normal function, which we call stagnation. Attempts to resolve the stagnation lead to the accumulation of metabolic heat to overcome it, reflected in the Tense and mild Robust Pounding qualities. If the body is unable to eliminate the heat—via the intestines, urine, skin, and Lung—some heat will then enter the blood, seen in the Blood Heat pulse. This can eventually progress to the Blood Thick, Hollow Full-Overflowing, and Rapid qualities that are pathognomonic of hypertension.

If unable to eliminate the heat, the body must provide fluids (yin) to balance it, which gradually depletes the yin, especially the Kidney yin, and the pulse qualities change to Tight and Wiry and perhaps slightly Rapid. At the blood depth, the Slippery quality will appear as a sign of turbulence, and later, as the heat affects the walls of the vessels, Rough Vibration at the blood depth, and finally a Ropy and Leather-Hard quality over the entire pulse will also appear. When heat accumulates, the blood begins to stagnate, a process that presents with the Choppy qualities, especially in blood-dependent areas such as the pelvis.

Over time, this effort depletes qi as well as yin, and the pulse qualities progress through those associated with the stages of qi deficiency, blood deficiency, and finally to the 'separation of yin and yang'.

BALANCE

Balance and stability in general refer to a condition in which all parts of a whole maintain a harmonious relationship with each other. Balance of the relationships among the different pulse positions is primarily a function of the Triple Burner. Stability refers to a consistency in function such as rhythm, rate, amplitude, and quality, and in the relationship of yin and yang.

Usually, whenever there is a great disparity between the pulse and other sources of diagnostic information, we are dealing with a more serious situation. Also the pulse that has widely different qualities at each position and burner as well as at each depth points to chaos in the Triple Burner, potentially the most serious of all disorders. The Heart is the emperor; the Triple Burner runs the empire.

ECOLOGY

Symptoms, and the pulse signs that accompany them, indicate not only that a problem exists but also inform us of the nature of the problem and the body's attempt to solve it. Thus diarrhea presenting with a pulse that reflects considerable heat may be an attempt by the organism to eliminate toxic heat that might damage the more critical yin (solid) organs. Instead of just stopping the diarrhea, we must look for the source of the heat.[8]

THE PREEMINENCE OF THE CARDIOVASCULAR SYSTEM IN THE DISEASE PROCESS

Dr. Hammer's experience over the past forty years has shown that the Heart and the Kidneys are the two systems that seem to bear the brunt of both constitutional deficits and self-abuse. Most significantly, the cardiovascular system shows the signs of depletion of qi, yin, and blood at an earlier age and to a greater degree than other systems, including the Kidney. Dr. Hammer has also observed that a large number of disorders—as diverse as gynecological, neurological, headaches, arthritis, as well as chronic fatigue syndrome—are due primarily to deficits in the Heart (cardiovascular) function.

This section on the cardiovascular system has been included because the ubiquitous finding of early Heart pathology with this pulse method has attracted the attention of those who use it. Considering that diseases of the heart and circulation are the single largest cause of death in this country, it must accordingly be regarded as the single most important pulse sign.

Pulse signs are the earliest indicators portending the development of disease. Using this subtle pulse system we can prevent most disease, including Heart disease, at inception or at very early stages.

4

Taking the Pulse: Methodology

Brandt Stickley, A.P.

PRELIMINARY CONSIDERATIONS

Factors to consider in taking the pulse in Contemporary Chinese Pulse Diagnosis include the timing and duration of the exam, the positioning of both patient and practitioner, and proper finger placement.

To perform an examination with adequate sensitivity to all of the messages the pulse may deliver initially requires 30–45 minutes and follow-up examinations of about five to ten minutes.[1] The patient as well as the practitioner should be rested and calm.

Within the limits of safety, the patient should be encouraged to refrain from taking medications and stimulants like coffee and tea. It is recommended that the patient be neither excessively full nor hungry. Always alert the patient to these requirements beforehand.

Though often neglected, the comfort of the practitioner as well as the patient is very important, especially during a prolonged examination of the pulse. Traditionally the pulse is taken with the patient's arms at the level of the heart, and this implies that the practitioner's arms be supported on the table as much as possible. The rolling movement necessary to access some pulse positions requires lifting the arm, but one must take care to remain comfortable.

Fig. 4-1 A Pulse Record

Contemporary Chinese Pulse Record

Date:	

Name:	Gender:	Age:	Hgt:	Wgt:	Occup:

Rhythm:	**Rate/min:** Begin: End: W/exertion: Chg: **Other Rates During Exam:**

First Impressions Of Uniform Qualities	DEPTHS
	 Floating:
	 Cotton:
	 Qi:
	 Blood:
	 Organ:
	   O-B:
	   O-S:
	 Wave:

Left Side: **Right Side:**	

PRINCIPAL POSITIONS	COMPLEMENTARY POSITIONS
L: DISTAL POSITION R:	L: NEURO-PSYCHOLOGICAL R:
	L: SPECIAL LUNG POSITION R:
	Pleura:
	HEART **Mitral Valve:** **Enlarged:** **Large Vessel:**
Pericardium:	
L: MIDDLE POSITION R:	L: DIAPHRAGM R:
	LIVER **ENGORGED** **Distal:** Ulnar: **Gallbladder:**
	SPLEEN-STOMACH **Esophagus:** Spleen: **Stom-pyl. Exten:** **Peritoneal Cavity/pancreas:** **Duodenum:**
L: PROXIMAL POSITION R:	**Large:** INTESTINES **Small:**
	L: PELVIS/LOWER BODY R:
THREE BURNERS **Upper:** **Middle:** **Lower:**	**COMMENTS** Δ = Change [1] → [5] = low → high degree

TAKING THE PULSE

The first and most important consideration is to find the principal impulse, which must be palpated where it imparts the strongest, clearest sensation. The failure to palpate the main impulse accounts for the majority of different (and often erroneous) findings among examiners. There can be some variations, medially or laterally, in the location of the artery, and taking the time to seek out the clearest impulse is essential.

We record the quality that appears at the highest amplitude. It is at this point that it is clearest and most accurate. We agree upon this standard because it facilitates the clearest communication among practitioners.

Another important distinction in Contemporary Chinese Pulse Diagnosis is the necessity of rolling the fingers to access some positions. The distal positions are felt by rolling the fingers in order to correct for the tendency of the middle burner (and sometimes the diaphragm) to expand and overtake the adjacent positions. Complementary positions also require rolling the fingers with specific location techniques.

Some complementary positions will have no qualities in the absence of pathology. These are the Large Vessel, Mitral Valve, Diaphragm, Liver Engorged, and Spleen positions. The Stomach-Pylorus Extension position should have the same quality as the right middle principal position. The Gallbladder, Pelvis/Lower Body, and Intestine positions must be assessed independently of their associated principal positions.

The Special Lung position, Neuro-psychological, and Pelvis/Lower Body positions inform us about the opposite organ: the left Special Lung position would reveal pathology in the right lung, the left Neuro-psychological position about the right side of the brain, and the left Pelvis/Lower Body position about the right ovary.

CONTEMPORARY CHINESE PULSE DIAGNOSIS TECHNIQUE

There are three stages to pulse examination: broad focus, closer focus, and closest focus. The broad focus includes the rhythm, rate, and qualities found uniformly over the entire pulse, including the Floating. The closer focus involves the qualities found uniformly at the different depths, sides, and burners. The closest focus is on the individual principal and complementary positions.

We begin with the broad and closer focus stages, using both hands: the practitioner's left hand palpates the patient's right wrist and vice versa. As the first step in any examination, both hands are used in order to access consistent messages on the entire pulse, to facilitate a clear comparison of both sides, and to deliver a picture of the qualities present over large segments of the pulse. Primary considerations such as the rate, rhythm, and wave form are best obtained by using both hands. Substances (qi, blood, yin, yang, essence), stability,

Heart-circulation, balance, strength, the Floating depth, and signs of potentially serious conditions can also be evaluated at this stage. The closest focus is later approached as a part of this global presentation rather than as a gathering of isolated pieces of information about specific organs, thus leading us to a more effective therapeutic strategy.

Within the first broad focus it is also possible to compare the pulse findings in relation to the overall body condition in terms of paradoxical findings. The Thin pulse in a man is a particularly important sign of possible serious disharmony. A very Wide pulse in a woman also suggests more concern.

One can also make necessary calibrations based on the broader focus or first impression that determine the assessment of other close focus findings. For example, if an overall Thin Pliable pulse has a relative widening or hardness in one position, or one finds a hardness in one position on an overall pliable pulse, both of these have different indications than the same finding on a normal pulse.

FINGER PLACEMENT

We recommend that one adhere to a pattern of finger placement using the scaphoid bone as the point of reference for the lateral edge of the index finger. Because some individuals may have anatomical differences of the ligamentous attachments of the radial styloid, the scaphoid bone proves a more reliable landmark for finger placement. The middle finger is placed at the middle or second position relative to the index finger, usually on or near the styloid process. The ring finger is placed proximally to the middle finger. Placing the thumb on the opposite dorsal aspect of the wrist at about LI-5 (*yáng xī*) enhances the practitioner's control.

For maximum sensitivity, position the fingers to use the area centered between the nail and the fingerpad. The practitioner must adjust her finger placement based on the relative size of the patient, spreading the fingers if the patient is large and compressing them if the patient is small. The radial artery is explored longitudinally in the middle and proximal positions, while the distal positions are examined horizontally, from lateral to medial aspects.

DEPTH AND LEVEL

FINGER PRESSURE AND NINE DEPTHS

Depth refers to the vertical dimensions of the pulse. It is important to develop the skill to accurately and consistently palpate the nine depths, especially the principal three: qi, blood, and organ. It is all too common to find practitioners exerting too little, too much, or too inconsistent pressure, all of which can distort the findings. The key to accurately finding the pulse depths is all in the wrist, hands, and fingers, and is a question of adjusting the pressure—a skill that we call 'calibrating'—that is best learned at a hands-on workshop.

The three depths are at prescribed and fixed locations, there being less than one thirty-second of an inch between the surface and the qi depth, and slightly less between the depths themselves. Proportional allowance should be made for the size of the individual, as the entire pulse is slightly deeper in a heavy person and more superficial in a thin person.

The Floating depth is the most superficial, found by simply laying the fingers on the skin above the radial pulse without pressure. The qi depth is the next most superficial, not necessarily found where the impulse is first evident, but in fact at a specific pressure. If nothing is found there we say that the qi depth is Absent. The blood and organ depths are found at precise locations below the qi depth. These depths are located according to the pressure applied to the radial artery, not according to the qualities that may or may not be present. These degrees of pressure are a relatively impartial tool by which the patient's pulse is subject to an unbiased measurement that can be objectively compared with every other patient and every other practitioner.

COMPLEMENTARY POSITIONS, QUALITIES, AND THE THREE DEPTHS

The three principal depths—qi, blood, and organ—do not apply to the complementary and distal positions, although there are some qualities that are felt more superficially, and others more deeply, in any one of these positions. It is necessary to move the fingers to explore various parts of the Special Lung, Gallbladder, Stomach-Pylorus Extension, and Pelvis/Lower Body positions. Particularly in the Special Lung position, different qualities may be found at the two depths and distally or proximally. Similarly, due to the ephemeral nature of findings at the Neuro-psychological and Mitral Valve positions, movement with a light touch, and patience, are required to assess them.

LEVEL

Level refers to the horizontal dimensions of the pulse from the wrist to the elbow that are associated with the upper, middle, and lower burners. Of considerable import is the tendency of the middle position (middle burner) qualities to dominate and expand into the adjacent positions, especially into the distal ones. There are anatomical, physiological, and energetic considerations for this expansion, and methodologically they require that one roll the fingers distally from the conventional upper burner position in order to accurately find the qualities in the upper burner. Remember that the distal positions are explored horizontally, from lateral (radial) to medial (ulnar), along the radial edge of the index finger.

QUALITIES

For the sake of uniformity the quality is assessed at the height of the wave or amplitude at the depth being assessed (qi, blood, organ) and where the impulse is strongest.

The classification of qualities is made according to their sensations:

- Hardness or pliability is a function of yin.

- Force (strength or weakness) is a function of qi or yang.

- Width (narrow or wide) is predominantly a function of blood and heat.

The degree of presence of a quality is measured on a scale from one to five, with one being the least degree and five the greatest, for example, Thin (1-5).

Again, certain uniform pulse qualities may obscure or conceal other qualities, or make *them more difficult to discern. Among these are the Robust Pounding, Uniformly Tense, very Rapid, very Slow, Muffled, Heavy Cotton, very Thin, very Tight, Ropy, very Deep, Interrupted, and Intermittent pulses. The same is true of certain medications and substances.

PROCEDURE

As already mentioned, the methodology of pulse examination is conducted in three stages: the broad focus, closer focus, and closest focus.

The pulse is accessed using the sensitive center of the area between the fingerpad and the nail of the fingertips, with the exception of those positions that require rolling of the fingers. Specific recommendations include:

- For the Special Lung position, use the flat fingerpad part of the index finger.

- For the distal positions, use the radial side of the index finger, which is rolled under the scaphoid bone, then its pressure is released slightly to access the upper burner. It is most important to distinguish the impulse coming from the middle burner, felt on the ulnar surface of the index finger, from the impulse coming from the upper burner, felt on its radial edge.

- For the Gallbladder and Stomach-Pylorus Extension positions, use the ulnar side of the middle fingers.

- For the Pelvis/Lower Body position, use the ulnar side of the ring (fourth) finger.

- For the Neuro-psychological, Mitral Valve, and Special Lung positions, use one finger alone.

Broad Focus

Gender and Age

Discussed in Ch. 3, these are primary considerations in relation to pulse findings, especially in the context of paradoxical findings.

Rhythm and Rate

True Arrhythmias and Pseudo-Arrythmias

By first simultaneously feeling the rate of the pulse on both wrists, one can note irregularities in the rhythm or differences in rate between sides and burners. Variations in rhythm include Changing Rate at Rest as well as the Intermittent and Interrupted qualities.

Usually, rates are Normal, Rapid, or Slow. It is noted that in present times the rate is more indicative of the heart and vascular circulation, or of emotional states, than of external pathogens like heat or cold.

The rate is also taken again at the end of the exam, with the patient in a seated position, and then immediately after exertion. To measure the pulse rate on exertion, have the patient vigorously rotate his arm at the shoulder ten to fifteen times, then take the pulse for ten seconds, and multiply by six. A substantial change in rate from rest and exertion, or lack of change, are significant indicators of Heart function (see Ch. 6 for more detail).

Pseudo-arrythmias include the Hesitant wave, Change in Amplitude, and Unstable qualities, all of which mimic true arrhythmias.

Uniform Qualities over the Entire Pulse

By taking the pulse at both wrists, one obtains a first impression of the uniform qualities on the whole pulse. This provides an overall assessment in terms of excess and deficiency, guided by questions such as: Is it Deep, Normal, or Superficial? Is it Thin or Wide, Pounding with or without spirit and force (Robust or Reduced)? Is it resilient or easily compressible, continuous or fragmented (Long, Scattered, or Short)? Or is it Feeble-Absent, Empty or Hollow Full-Overflowing, Flooding Excess or Flooding Deficient, or balanced or unbalanced among the three depths and six principal positions?

Qualities found uniformly over the pulse include the following: Floating, Tense, Tight, Pounding, Thin, Cotton, Deep, Smooth and Rough Vibration, Choppy, Leather-Hard, Slippery, Reduced Substance, Ropy, Muffled, Spreading, Change in Amplitude, or Qualities, Blood Heat, Blood Unclear, Blood Thick, Hollow Full-Overflowing, Suppressed, Flooding Excess, Flooding Deficient and Hesitant Wave.

Iatrogenic-related Qualities

Pharmaceuticals can affect the pulse in a number of ways. Some commonly used diuretics are associated with the Suppressed quality in which the wave seems cut off. Some cardiac and antihypertensive medications cause the Robust Pounding quality at the organ depth (usually due to excess heat) and diminished at the blood and qi depths. Steroids usually cause the pulse to become Slippery. Antidepressants reduce or eliminate the Cotton quality, and the Muffled quality may be associated with antipsychotic drugs. Beta-blockers and calcium channel blockers can slow the pulse rate dramatically and even cause different rates at different positions.

Stability or Instability

Large Changes in Quality as well as the Empty quality found on one or both sides suggest a state of extremely compromised qi function characterized by chaos (the 'qi wild' condition).[2] Consistent Changes in Amplitude over the entire pulse are associated with the Heart; these can be distinguished from the inconsistent Changes in Amplitude related to Liver qi stagnation.

Width and Hardness

As previously noted, the evaluation of the hardness or pliability of qualities must be made with an overall allowance for the general width of the pulse. Some general aspects of width and hardness can be considered normal. Women's pulses tend to be Thinner and Tighter (harder) than men's, which tend to be Wider (Tense) and more pliable. The organ depth should normally be the most substantial and wide, which decreases as one releases pressure to the blood and qi depths.

Fig. 4-2 Wave comparisons

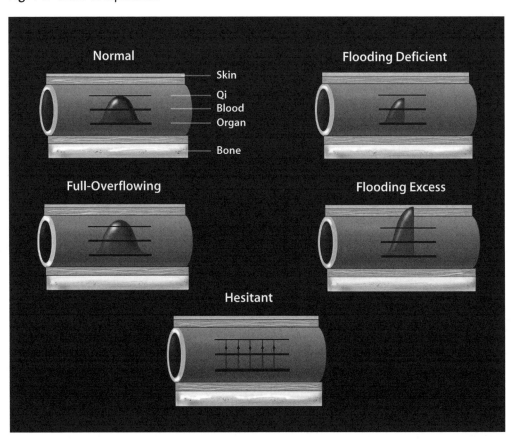

Wave Form

The Normal wave form resembles a sine or bell curve that stays between the organ and qi depths. Unusual wave forms include the Hollow Full-Overflowing, Flooding-Excess, and Flooding-Deficient qualities, the Suppressed quality, and the Hesitant quality. The Hollow Full-Overflowing quality has the correct shape but exceeds the qi depth. The wave form should be evaluated at the height of the amplitude.

CLOSER FOCUS

Uniform Qualities on the Left Side

The most common uniform qualities to be found on the left side are Tense, Tight, Yielding, Spreading, Diffuse, Reduced Substance, Smooth and Rough Vibration, Deep, Feeble, Hollow, Hollow Full-Overflowing, Slippery, Choppy, Change in Amplitude, and Cotton. A slightly Feeble Deep quality with a Thin Tight quality at the pulse's most superficial aspect is found when the 'nervous system' affects the 'organ system'. When the etiology is moderate and persistent worry, superficial Smooth Vibration is found over the entire left side. Rough Vibration on the left side only is a sign of parenchymal damage to the vital yin organs, the Heart, Liver, and Kidney.

Uniform Qualities on the Right Side

The common qualities found uniformly on the right side are Tense, Tight, Yielding, Reduced Substance, Deep, Feeble, and Cotton. A Slippery quality may also be encountered uniformly, but much less often. A Thin and Tight quality at the pulse's most superficial aspect is found when a person eats too quickly.

Amplitude Alternating between Sides

When palpating both left and right radial arteries simultaneously, the amplitude may seem at first to increase and decrease on only one side, and then reverse sides. This is most often associated with a current, significant interpersonal conflict, and also (but less frequently) associated with a situation in which the person has worked or exercised beyond their capacity for a period of weeks prior to the examination.

Qualities Alternating between Sides

When the qualities on the left and right sides switch places over the course of the examination, this is a sign of the separation of yin and yang and a serious 'qi wild' condition (see Ch. 6 for more detail).[3]

Depths

While we commonly speak of three principal depths, there are actually nine

Fig. 4-3 The nine depths

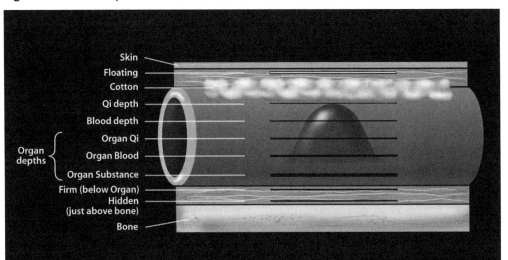

depths in our system of pulse examination (Fig. 4-3). These include, above the qi depth, the Floating depth (quality) just below the skin, and the Cotton depth (quality) just below that; the qi depth; the blood depth; the organ depth (with three subdivisions); the Firm depth (quality) between the organ depth and the bone; and the Hidden depth (quality) just above the bone.

The importance of accurately palpating the depths at their precise locations cannot be overstated. Located only slightly apart from each other, the depths are accessed by very small increases or decreases in pressure from the wrists, and therefore the fingers. The movement is all in the wrists and must be demonstrated repeatedly to truly master the technique. This movement is one critical aspect of properly identifying the presence or absence of pulse qualities, some of which are defined by the absence of sensation at, for example, the qi depth, or both qi and blood depths. The greatest substance and width is ordinarily found at the organ depth. As pressure is released, the pulse should become less wide with less substance. The lightest and least wide sensation is found at the qi depth.

Above the Qi Depth

The qualities found above the qi depth are Floating, Flooding Excess, Hollow Full-Overflowing, and, most often, Cotton. The Floating qualities are accessed at or slightly below the skin with very gentle pressure at the Floating depth. The Cotton quality is the amount of resistance in the connective tissue between the skin and the qi depth at the Cotton depth, or to the side of the pulse with those wave forms that exceed the qi depth (Flooding Excess etc.).

Qi Depth

All three positions are palpated with all three fingers, checking for the presence or absence of qualities at the qi depth. The most common qualities are Tense, Tight, Thin, Yielding, Diminished or Reduced Substance, Absent, Slippery, and Smooth Vibration.

Blood Depth

The blood depth manifests patterns of deficiency or excess. Deficiency is felt by gradually increasing the pressure from the qi to the blood depth. If the qi depth is Absent and the blood depth is Spreading (Separating), there is deficiency of both qi and blood. If both the qi and blood depths are Absent and the organ depth is present, this demonstrates a more advanced deficiency of qi and blood; and a Thin quality indicates that the blood deficiency is greater still. If the qi depth is present, the blood depth Separating or Absent, and the organ depth separates under pressure, the quality is Empty. If the qi depth is intact and the blood depth separates or disappears under pressure, yet the organ depth is clearly felt upon further pressure, this is the Hollow quality, a sign of blood deficiency or hemorrhage (see Chapter 9).

Fig. 4-4 Pulse Positions

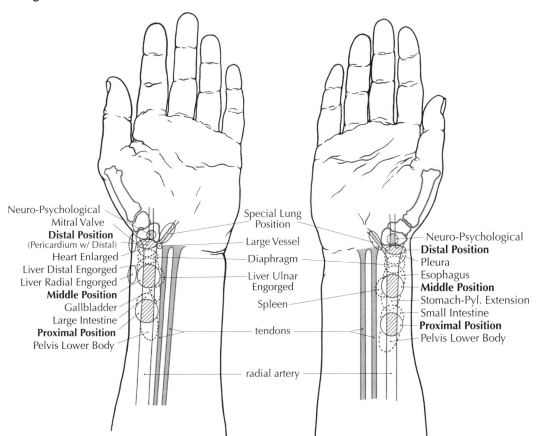

Neuro-Psychological
Mitral Valve
Distal Position
(Pericardium w/ Distal)
Heart Enlarged
Liver Distal Engorged
Liver Radial Engorged
Middle Position
Gallbladder
Large Intestine
Proximal Position
Pelvis Lower Body

Special Lung Position
Large Vessel
Diaphragm
Liver Ulnar Engorged
Spleen
tendons

Neuro-Psychological
Distal Position
Pleura
Esophagus
Middle Position
Stomach-Pyl. Extension
Small Intestine
Proximal Position
Pelvis Lower Body

radial artery

Excess patterns in the blood are felt by compressing the pulse to the organ depth and then gradually releasing pressure toward the surface. Normally the pulse diminishes in size and strength as pressure is released. If the pulse fills out in the blood depth, and then diminishes at the qi depth, a disharmony (and pulse quality) such as Blood Unclear or Blood Heat is present. If the substance of the pulse does not diminish as pressure is released toward the qi depth, the condition (and pulse) is regarded as Blood Thick, and if the pulse increases in substance above the qi depth with a sine wave, the quality representing this increasing heat in the blood is Hollow Full-Overflowing.

Organ Depth

At the organ depth the pulse should be most substantial and reflect both the functional and material aspects of the organs. Qualities found uniformly at the organ depth are Taut, Tense, Tight, Thin, Diffuse, Reduced Substance, Feeble-Absent, Slippery, Choppy, Pounding, Rough Vibration, and Separating.

Within the organ depth, through a careful sense of touch, one can find a qi, blood, and more material substance (yin) layer, the latter of which equates with the biomedical concept of parenchyma. Strong evidence of retained pathogens can be found at the organ-blood (O-B) and organ-substance (O-S) depths.

Below the Organ Depth

The qualities Firm and Hidden are found below the organ depth: the Firm quality is found between the organ depth and the bone, and the Hidden quality just above the bone.

Fig. 4-5 Both hands

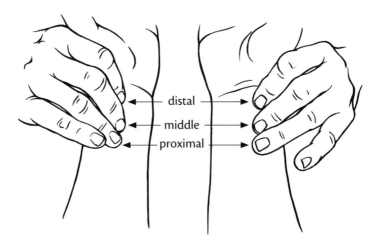

Fig. 4-6 Left Special Lung position

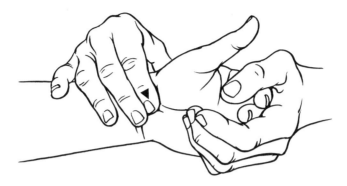

CLOSEST FOCUS

Left Principal and Complementary Individual Positions

Left Special Lung Position

The left Special Lung position is found at a small branch of the radial artery (superficial palmer) approximately between the acupuncture points LU-9 *(tài yuǎn)* and PC-7 *(dà líng)*. A light touch using the pad of the right index finger is employed to feel this small branch medial to the radial artery. The left Special Lung position reveals the status and history of the material right lung and the location of disharmony in the energetic right Lung. The right Special Lung position gives us information about the left lung. The qualities found here are Tense, Tight, Wiry, Narrow, Restricted, Slippery, Vibration, Floating, Inflated, Muffled, Restricted, Change in Amplitude, Absent, and Choppy.

Left Neuro-psychological Position

The right index finger is used to find the left Neuro-psychological position in, on, or around a truncated depression on the scaphoid bone just distal to the principal position. Dr. Shen used this position but never fully developed its interpretation. Some conclusions have been made about its interpretation, and further associations have yet to be explored. It is correlated with the central nervous system and the head. Qualities found at this position are Smooth Vibration, Choppy, Doughy, Change in Amplitude, Tight, Slippery, Smooth and Rough, Robust Pounding, and Muffled. The Smooth Vibration quality found here was associated by Dr. Shen with 'Heart nervous' qi agitation; and a Choppy quality may be felt in a person with head trauma. The undifferentiated or Doughy quality has been tentatively linked with neurological problems, including headache. (See Ch. 12.)

Fig. 4-7 Left Neuro-psychological position

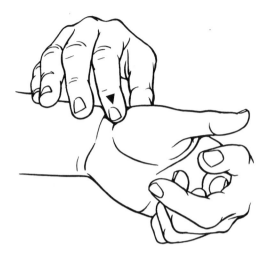

Left Distal, Pericardium, and Large Vessel Positions

Within the left distal position, another distinct quality is sometimes ascertained by rolling the edge of the index finger from the lateral to the medial aspect of the left distal position and back again, from medial to lateral. This is the Pericardium position, which is located in the center of the left distal position. A sharp Tight quality is most commonly found in the Pericardium position and this is sometimes accompanied by Slipperiness.

Rolling the index finger medially toward the ulna also accesses the Large Vessel position. At the intersection of the tendon of the flexor carpi radialis and the scaphoid bone is a hole or cave-like place that is palpated by the lateral distal

Fig. 4-8 Left distal position

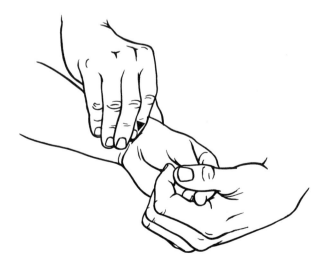

edge of the index finger. While both qualities are rare, most commonly found here is an Inflated quality (indicating aneurysm) or much less often, a Tense-Tight Hollow Full-Overflowing quality (indicating cardiac hypertension).

Fig. 4-9 Large Vessel position

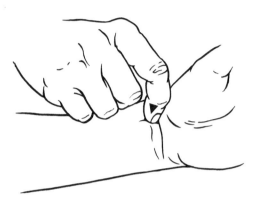

Mitral Valve Position

Using the right index finger and an especially light touch, the Mitral Valve is accessed on the muscle-ligament connecting the styloid process and the scaphoid bone. The most commonly found qualities here are Vibration and Slipperiness. Like the Neuro-psychological position, the qualities here are ephemeral, subtle, and sometimes moving around the position.

Fig. 4-10 Mitral Valve position

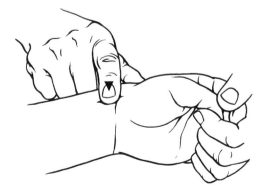

Diaphragm Positions

The Diaphragm positions are found on both wrists between the distal and middle positions. They are accessed as the index finger is rolled proximally from just below the distal position and the middle finger is rolled distally from the middle position.

Commonly found in the Diaphragm position, the Inflated quality will be perceived as a sensation of the fingers rolling uphill from a distal to proximal direction and then downhill proximally into the middle position. Mild inflation [2] is considered normal. Greater than two [3-5] is an indication of qi stagnation in the chest and diaphragm area. An Inflated quality larger than three [3] on the left side is associated with the suppression of tender feelings that have been replaced by anger, as in the withdrawal of one's affections in the dissolution of a relationship. The absence of or very low Inflation at the left Diaphragm position indicates either an absence of close relationships or very harmonious ones.

Inflation on the right side is usually a measure of lifting, again with greater than two indicating lifting beyond a person's ability (qi). However, when the emotional conflict is great, as noted above for the left Diaphragm, it can manifest as an excessively Inflated quality on the right side as well.

Heart Enlarged, and Distal Liver Engorgement Positions

The presence of Heart Enlarged (the condition and its associated pulse) is discernible when the distal aspect of the left Diaphragm position is either more Inflated or Rougher than the proximal aspect.[4]

Fig. 4-11 Heart Enlargement position

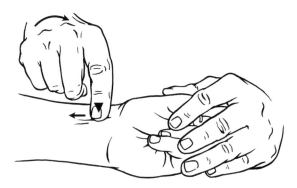

The presence of distal engorgement of the Liver can be discerned using the right middle finger when the proximal aspect of the left Diaphragm position is either more Inflated or Rougher than the distal aspect.

Fig. 4-12 Distal Liver Engorgement position

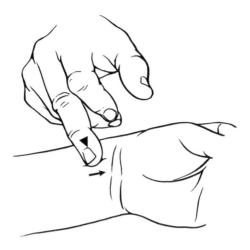

Principal Left Middle Position

The left middle position is palpated with the right middle finger. It is imperative that one locates the principal impulse, which is often quite medial. Common qualities found here are Tense, Tight, Wiry, Thin, Pounding, Hollow Full-Over-flowing, Flooding Excess, Slippery, Deep, Feeble, Empty, Hollow, Vibration, Diffuse, Reduced Substance, Choppy, Muffled, and Changes in Qualities and Amplitude. Qualities such as Blood Unclear, Blood Heat, and Blood Thick may also be best palpated here as one releases one's finger from the organ to the qi depth, reflecting the relationship of the Liver and its storage of blood.

Fig. 4-13 Left middle position

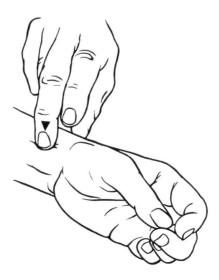

Ulnar Engorgement of the Liver

The following two Engorgement positions can measure blood stagnation of the Liver. From the principal position, one rolls the middle finger toward the flexor carpi radialis tendon to lightly palpate this position. Ulnar Engorgement is detected when a very superficial Inflated quality is felt with the portion of the finger next to the nail. As it is found in a relatively confined space, the Inflated quality can be quite subtle.

Fig. 4-14 Ulnar Liver Engorgement position

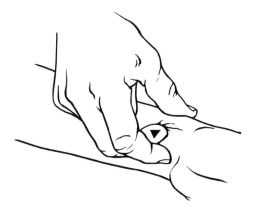

Gallbladder Position

To find the Gallbladder position, one lays the entire right middle finger proximal to the left middle position medially along and on top of the artery. The sensation is felt approximately at the ulnar side of the distal interphalangeal joint, although one may have to roll the finger medially and laterally to find the strongest impulse. Common qualities include Tight, Tense, Wiry, Inflated, Slippery, Robust Pounding, Choppy, Muffled, and Change of Amplitude.

Fig. 4-15 Gallbladder position

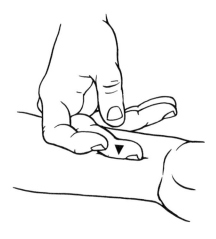

Left Proximal Position

The left proximal position is evaluated by placing the right ring finger adjacent to the middle finger. The principal position is felt with the right ring finger, which may be rolled medially to follow the course of the artery and to access the main impulse.

Common qualities include Tense, Tight, Wiry, Reduced Substance and Pounding, Deep, Feeble-Absent, Muffled, Choppy, and Changes in Qualities and Amplitude. The harder qualities in this position suggest Kidney yin-essence deficiency, overriding and masking the more pliable ones, which suggest Kidney qi and yang deficiency. The Wiry quality can indicate more severe essence deficiency, early diabetes, hypertension, or pain in the lower back or pelvis area.

Fig. 4-16 Left proximal position

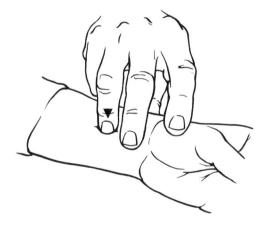

Large Intestine Position

The Large Intestine position is found by rolling the right ring finger distally and very medially from the principal left proximal position toward the flexor carpi radialis so that it is vertical, and then tilting the hand distally at a 30° angle. In this manner, the radial edge of the ring finger is used to differentiate between qualities at the Large Intestine position rather than those of the principal left proximal position. Common qualities include Tense, Tight, Slippery, Biting, Rough Vibration, Inflated, Choppy, Change of Amplitude, and Muffled.

Left Pelvis/Lower Body Positions

The Pelvis/Lower Body is found on both wrists. To find the left position, lay the entire ring finger proximally from the LPP along the artery. To feel a sensation at approximately the distal interphalangeal joint, one may have to roll the finger medially and laterally to search out the principal impulse. Choppy, Slippery, Tight, Tense, Muffled, and Change in Amplitude are all commonly found qualities at this position.

Fig. 4-17 Large Intestine position

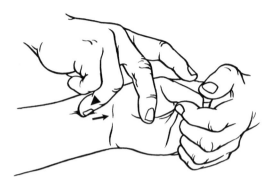

Fig. 4-18 Left Pelvis/Lower Body positions

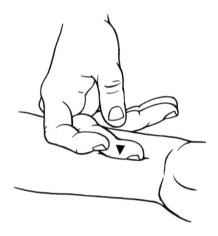

Right Principal and Complementary Positions

Right Special Lung Position

On the right wrist, first to be palpated is the Special Lung position, which is found the same way as that on the left (LU-9 to P-7) but using the flat pad of the left index finger. By the same qualities seen at the left, the right Special Lung position reveals the status and history of the material left lung (and simultaneously the location of disharmony in the energetic left Lung) including its medial, lateral, upper, and lower aspects, each of which can be accessed by rolling the finger in the appropriate direction. (Refer to Fig. 2-1 in Ch. 2 for more detail.)

Right Neuro-psychological Position

Using the left index finger, the right Neuro-psychological position is accessed in the same manner as the corresponding position on the left wrist, with similar qualities and interpretation.

Fig. 4-19 Right Special Lung position

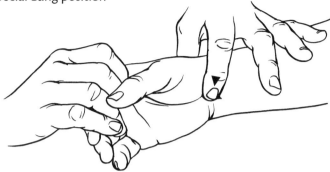

Fig. 4-20 Right Special Lung position, another view

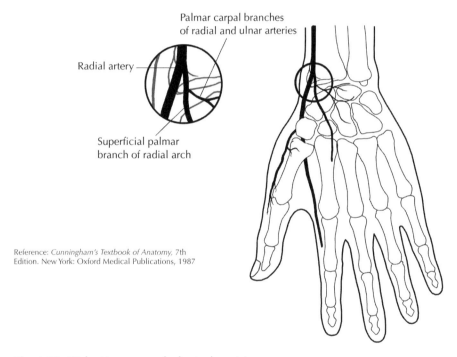

Palmar carpal branches
of radial and ulnar arteries

Radial artery

Superficial palmar
branch of radial arch

Reference: *Cunningham's Textbook of Anatomy,* 7th
Edition. New York: Oxford Medical Publications, 1987

Fig. 4-21 Right Neuro-psychological position

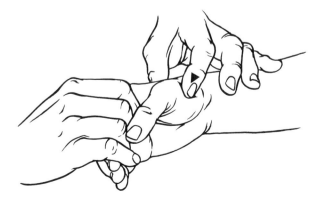

Right Distal (regular Lung) Position

This position is accessed in the same manner as the left distal position, but by using the left index finger, rolled distally and slightly radially toward and slightly under the right scaphoid bone. Common qualities found in this position are Tense, Inflated, Tight, Wiry, Slippery, Vibration, Choppy, Floating, Feeble-Absent, Muffled, and Changes of Amplitude and Qualities. If the Dead quality is encountered, it is usually associated with lung cancer.

Fig. 4-22 Right distal position

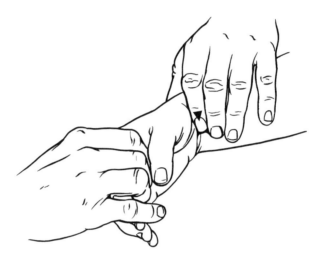

Right Diaphragm, Pleura, and Esophagus Positions

For the Right Diaphragm position, the left index finger is rolled proximally from the distal position and the middle finger is rolled distally from the middle position. Commonly found in the Diaphragm position, the Inflated quality will be perceived as a sensation of the fingers rolling uphill, moving from the distal to proximal and vice versa. Mild inflation [2] is considered normal. If more significant, it is an indication of qi stagnation in the chest and diaphragm area. An Inflated quality larger than three [3] is associated with lifting beyond a person's energy, and less often with suppressed emotions with respect to an interpersonal separation.

The presence of a pleural condition at the Pleural position (acute or chronic) is discernible when the distal aspect of the left Diaphragm position is either more Inflated or Rougher than the proximal aspect.

The presence of esophageal qi stagnation is discernible when the proximal aspect of the right Diaphragm position is either more Inflated or Rougher than the distal aspect. A Slippery quality instead of a Rough quality is a sign of esophageal food stagnation.

Fig. 4-23 Pleura position

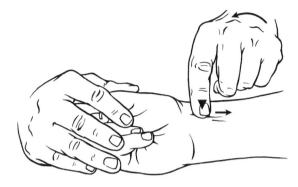

Fig. 4-24 Esophagus position

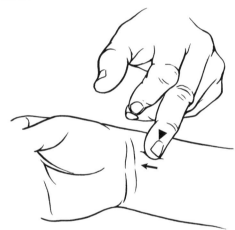

Right Middle Position

Principal Right Middle Position

Using the left index finger this position is accessed in the same manner as the corresponding position on the left wrist. Harder qualities (Tense, Tight, Robust Pounding) at this position indicate Stomach heat; the more pliable qualities (Spreading, Deep, Reduced Substance, Diffuse, Reduced Pounding, Feeble-Absent, and Empty) indicate Spleen deficiency. Both harder and more pliable qualities can be felt concurrently as Changing Qualities representing the presence of both severe Stomach and Spleen pathology respectively. The Muffled quality is associated with a neoplastic process.

Spleen Position

Place the left middle finger on the right middle position, and roll it medially and superficially toward the ulna to access the Spleen position. This is found between the vessel and the flexor carpi radialis, felt by the area of the finger next to the nail as a very superficial Inflated quality.

Fig. 4-25 Right middle position

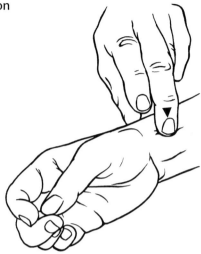

Fig. 4-26 Spleen position

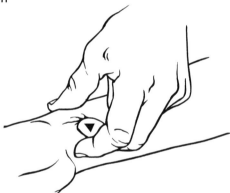

Stomach-Pylorus Extension & Duodenum Positions

The Stomach-Pylorus Extension position is palpated by laying the entire left middle finger on the vessel proximally and medially from the right middle position in the same manner as the Gallbladder position on the left side. To find the exact position, one must roll the finger medially and laterally until one palpates the principal impulse.

Tense, Tight, Choppy, Slippery, Inflated, Muffled, Biting, Rough Vibration, Choppy, and Change of Amplitude qualities are found here. More rarely, a Hollow or Slippery quality may be found in cases of stomach duodenal ulcers.

Pathology in the duodenum is present when the quality in the Stomach-Pylorus Extension position and in the Small Intestine position are the same, often Tight and/or Slippery, indicating a duodenal ulcer and/or energetic disharmony in this area. An Inflated quality here signifies a less severe energetic and physical pathology.

Fig. 4-27 Stomach-Pylorus Extension position

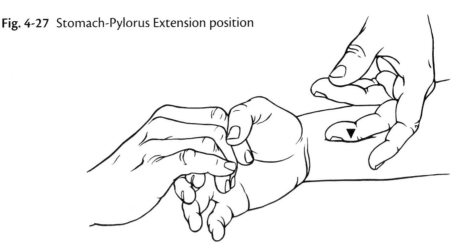

Peritoneal-Pancreatic Position

When both the Ulnar Engorgement and Spleen positions are present, usually Inflated, this suggests a problem in the peritoneal cavity. Pancreatic inflammation or tumor, depleted enzymatic activity, other kinds of tumors in the cavity (including intestinal), or ascites are all associated with this finding.

Right Proximal Position

Principal Right Proximal (Bladder) Position

The right proximal position is evaluated by placing the left ring finger adjacent to the middle finger. We interpret this position to represent deficient Kidney yang issues manifested by the pliable qualities (Reduced Substance, Feeble-Absent, Changing Qualities and Amplitude). However, yin deficiency, or less often, severe pain, may also be evident here with the harder qualities of Tight or Wiry overriding the pliable ones. If there is infection present in the bladder or acute fulminating infection of the small intestine or pelvic organs, the sensations in this position are excess qualities such as Flooding-Excess and Robust Pounding (graded 3+ to 5).

Fig. 4-28 Right proximal position

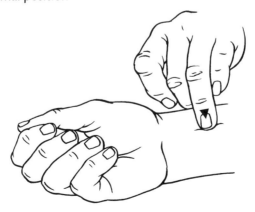

Small Intestine Position

The Small Intestine position is accessed on the right proximal position by rolling the ring finger distally and very medially toward the right middle position. The usual qualities found here are Tense, Tight, Biting, Slippery, Robust Pounding, and Muffled. Rough Vibration, Inflated, and Choppy qualities are also sometimes encountered.

Fig. 4-29 Small Intestine position

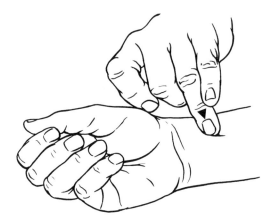

Right Pelvis/Lower Body Position

The right Pelvis/Lower Body position is palpated in the same way as the corresponding position on the left side, except that the practitioner lays the entire left ring finger down proximally on the vessel. To find the exact position one must roll the finger medially and laterally until one palpates the principal impulse. As on the left wrist, qualities frequently found here are Tense, Tight, Slippery, Muffled, Change in Amplitude, and Choppy.

Fig. 4-30 Right Pelvis/Lower Body position

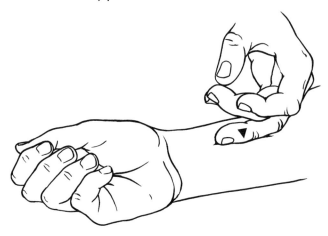

Similar Qualities found Bilaterally at the same Position (Burner)

The simultaneous appearance at one position, or burner, of the same quality on both sides has a special significance, detailed in Ch. 14 and in Table 14-1. Some of the more common qualities found bilaterally are Floating, Cotton, Hollow Full-Overflowing, Inflated, Flat, Tense, Tight, Wiry, Slippery, Thin, Feeble-Absent, Empty, Hollow, and Vibration.

Musculoskeletal Positions

By rolling the fingers to the radial side of the area between the burners one can detect musculoskeletal disorders. The Tight quality usually signifies pain in these areas. Distally and radially from the distal pulse positions, one can access the neck position. Radial to the area between the distal and middle positions is the shoulder girdle position. The area radial to and between the middle and proximal positions reflects the hip, and radial to the area between the proximal and Pelvis/Lower Body positions reflects the position of the knees.

Rate on Exertion

At the end of the examination, after taking the resting rate, the patient is asked to rotate one arm at the shoulder vigorously, immediately after which one takes the rate for ten seconds and then multiplies this figure by six to get the rate on exertion. It is helpful to repeat the procedure twice, taking an average of the results, due to the possibility of error. This is a measure of Heart qi, yang, and blood deficiency (see Ch. 12 for more details).

The Pulse and Psychology

Each 'focus' (broad, closer, and closest) reveals psychological conditions. At the broad focus, psychological issues such as Heart shock (Rough Vibration over the entire pulse) and Heart qi agitation (Change in Rate at Rest) manifest here. At the closer focus, examples are the Cotton quality (resignation) and 'nervous system tense' (Tight and Thin at the qi depth). At the closest focus, each quality has a psychological implication (see Table 15-1).

PULSE EVALUATION FOLLOWING TREATMENT WITH NEEDLES

Dr. Shen was very clear that in his experience (and also in Dr. Hammer's), evaluation of the pulse using this system immediately after a treatment is inaccurate and not useful until several days have passed due to the ongoing changes set in motion by the introduction of needles.

A REMINDER

The best therapeutic results are achieved by recognizing that the information gathered from the larger picture is often the pattern that must be resolved first if the therapy is to have lasting significance. This information includes the rhythm and rate, first impressions and qualities that are common or uniform over the large segments, the three depths, and signs of instability or chaos.

5

Classification and Nomenclature of Pulse Qualities

Ross Rosen, L.Ac.

THIS CHAPTER FOCUSES ON the style and format of the classification and nomenclature of the pulse qualities, described in detail in Chs. 6 through 11. We begin with a discussion of the Normal pulse, a baseline from which all others are a departure.

Because this chapter is concerned with qualities, it is important to remember that these are recorded as they appear at the principal impulse and at the highest amplitude at each depth. It is at these places that pulse qualities are clearest and most accurate. We agree upon this standard because it facilitates the most lucid communication among practitioners.

THE NORMAL PULSE

The Normal pulse provides us with a sensitive, precise, and measurable standard of health, enabling us to detect early deviations from health, and thereby to prevent disease.

ATTRIBUTES OF THE NORMAL PULSE

Rhythm

Consistently regular.

Stability

The qualities and amplitude are consistent over time and in each position.

Rate

Consistent with age (see Ch. 7). The pulses of women and children tend to be more Rapid than those of men. Athletes generally have Slower pulses. The rate should be assessed by a 'kinetic' self-winding watch with a second hand rather than by the patient's or practitioner's respiration, which can be inconsistent and therefore unreliable.

Wave forms

The Normal wave is a sine wave that begins at the organ depth and gradually rises to the qi depth, then subsides again to the organ depth.

Fig. 5-1 Normal pulse wave

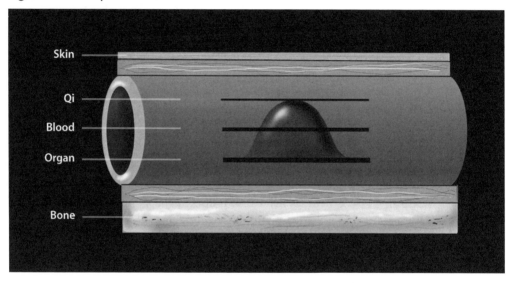

Volume

Moderate strength with spirit, depending on body build.

Buoyancy

Resilient, compressible, elastic, and with Robust Substance. The Normal pulse in a child (and a vegetarian) tends to be more Yielding, in a woman more Thin, and in a man more Wide.

Shape

Long and continuous, flowing smoothly with no turbulence. Pregnant women usually have more Slippery and more Rapid pulses.

Balance

Depth

Depth is balanced between superficial, middle, and deep. The qi depth is the

Table 5-1 Characteristics of the Normal pulse

Following are some characteristics of the Normal pulse,
which serves as a baseline and standard for health.

1. **Rhythm**

   Consistently regular

2. **Stability**

   The qualities and amplitude are currently steady overall and
   in each position and over time.

3. **Rate**

   Consistent with age

   AGE AND RATE ACCORDING TO DR. SHEN:

AGE		RATE PER MIN.
Birth →	4	84–90
4 →	10	78–84
10 →	15	78–80
16 →	40	72–78
41 →	50	72
51 →	70	66–72

4. **Wave**

   Sine curve

5. **Volume**

   Moderate strength and spirit, depending on body build

6. **Buoyancy**

   Resilient, compressible, elastic, with Robust Substance

7. **Shape**

   Long and continuous with no turbulence

8. **Balance**

   DEPTH

   - Balanced among superficial, middle, and deep
   - Qi depth is lightest, increasing in substance until the organ depth,
     which is greatest in substance and therefore has 'root'
   - Deeper in heavy people and more superficial in thin people

   POSITION

   - Middle position overflows into distal and proximal positions
   - Distal position most confined
   - Middle position least confined
   - Proximal position moderately confined

lightest, increasing in breadth and strength as the organ depth is approached. Heavy people have Deeper pulses, and thin people more Superficial. In the Normal pulse there should be no sensation felt above the qi depth.

Position

The relationship of one position to another is even and balanced. Normally, the qualities of the middle positions tend to overflow into the other positions. (See Table 5-1.)

NORMAL CHARACTERISTICS RELATED TO QI, SPIRIT, AND ESSENCE

Stomach qi

Stomach qi is equated in the literature with the true or upright qi of the body, a summation of the organism's global ability to function. In this context, balance, stability, and moderation are more specific and familiar terms used here with Contemporary Chinese Pulse Diagnosis to delineate the more global Stomach qi.

We assess the Stomach ('earth') and its associated complementary positions (see Chs. 4 and 12) at the right middle position, and the uniform qualities and volume on the right side or 'digestive system' (see Ch. 14). (For more detail on how the literature views this quality, see the source text.)

The balance attributed to 'earth' on the pulse and in the organism is mediated through the 'internal duct' of the Triple Burner, and is evaluated by the balance of individual qualities among the burners and the individual positions (see Ch. 12). The integrity of the Spleen, Stomach, Liver (moves the qi in all organs, and normally downward in the digestive system) and Triple Burner qi is essential to the digestion, assimilation, transportation, and storage of all the organism's qi, blood, yin, and essence, apart from what is inherited from the ancestral qi.

Spirit

In the Contemporary Chinese Pulse Diagnosis model, spirit is measured by the amplitude of the pulse, a function of its volume or yang force. (Again, please refer to the source text for more detail on how the literature views this quality.)

Essence ('root')

Contemporary Chinese Pulse Diagnosis associates essence or 'root' with Kidney qi. As explained in Ch. 2, there is both yin and yang essence. Deficiency of yin-essence is marked by a Tight-Wiry pulse (Tight reflects the yin and Wiry reflects the essence), usually in the proximal positions, and yang-essence deficiency by a Feeble/Absent or Empty quality in the proximal positions, and possibly a Doughy quality at the Neuro-psychological positions (a subject of continuing investigation). (Further explanations in the literature can be found in the source text.)

Seasonal Variations

Contemporary Chinese Pulse Diagnosis finds seasonal variations only in those rare instances where a person has little disharmony. Dr. Shen did not mention these. Subtle seasonal changes are lost in the overwhelming presence of pulse patterns and qualities representing severe disharmonies and pathologies. (Further discussion can be found in the source text.)

Gender Variations

With a relatively Normal pulse, Dr. Hammer's past experience indicates that the pulse is somewhat stronger on the right side in women and on the left side in men. Pathology can of course easily alter these tendencies.

Age

Contemporary Chinese Pulse Diagnosis finds that before the age of about eighteen, the presence of extraordinarily unstable qualities, indicative of severe disharmony and chaos, are actually signs of rapid physiological growth and change, and not of pathology. This must be kept in mind when assessing the pulses of young people. In addition, the pulse tends to be more pliable in young patients.

In cases of disease etiologies that occurred before birth or at delivery and early infancy, all of the pulse positions might be relatively unremarkable except the left distal (Heart) and proximal (Kidney) positions. If the disease etiology occurred after this early period, any pulse position may show signs of excess or deficiency depending upon the nature of the insult and the initial vulnerability of the organism. (Other views reflected in the literature can be found in the source text.)

Pregnancy

In Contemporary Chinese Pulse Diagnosis, according to Dr. Shen, "If a woman's left *chí* [proximal] pulse is slippery (and both *chí* and *cùn* [distal] pulses are a little tight), and in addition she has missed her menstruation, it is a sign of pregnancy." In pregnancy, from about three days to three months, the entire pulse is usually very Slippery. If the fetus is a boy, according to Dr. Shen, there is a very Tense left distal position; if the fetus is a girl, there is no special change.

Richard Van Buren argues to the contrary, that the fetus is a boy if the left proximal position is very Tight, and a girl if the right proximal position is very Tight. Dr Hammer has found this latter view to be 90 percent accurate. According to Dr. Shen, a miscarriage is heralded by a suddenly Rapid rate, with either a Feeble-Absent or very Tight left proximal position; this is accompanied by dark vertical lines on the tongue, and pain in the low back and abdomen.

ABERRATIONS FROM THE NORMAL PULSE

The Normal pulse (rarely observed due to the enormous stresses of modern life) is a sensitive barometer capable of guiding the practitioner to an accurate assessment of those aspects that need to be addressed by the patient in order to return to harmony. Medications often render the pulse seemingly uniform and mistakenly Normal, but the more experienced hand will notice the top of the Normal pulse wave to be flattened (Suppressed) and disharmony still discernible.

Other pulse qualities (see Ch. 4) can appear to be Normal due to their uniformity. Commonly, these are the uniformly Tense pulses associated with what Dr. Shen termed the 'nervous system tense' condition, or the Hollow Full-Overflowing pulse associated with excess heat in the blood (see Chs. 8, 10, 11, 13, and 14 for further discussion). Uniformity can also be a sign of pretense during which, for a short period, a person can obliterate the subtleties of the pulse to protect themselves from the detection of hidden problems and perceived weaknesses.

Deviations from normal are indicated on the pulse record in degrees of severity using a scale of one to five, with five revealing the greatest deviation from normal and the greatest degree of abnormality. The numbers on the pulse record are placed next to the quality inside brackets, for example, Rough Vibration [5].

CLASSIFICATION AND NOMENCLATURE OF PULSE QUALITIES

The differences in Chinese medical terminology are exemplified in the variety of terms adopted by various writers to describe the qualities of the pulse over the centuries (see Table 1-1 in Ch. 1).

In Contemporary Chinese Pulse Diagnosis, pulses are classified by their sensations (see Table 5-2), one lastingly valuable medium by which the body communicates its inner condition to the outside world. This is the necessary first and irreplaceable step without which didactic discussion is merely speculation. Interpretation is vitally important, but only after sensation is correctly identified. And that can only be done with repeated hands-on training.

These sensations are called qualities. A detailed discussion of each of the qualities can be found in the source text, *Chinese Pulse Diagnosis, A Contemporary Approach*; the more important defining characteristics are also described in this handbook. (For the sake of completeness, we also include in Table 5-3 a classification according to condition.)

ORIENTATION TO THE STYLE USED IN THE CLASSIFICATION OF QUALITIES

The style used in this book for the written expression of the qualities and their combinations requires some explanation. For example, we write the combination Yielding Empty Thread-like without separating the individual qualities with commas. Contemporary Chinese Pulse Diagnosis doesn't use the serial comma because we prefer to retain the sense of their flow as they cascade into each other, as they are experienced simultaneously. The exception is the qualities defining rate—Rapid and Slow—which are set off from other qualities by 'and' or 'with' in order to emphasize the importance of rate in the overall pulse picture. For example, we say Yielding Hollow Full-Overflowing and Slow, which has a totally different etiology from that of a Rapid rate with the same qualities.

A few qualities are hyphenated, such as Full-Overflowing, which stems from the use by Dr. Shen of the term Overflowing for the sensation called Full in the literature.

THE NINE PRINCIPAL CATEGORIES OF QUALITIES

Table 5-4 at the end of this chapter illustrates the nine principal categories of qualities, of which the other qualities are subsidiaries. They are Rhythm, Stability, Rate, Volume, Depth, Width, Length, Wave and Shape.

FORMAT FOR PRESENTATION AND DISCUSSION OF THE QUALITIES

Except for rate and rhythm, discussion of qualities in this handbook will be presented in the following manner: Category (the quality's larger context), Sensation (as actually felt), General Interpretation (drawn from the ideas of Dr. Shen, Dr. Hammer, and others), Combinations, Positions (which includes qualities found bilaterally at the same position, left side, right side, and at the individual positions, including principal and complementary positions).

Again, after each quality on the pulse form will be a number in brackets, from one to five. This is a measure of the extent to which a quality is present on the pulse, with one being the minimum and five the maximum. These numbers also generally reflect the seriousness of the condition related to that quality.

Table 5-2 Qualities classified according to sensation (Hammer)

Normal quality
Moderate
Languid
Leisurely-relaxed
Slowed down
Long
Wide Moderate

Rhythm
At rest:
    Rate measurable without missed beat
        Change in Rate at Rest
            Occasional
                Small
                Large
            Constant
                Small
                Large
    Rate measurable with missed beat
        Intermittent
            Constantly Intermittent
                Frequently missed beats
                Infrequently missed beats
            Inconsistently Intermittent
            Interrupted
    Rate not measurable
        Interrupted
            Constant
            Occasional
            Sudden Transient
            Literature:
                'hurried'
                'knotted'
On exertion:
    Large increase in rate
        Constant
        Occasional
    Small increase, no change, or decrease
    in rate
        Small increase
        Same rate or decrease

Pseudo-Arrhythmia
Hesitant Wave
Large Change in Amplitude and Width
Unstable

Stability
Qi:
    Entire pulse
        Circulation
            Occasional Change in Amplitude
            (Liver Qi Stagnation)
            Consistent Change in Amplitude
            (Heart-Circulation qi deficiency)
        'Qi wild'
            Burners and positions vary
              greatly in qualities
            Empty
            Empty Thread-like
            Leather
            Minute
            Change in Quality
            Qualities Shifting from Side to
              Side
            Scattered
            Yielding Hollow Full-
              Overflowing and Slow
            Yielding Hollow Full-
              Overflowing and Rapid
            Sides vary greatly in substance
            Muffled
            Empty Interrupted-Intermittent
            Yielding Hollow and Interrupted-
              Intermittent
            Very high fever and very low rate
            Very low fever and very high rate
    Single position (Separation of yin and
    yang)
        Extreme Qi, Yin, Blood & Essence
        Deficiency of a Yin Organ
            Empty
            Change in Quality
            Change in Width
            Change in Amplitude
            Unstable
            Nonhomogeneous
Blood:
    Circulation out of control at individual
      positions
        Leather-Hollow
            Rapid
            Slow

Out of control over entire pulse
  Very Tense or Tight Hollow Full-
    Overflowing
Circulation erratic over entire pulse
  Constant Change in Amplitude and
    Intensity
  Change in Amplitude and Intensity
    shifting from side to side

Rate
Rapid:
  Bounding
Slow:
  Mildly slow
  Moderately slow
  Very Slow
Right and left side:
  Pulses vary in rate

Volume
Robust:
  Hollow Full-Overflowing
  Robust Pounding
  Flooding Excess
  Inflated
    Inflated Yielding
    Inflated Moderately Tense
    Inflated Very Tense
Reduced:
  Suppressed Wave at qi depth
  Suppressed Pounding
  Yielding at qi depth
  Feeble at qi depth
  Absent at qi depth
  Spreading at blood depth
  Yielding Partially Hollow at blood depth
  Flooding Deficient (Retarded, 'push
    pulse')
  Diffuse
  Reduced Substance
  Reduced Pounding
  Deep
  Flat
  Feeble
  Absent
  Muffled
  Dead

Depth
Superficial:
  Floating
    Yielding
    Tense
    Tight
    Slippery
    Vibrating
  Cotton
  Empty
  Yielding Empty Thread-like
  Leather-Empty (drum-like)
  Scattered
  Minute
  Hollow
    Yielding Partially Hollow
    Leather-Hollow
      Rapid Rate
      Slow Rate
    Hollow Full-Overflowing
    Hollow Interrupted-Intermittent
Submerged:
  Deep
  Firm (primarily in literature)
    Firm Tense
    Firm Yielding
  Hidden (primarily in literature)
    Hidden Tense
    Hidden Yielding

Width
Wide:
  Blood
    Excess (entire pulse)
      Least Wide
        Blood Unclear
      Less Wide
        Blood Heat
      Moderately Wide
        Blood Thick
      Extremely Wide
        Tense Hollow Full-
          Overflowing
    Deficient (individual position)
      Leather-Hollow

Sudden severe hemorrhage
Rapid rate: imminent
Slow rate: recent
Organ
Excess (usually one position)
Extremely Wide
Flooding Excess
Deficient
Less Wide
Diffuse
Moderately Wide
Yielding Hollow Full-
Overflowing
Yielding Ropy
Narrow:
Thin
Thin Tight
Thin Yielding
Yielding Empty Thread-like

Length
Extended
Long
Long Robust Pounding
Diminished:
Restricted
Short 'brief'
Short Yielding
Short Tense
Bean (Spinning)

Shape
Fluid:
Slippery
Pseudo-Slippery
Non-fluid:
Hard
Taut
Tense
Tight
Wiry
Ropy
Ropy Yielding
Ropy Tense

Ropy Tight
Leather (Drum-like)
Uneven
Choppy
Vibration
Smooth
Rough
Nonhomogeneous
Doughy

Modifiers
Reduced or Robust
Rough
Smooth
Subtle
Biting
Ephemeral
Separating

Wave
Normal
Hollow Full-Overflowing
Flooding
Excess
Deficient
Hesitant
Suppressed

Miscellaneous qualities
Split
Nonhomogeneous
Bean (Spinning)
Doughy
Amorphous
Collapsing
Electrical
Leisurely

Anomalous
Three Yin or Hidden Left Side *(sān yīn mài)*
Transposed *(fǎn quán mài)*
Ganglion
Local trauma
Split vessel
Multiple radial arteries

Table 5-3 Qualities classified according to Chinese condition (Hammer; see also source text)

1. Normal
   Moderate
   Languid
   Leisurely-relaxed
   Slowed down
   Long
   Wide Moderate

2. Deficiency
   A. Qi and yang
      Yielding at qi depth
      Feeble-Absent at qi depth
      Spreading at blood depth
      Flooding Deficient Wave
      Diffuse
      Reduced Pounding
      Reduced Substance
      Deep
      Flat
      Feeble
      Absent
      Firm Deficient
      Hidden Deficient
      Short Yielding
      Muffled
      Dead
   B. Parenchymal damage
      Nonhomogeneous
      Restricted
      Rough Vibration
      Muffled
      Dead
      Bean (Spinning)
   C. Blood deficiency
      General
         Spreading
         Yielding Partially Hollow
         Thin
            Thin Yielding (blood and qi
               deficiency)
            Thin Tight (blood and yin
               deficiency)
         Deep
         Leather
      Heart blood deficiency
         Rate Increases Excessively on
            Exertion
   D. Yin (deficient heat)

General
   Tight
   Wiry
   Ropy Tight
   Very Tight (Hollow) Full-
      Overflowing
Heart
   Hesitant Wave
   Tight at Pericardium or left distal
      position
   E. Essence
      Leather
      Wiry
      Doughy at Neuro-psychological
         positions
   F. Internal wind
      Floating Tight (blood and yin deficiency)

3. Stability
   A. Heart qi agitation (entire pulse)
      i. Mild Heart qi agitation
         Smooth Vibration
      ii. Moderate Heart qi agitation
         Occasional Change in Rate at Rest
      iii. Severe Heart qi agitation
         Constant Change in Rate at Rest
         Occasionally Intermittent/
            Interrupted
      iv. Severe Heart shock
         Rough Vibration and Tight over
            entire pulse
         Bean (Spinning) at distal (positions)
      v. Heart qi and blood deficiency
         a. Change in Rate
            Change in Rate on Exertion
               Heart blood deficiency
                  Large increase
               Slight Heart qi deficiency
                  Very small increase
               Heart qi deficiency
                  Stays the same
               Heart yang deficiency
                  Decrease
            Constant Change in Rate at Rest
               Moderate Heart qi deficiency
         b. Change in Amplitude over entire
            pulse
               Moderate Heart qi deficiency

    c. Rough Vibration at left distal
      position
    Heart qi deficiency and parenchymal
      damage
  vi. Heart yang deficiency
    Moderate
      Heart Large
    Severe
      Rate stays same or decreases on
        exertion
    Very Severe
      Intermittent/Interrupted Yielding
      Hollow
B. 'Qi wild' (entire pulse)
  Burners and positions vary greatly in
    qualities
  Change in Amplitude
  Empty
  Yielding Empty Thread-like (yin and
    yang deficient)
  Leather (essence, yin, blood)
  Minute (yang, qi, blood)
  Change in Qualities
  Change in Qualities and/or Substance
    from side-to-side
  Muffled
  Scattered (exhaustion of yang)
  Yielding Hollow Full-Overflowing
    Rapid
    Slow
  Yielding Hollow and Interrupted/
    Intermittent
C. Separation of Yin and Yang (individual
  positions)
  Nonhomogeneous
  Unstable
  Empty
  Change in Amplitude
  Change in Intensity
  Change in Quality
D. Fear/terror
  Bean (Spinning)

4. Stagnation
A. Qi
  i. External
    Wind
      Floating Tense
    Wind-cold
      Floating Tense and Slow

    Wind-heat
      Floating Yielding and Rapid
    Wind-damp
      Floating Slippery
    Cotton
  ii. Internal
    Medications
      Suppressed
    Liver qi stagnation
      Taut
      Occasional Change in Intensity
    Liver qi stagnation and excess heat
      Tense
    Qi trapped in organ
      Inflated Yielding Tense
    Qi trapped outside of organ
      Flat
    Qi very stagnant (obstructed) within
      organ
      Restricted
    Liver wind
      Tight Floating
    Qi unable to circulate between
      organs or burners
      Short (excess and deficient)
    Stagnation in hollow organ due to
      obstruction or in any organ due to
      trauma or shock
      Bean (Spinning)
    Stagnation at cellular-molecular-
      chromosomal level (absolute yin)
      Muffled
      Dead
B. Blood and circulation
  i. Blood out of control (Hollow
    [scallion])
    Leather-Hollow
      Hemorrhage from yin organ
    Very Tense/Tight Hollow Full-
      Overflowing
      Potential brain hemorrhage
        (stroke)
    Yielding Partially Hollow
      Gradual slow hemorrhage
  ii. Blood stagnation
    Tissues
      Choppy
      Liver Engorgement positions
        present
      Inflated Very Tense

Vessels
  Slippery at blood depth
  Rough Vibration at blood depth
  Ropy Tense
Cellular–Molecular Level
  Muffled
  Dead
iii. Circulatory system
  Heart qi agitation and excess heat
    Too Rapid
  General qi or Heart qi deficiency
    Too Slow
  Blood toxicity
    Deep and very Slow
    Blood Unclear
  Excess Heat and turbid blood
    Robust Pounding at blood depth
    Wide Excess
      Blood Heat
      Blood Thick
    Tense Hollow Full-Overflowing
    Slippery at blood depth
  Vessel walls damaged
    Separation of yin-yang in vessels
      Ropy Yielding
      Ropy Tense
    Rough Vibration at blood depth
C. Essence
  Proximal positions very Taut
D. Excess Heat
  External
    Floating Yielding and Rapid
  Internal
    Very Long
    Inflated Moderately Tense
    Tense
    Pounding with Force
    Flooding Excess Wave
    Ropy Tense
    Very Tense Hollow Full-Overflowing
E. Damp
  Slippery
F. Cold
  i. External
    Floating Tense and Slow
  ii. Internal
    Very Tight/Wiry
    Firm Excess
    Hidden Excess
    Short Excess

G. Wind
  External
    Floating Tense
  Internal
    Floating Tight (excess heat)
H. Food
  Esophagus position: Slippery
  Short Excess
  Bean (Spinning): intestinal obstruction
    w/severe pain
I. Parenchymal damage
  Rough Vibration at individual positions

5. Systems
  A. 'Nervous system'
    i. Tense
      Entire pulse Tense (consistently)
        Constitutional
          Slow rate
        Non-constitutional
          Normal or Rapid rate
    ii. Weak
      Early
        Yielding Floating and Rapid
        Smooth Vibration
      Middle
        Tight and Pounding just above
          organ depth
        Rapid
      Late
        Feeble-Absent
  B. 'Circulatory system'
    Very Slow rate
    Consistent Change in Intensity
  C. 'Digestive system'
    Eating too rapidly
      Right side
        Very Tight at surface of pulse
    Eating irregularly
      Right side
        Reduced Substance → Feeble-
          Absent
  D. 'Organ system'
    Entire left side
      Deep Feeble-Absent → Absent

6. Pain
Early: Tight-Wiry and Rapid
Profound with fear: Bean (Spinning)
With blood stasis: Choppy Wiry

Table 5-4 Nine principal categories of qualities

FUNCTION	SENSATION	TONGUE	PATHOLOGY
■ 1. Rhythm			
Most critical measure of Heart function	Regular	Normal	Heart and circulation normal; Heart qi relatively strong
Pivotal quality since Heart is 'emperor'	Arrhythmic	Pale	Heart relatively weak
		Red purple	Blood stagnation
	Arrhythmic Hollow	Pale	'Qi wild'
■ 2. Stability			
Balance and/or contact between yin and yang in either the entire organism or within one organ system	Yielding Hollow Full-Over-flowing over entire pulse Change in Qualities/Amplitude over entire pulse	Pale, swollen, wet	'Qi wild'
Stability is necessary for even minimal function	Inconsistent Change in Amplitude over entire pulse	Red, dry	Qi Stagnation, 'nervous system' imbalance
Instability indicates severe dysfunction	Consistent Change in Amplitude over entire pulse	Red purple pale, wet	Blood circulation function of Heart impaired
	Change in Amplitude, Qualities at one position	Depends on yin organ system	Severe organ, qi, blood, yin deficiency ('qi wild')
	Unstable impulse changing position	Depends on yin organ system	Very severe organ, qi, blood, yin deficiency (separation of yin and yang)
	Leather-Hollow	Variable	Blood out of control, hemorrhage

FUNCTION	SENSATION	TONGUE	PATHOLOGY

■ 3. Rate

FUNCTION	SENSATION	TONGUE	PATHOLOGY
Activity of Heart and circulation	1. Rapid: Heart shock 2. Slow: Heart qi deficiency	1. Coating thin, yellow red tip; vertical line 2. Pale underneath; vertical line	1. Increased activity of Heart/circulation 2. Decreased activity of Heart/circulation
Heat and cold 1. Heat	1. Rapid, Robust Pounding a. Very Rapid b. Slightly Rapid	1. Coating thick yellow, body very red 2. Coating thin yellow, patchy, dry; body thin, red	1. Heat from excess 2. Heat from deficiency
2. Cold	2. Slow a. Acute: slightly Slow b. Chronic: very Slow	1. Coating thin white, body normal 2. Coating white and wet, body pale and swollen	1. Acute, external pathogenic factor 2. Chronic qi-deficient cold

■ 4. Volume

FUNCTION	SENSATION	TONGUE	PATHOLOGY
Spirit	Amplitude		
Functional heat	1. Robust	Red body	Excess yang
Yang force	a. Excess	Red body	Excess heat in qi & blood
	i. Full-Hollow Overflowing	Red body	Excess heat in qi & blood
	ii. Flooding Excess	Red body	Excess heat in yin organs
	iii. Pounding	Red body	Excess heat in yin organs
	b. Moderately Inflated	Normal, slightly red and swollen in one area	Heat or qi trapped in organ or area
	2. Reduced a. Flooding Deficient	Coating thin white, body pale	Overwork: moderate qi deficiency
	b. Feeble Deep c. Absent	Coating thin white, body swollen, wet	b. Severe qi deficiency c. More severe qi deficiency

FUNCTION	SENSATION	TONGUE	PATHOLOGY

■ 5. Depth

FUNCTION	SENSATION	TONGUE	PATHOLOGY
Location and stage of disease process	1. Superficial a. Floating: stagnant qi b. Cotton: stagnant qi	Coating thin, patchy, white, normal	a. External pathogenic factor b. Superficial qi stagnation due to trauma, resignation
	2. Deeper a. Deficient qi i. Deep: mild ii. Hidden: very deficient	Coating and body depend on type and degree of deficiency	Disease is deeper, internal, and/or later-stage chronic deficient
	b. Excess qi Hidden Excess	Coating/body depend on nature of excess	Stagnation due to sudden severe excess

■ 6. Width

FUNCTION	SENSATION	TONGUE	PATHOLOGY
Activity & condition of substance: primarily blood (some qi) i. Excess	Intensity		
a. Toxicity	a. Slightly Wide	Normal	a. Blood unclear
b. Heat	b. Moderately Wide	Body red	b. Blood heat
c., d. Heat and viscosity	c., d. Very Wide	Body red	c. Blood thick
ii. Deficiency	Thin	Body pale	Blood deficient

■ 7. Length

FUNCTION	SENSATION	TONGUE	PATHOLOGY
Condition of qi and circulation of qi between organs and burners	1. Long	Normal	Normal
	Long Robust Pounding	Body slightly red	Heat from excess
Type and degree of disease activity	2. Short: a. Excess	Depends on type of stagnation	a. Stagnation of qi, phlegm, food, blood
	b. Deficiency	Body pale	b. Qi deficiency

FUNCTION	SENSATION	TONGUE	PATHOLOGY
■ 8. Wave			
Variable	1. Normal	1. Normal	1. None
	2. (Hollow) Full Overflowing	2. Body red and dry	2. Heat from excess and deficiency in the blood
	3. Flooding Excess	3. Body very red and thick, coating w/raised papillae	3. Heat from excess in organ
	4. Flooding Deficient	4. Pale, swollen, wet	4. Qi deficiency
	5. Hesitant	5. Dry, bright red & shiny, raised red on end	5. Obsessive, mono-maniacal
■ 9. Shape			
Elasticity			
1. Fluid (yielding): excess yin	Slippery	Coating wet	Damp stagnation
2. Static (hard)			
a. Excess:			
Qi	Taut	Normal	Qi stagnation
Qi and heat	Tense	Body slightly to very red	Qi stagnation and heat
Blood	Choppy	Red-purple	Blood stagnation
Heat in blood vessels	Ropy	Red, dry	Heat: vessels lose elasticity; yin-essence deficiency
b. Deficiency:			
Yin	Tight	Coating dry, red patchy	Heat from deficiency
Yin-essence	Wiry, Leather	Very dry, red, thin to no coating	Heat from extreme deficiency
Qi	Diffuse Feeble-Absent	Pale, swollen, wet	Deficiency of qi-yang
	Empty Thread-like		Instability
	Scattered		Separation of yin/yang
	Minu te		
c. Parenchymal damage	Rough Vibration		Parenchymal damage
	Nonhomogeneous		
	Muffled		

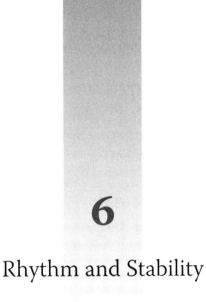

6

Rhythm and Stability

Ross Rosen, L.Ac.

ISSUES OF RHYTHM (see Table 6-1 and Figs. 6-4a & b at end of the chapter) occur over the entire pulse, at all three positions bilaterally. Issues of stability (Fig. 6-5, end of chapter) can involve the entire pulse, or just individual positions. Both relate to mind and emotion and the nervous system.[1] We consider the Heart to control the mind, therefore rhythm problems concern Heart function.

RHYTHM

The integrity of the rhythm is the single most important facet of pulse diagnosis. Rhythm primarily, and rate secondarily, are reflections of cardiac function. The Heart is the emperor, and with rare exceptions, the rhythm and rate are the overriding considerations in diagnosis and treatment and overshadow all other findings.

A few points should be noted. All shock, especially emotional, affects the Heart. All sudden physical trauma is a shock to the Heart directly as well as the circulation that secondarily depletes Heart qi. With Heart shock, there is ultimately disharmony between the Kidney and Heart; and one Heart condition can lead to another. For example, prolonged but mild excess heat in the Heart can cause Heart qi agitation, and either condition can lead to more serious Heart disorders.

Dr. Hammer translated the Heart conditions described by Dr. Shen (see Glossary) into terms that reflect the more familiar diagnostic patterns of Chinese medicine and allow a greater understanding of the pathologies.

CLASSIFICATION OF ARRHYTHMIAS

Arrhythmias—or changes in rhythm—are classified in accordance with the following parameters:

- Does the change in rhythm occur at rest or on exertion?
- Is the rate measurable?
- If measurable, are there missed beats?
- If there are missed beats, do they occur regularly after the same number of beats (Intermittent) or inconsistently (Interrupted)?
- How often does the irregularity occur?
- If there are no missed beats, is the change occasional or constant, large or small?

The changes discussed in this chapter are independent of, and easily distinguished from, the small changes in rate normally recorded with the breath, increasing with inhalation and decreasing with exhalation.

CHANGES IN RHYTHM AND RATE AT REST

Rate measurable without missed beats

The speeding up and slowing down of the rate can be occasional or continual, small or large, and is associated with moderate to severe degrees of Heart qi agitation and Heart qi deficiency.

According to Dr. Shen, all changes in rate involve the Heart and are also

Table 6-1 Terms of the Heart

DR. SHEN'S HEART PATTERNS*	DR. HAMMER'S TERMS
Heart vibration	Mild Heart qi agitation
Heart tight	Moderate Heart excess heat and qi agitation
Heart nervous	Severe Heart qi agitation
Heart large	Heart qi deficiency
Heart disease	Heart yang deficiency
Heart closed	Heart qi stagnation
Heart full	Qi trapped in the Heart
Heart weak	Heart blood deficiency
Heart small	Heart blood stagnation

*See Glossary

intimately intertwined with the 'nervous system'. An unstable 'nervous system' (essence) that controls the brain (marrow) destabilizes the Heart (that controls the mind), and this loss of Heart stability in turn causes the 'nervous system' to become unbalanced. Mood and qi are constantly changing, one moment up and the next moment down, ultimately compromising all physiology.

Over time, symptoms of emotional instability increase in frequency and intensity. If the Change in Rate at Rest is consistent, this signifies Heart qi deficiency. Change in Rate on Exertion reflects either Heart blood deficiency if the rate exceeds 20 beats/min, or Heart qi deficiency if the rate stays the same or decreases slightly, and Heart yang deficiency if it decreases considerably.[2]

Etiological events for these patterns usually occur before age twenty; the more consistent the rate change, the earlier or greater the triggering incident(s). Worry causes the least degree of rate change, and shock greater. Scarlet fever (strep throat) in childhood can lead to rheumatic heart disease and can cause a much greater degree of change in rate due to Heart qi deficiency. Constitutional Heart qi deficiency predisposes an individual to all arrhythmias.

With severe Heart qi agitation the rate is usually Rapid, especially when due to shock. If the true qi (the terrain) is deficient, the rate will be more Rapid immediately after a shock and during the early stages. Later, if the stress is protracted, the Rapid rate depletes the Heart qi and the rate slows, except in times of acute stress when it may temporarily increase. The rate tends to be more stable and closer to normal when the true qi is stronger.

CHANGE IN RATE AT REST   The rate continuously speeds up and slows down, independent of respiration.

OCCASIONAL CHANGE IN RATE AT REST   Over time this quality manifests as a Change in Rate at Rest sometimes and as a Normal rhythm at other times. It reflects a higher degree of agitated Heart qi (discussed in Chs. 12 and 15) than the Hesitant wave or Tight quality at the left distal (Pericardium) position. This pattern of Occasional Change in Rate at Rest is less serious than when the change is constant.

SMALL CHANGE IN RATE AT REST   When due to worry, the rate generally feels more stable, changing less often and Slower than when the etiology is shock. If constitutionally strong the left distal (Pericardium) position can be slightly Tight. With the same stress (worry, shock), if the Heart is constitutionally weak the left distal position can be more Feeble, and the entire pulse less Rapid.

There are three sources of agitated Heart qi: excess heat that begins with qi stagnation, yin deficiency false heat, and mild shock (see also Chs. 12 and 15).

Excess Heat

If all of the yin organ systems are equally strong, tension affects the Liver first, causing qi stagnation to contain the associated emotions, hyperactivity of the peripheral nerves. If the Liver is unable to overcome the stagnation, the accumulating Liver excess heat may affect the most vulnerable organ. If this vulnerable organ is the Heart, the excess heat from the Liver can cause severe Heart qi agitation, including palpitations at rest.

Yin Deficient False Heat

Moderate Heart qi agitation can be considered an intermediate stage of Heart yin deficiency in which the diminished yin causes the nerves of the Heart to become slightly dry, easily excited, agitated, and thus unstable. The rate is not as Rapid as when associated with excess heat.

It may be caused by emotional shock to the Heart, producing a sudden Heart yin deficiency as profound as the degree of shock; or prolonged Heart qi stagnation. Excess heat will accumulate in the Heart, which drains the compensating yin if the metabolic heat cannot move the qi stagnation. When due to long-term worry, the Change in Rate at Rest will probably be accompanied by a Smooth Vibration.

Symptoms with Small Change in Rate at Rest

The most common symptom associated with this pulse is a mild roller coaster feeling in which the mind races out of control, with alternating high and low moods, difficulty in focusing thoughts and actions, constant self-doubt, and indecisiveness.[3] Other symptoms include nervousness and agitation with moderate to intense stress; fatigue after strenuous exertion; mild sporadic and non-persistent palpitations upon heavy exertion; sleeping lightly and waking easily, then quickly returning to sleep, thus tending to be up and down all night; and occasional tiredness in the morning. The tongue and eyes are normal.

LARGE CHANGE IN RATE AT REST   The entire pulse feels as if it is beating with a slightly syncopated irregularity, however there are no truly missed beats and the rate is discernible.

This is the more severe form of Heart qi agitation. Its less dangerous form is seen in younger persons; the more serious form occurs in individuals where Heart qi agitation has progressed into Heart blood deficiency that is most often associated with prolonged worry. Large Change in Rate at Rest is often seen in borderline psychological states.

Large Change in Rate at Rest results from shock due to a sudden, moderate to large fright, or due to major physical trauma involving fright between the ages of fifteen and twenty. Constitutional Heart qi deficiency plus working beyond one's energy for a long period of time can also result in a larger change in rate.

Individuals with this pulse constantly change their minds, have severe mood swings and a more persistent roller coaster feeling. They have difficulty in focusing thoughts and actions, experience self-doubt and indecisiveness, and their lives are characterized by impotence, turmoil, and disarray. Most are anxious, easily frightened, always worried, nervous, and insecure. They suffer persistent, moderate to severe palpitations upon light exertion, wake easily and often throughout the night (although quickly return to sleep), and wake tired. Infants who experienced shock at birth or during the first few months are up and down all night.

Tongue shape is normal or slightly thin, perhaps with a shallow, central furrow if the origin is constitutional. The body is slightly red, especially the tip; a bright red color might shine through. The coating is thin, dry, and yellow. In severe cases there can be a patchy loss of tongue coating, with a dark red body in the denuded areas. The eyes often show a confluence of blood vessels under the lid. If shock occurred in utero, at birth, or in early childhood, a bluish hue may be evident on the face.

CONSTANT CHANGE IN RATE AT REST   This quality consistently speeds up and slows down without missing a beat and is a sign of mild to moderate Heart qi deficiency. A small change is less serious, while a large change is more serious. Both are less dangerous than the Interrupted or Intermittent qualities.

Mild to moderate Heart qi deficiency

The pulse has constant Changes in Rate at Rest with the left distal position showing Changes in Amplitude or Qualities, Rough Vibration, and/or Slipperiness, and later Deep or Feeble qualities.

With Constant Change at Rest the process has reached only to the point of mild to moderate Heart qi deficiency, if the changes are small or moderate, and moderate to severe Heart qi deficiency if the changes are large. Constant Change at Rest is also a sign of concomitant severe Heart qi agitation.

All of the etiologies listed in the next paragraph lead to a gradual and (much later) extreme weakening of Heart qi and yang until the Heart qi can no longer control the circulation.

Precipitating conditions may include prolonged Heart qi agitation, Heart blood deficiency, Heart qi stagnation, and trapped qi in the Heart. Other causes are inherited predisposition; congenital Heart qi deficiency; physical work beyond one's energy as a child and pre-adolescent; childhood malnourishment; unresolved shock to the Heart and circulation early in life due to severe emotional trauma; and excessive and prolonged abuse of alcohol, drugs, and nicotine. Repressed, profound anger exacerbates all of the above.

Individuals with this pulse can experience symptoms of mild chest pain, fatigue, shortness of breath upon exertion, increasing coldness in the body, especially the limbs which may also have very mild pitting, dependent edema. They may also experience difficulty breathing lying flat, requiring sleep to be only in a slightly raised position; palpitations upon exertion; numbness of the upper limbs; and occasional spontaneous cold perspiration during the day upon minimal exertion. If chronic, anxiety and vulnerability follow their entire lives, with poor concentration, forgetfulness, and lack of focus (also found less seriously with Occasional Change in Rate at Rest).

The tongue is pale with a red tip, wet with a deep, central furrow with swelling alongside it. The insides of the lower eyelids are pale and show confluence rather than distinctness of the blood vessels. The face is pale; if due to constitutional or congenital causes, perhaps green-blue on the chin or around the mouth. The nails may be concave, and in the most serious cases, the fingertips are clubbed.

Wide variation in rate over short time

These rate changes at rest must be distinguished from instances when the rate is very different when taken at different times during a pulse examination, but is not changing faster and slower as we hold the pulse. The former indicates Heart qi deficiency. Heart qi is too deficient to maintain rate stability over the course of the approximately one hour needed for the initial assessment such that taking the pulse after five minutes might be very different than when taken after ten and again after fifteen minutes, and so on.

MISSED BEATS

Rate measurable with missed beats

This classification includes the Intermittent and Interrupted pulse qualities. Intermittent defines a pulse with missed beats, a regular cadence, and a usually measurable rate—as opposed to an Interrupted pulse whose rate cannot always be measured. Dr. Shen called the Intermittent quality the "pulse that stops suddenly."[4] Typically, Heart function is implicated as the major etiology, as well as the condition of the upright, true, or Stomach qi. Individuals with these pulse qualities are vulnerable to emotional shock. These qualities are signs of danger, the Interrupted quality with unmeasurable rate being the most serious.

INTERMITTENT This pulse stops on a regular basis (frequent or infrequent) and can also be described as delayed or syncopated. The Intermittent quality can be constant or inconsistent. If it is constant and beats are frequently missed (the more frequent, the more serious the condition), it represents Heart qi, blood, and yang deficiency. Symptoms associated with this quality can include severe oppressive chest pain (angina), extreme fatigue, and shortness of breath upon exertion. Patients also experience coldness in the body, especially in the limbs, and have pitting, dependent edema. If the pulse is inconsistently Intermittent, it reflects a serious Heart qi agitation ('Heart nervous') and/or Heart blood deficiency ('Heart weak'), usually due to shock or trauma. For etiology and additional signs that present with the Intermittent quality, please refer to Ch. 6 in the source text.

INTERRUPTED   This pulse quality misses beats irregularly. If one is able to assess the rate, it is a sign of moderate to severe Heart qi deficiency. If it occurs occasionally, it indicates moderate Heart qi agitation and mild Heart qi deficiency. If it occurs constantly, it is a sign of moderate to severe Heart qi deficiency. If one is unable to assess the rate, the situation is more serious. If the pulse is constantly Interrupted with no measurable rate, the condition is severe Heart qi and yang deficiency, most likely with Heart blood stagnation and phlegm misting the orifices. (Please refer to the section on stability in Ch. 6 of the source text for details of combinations such as Empty Interrupted and Yielding Hollow Interrupted.)

CHANGES IN RATE ON EXERTION

The pulse rate should normally increase about 12-20 beats per minute on vigorous exertion, such as rotating one arm vigorously at the shoulder for approximately 10 revolutions.

LARGE INCREASE IN RATE ON EXERTION   Change in Rate on Exertion greater than 12-20 beats per minute indicates Heart blood deficiency, the greater the increase, the more severe the condition. Usually the left distal position is also Thin and either Tight (with yin deficiency) or Yielding (with qi deficiency).

Unresolved Heart qi agitation, especially due to prolonged worry, will evolve into Heart blood deficiency and later qi deficiency. With this etiology, the left distal and even larger parts of the pulse will have Smooth Vibration and again be either Thin and Tight or Thin and Yielding. When predisposed by constitutional Heart qi deficiency due to either shock received in utero, during birth, or early life, or due to prolonged excessive work beyond one's energy level, the left distal and proximal positions will probably be Feeble-Absent, and the remainder of the pulse can be normal if there is no other pathology.

The principal symptoms are feelings of weakness and cold along with fatigue to the point of exhaustion. Other symptoms are steady sleep for a few hours followed by early morning waking and little difficulty returning to sleep; poor concentration, memory, attention and forgetfulness; tiredness in the morning; palpitations upon mild to moderate exertion; and slight cold and numbness in the extremities.

The tongue may show a central furrow, the depth of which correlates with the length of time the condition has existed. If the etiology is primarily constitutional, the furrow is shallower than when the etiology is due to life experience, or a combination of both. The insides of the lower eyelids are pale.

Constant Large Increase in Rate on Exertion reflects a more serious Heart blood deficient condition compared with occasionally occurring increases.

INCREASE IN RATE ON EXERTION LESS THAN 12 BEATS/MINUTE   A Change in Rate on Exertion of less than 12 beats per minute indicates Heart qi deficiency:

the smaller the increase, the greater the Heart qi deficiency.

DECREASE IN RATE ON EXERTION   If the Rate on Exertion remains the same or the rate is less than at rest, Heart yang deficiency is indicated.

PSEUDO-ARRHYTHMIAS

Certain qualities and wave forms mimic arrhythmias. Examples include Changes in Amplitude and the Unstable quality, which are discussed in the section on stability. Another such quality is the Hesitant Wave.

Fig. 6-1 Hesitant Wave

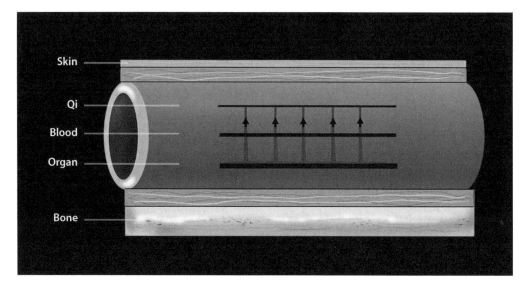

Hesitant Wave

This quality (Fig. 6-1) is associated with mild Heart yin deficiency and is characterized by the absence of a sine wave. It seems to be missing a beat because there is an apparent space between impulses due to the loss of a sine wave and the abruptness of the beat.

It occurs only over the entire pulse. The Hesitant Wave has lost its normal sine wave form and so the flow to and from the wave peak becomes sharp and abrupt, instead of being a gradual rise and fall. The quality feels as if it were faltering or balking, yet not missing a beat.

This quality occurs when an individual has a tendency to ruminate or think incessantly about one subject (often health or work), distinguished from a general tendency to worry, which is expressed by a Smooth Vibration. In the early stages, except for the symptom of worry or difficulty in falling asleep, there are no other related signs or symptoms. Later the individual has a strong sense of malaise and a feeling of being unable to keep up with the pace that they have set for themselves. Individuals with this pulse quality often collapse suddenly, physically and/or emotionally. The Hesitant quality is a form of the mental type of 'push pulse', distinguised from the Flooding-Deficient quality, the physical 'push pulse'.

STABILITY

The concepts of 'qi wild' and 'blood circulation out of control' are not included in the conventional Chinese medicine curriculum, despite being the most important aspects of Chinese pathology. They involve an entire range of disharmony and pathology that is rampant in our time and which many practitioners are unprepared to diagnose and treat[5] (see Fig. 6-5 at the end of this chapter).

Growth and Change

With regard to stability, we have observed that chaos is not exclusively pathological and that we find significant pulse instability in people who are in the process of changing positively. Personal growth in students attending Dragon Rises College of Oriental Medicine is impressive, and we often observe this pulse instability during this period of change and growth. Children's pulses characteristically change from day to day and often display 'qi wild' qualities and patterns whose significance is only that they are growing and changing daily.

Obfuscation

We have learned over time that some people can obscure the messages that the pulse communicates in a variety of ways, the most common of which is to constantly change qualities so no one quality persists, and within seconds it changes to another throughout the examination. Thus far, when presented with this finding, patients have revealed issues in their lives that they wished to conceal.[6] Other chaotic pulses can do the same.

'Qi Wild' Condition

'Qi wild' (*sān mài* 散脉), literally 'scattered pulse,' is a condition of extreme functional weakness and chaos in which, for one reason or another, the yin and yang have separated—lost operative contact in many yin organs—and are thus unable to support each other. This is a dangerous sign in which the immune system is injured and the body has little power to resist serious and fast spreading disease; it can occur within six months to three years unless intervention occurs. It is especially disruptive to the 'nervous system', which depends on the organized integrity of the lighter, fast-moving qi energies.

Yin, the material energy of the universe, is like a gravitational force that holds the more effervescent yang energies. If drained, the lighter yang energies wander aimlessly to all parts of the organism, unable to function effectively without the organizing force of the yin. The result is physiological disarray in which the orderly circulation of yang to the channels and the organs is disrupted, impairing their ability to function.

Sources for the correct pinyin and Chinese characters vary from Dr. Shen's (*sān mài* 散脈, literally 'scattered pulse') to that of Wen-Huai Chang and Brandt Stickley (*qì luàn* 氣亂).

Qualities associated with the 'qi wild' condition

The 'qi wild' condition affects the entire organism, and its pulse qualities characterize the entire pulse. These qualities include the Empty Interrupted-Intermittent, Yielding Hollow Interrupted-Intermittent, Empty, Yielding Hollow Full-Overflowing, Leather, Empty Thread-like, Scattered, Minute, and Change in Qualities. The pulse rate is usually Slow except when temporarily under stress.

Another, less obvious, sign of a 'qi wild' disorder is when the pulse qualities vary greatly at the burners and individual positions. This is a sign of a serious disruption of the harmonizing function of the Triple Burner, including that between the right and left brain (corpus collosum), leading to physiological anarchy and often associated with serious autoimmune and mental diseases (especially bipolar).

Still another rare 'qi wild' sign is a Change in Qualities from side to side, also observed with chronic autoimmune disorders. The qualities on the left and right sides periodically change places. Empty Interrupted or Empty Intermittent and Yielding Hollow Interrupted or Yielding Hollow Intermittent are the most serious pulse signs of current or impending disease.

Related signs and symptoms

The tongue is only slightly pale, but with the collapse of the yin organ system the tongue is very pale and often without color in some areas. Some tongues seem to have a flabby, milky-white appearance with loss of balanced or coherent shape, usually associated with extreme fatigue and enfeeblement, often with life-threatening diseases (cancer), even in young people.

Etiology

These associated 'qi wild' pulse qualities are linked to problems that begin in early life, the earlier the more serious, including:

■ In utero insults that include a myriad of physical and especially psychological insults to the mother during pregnancy and at birth that interdict Kidney essence and source qi.

■ Environmental deprivation (food, shelter, clothing) during childhood. This pulse is typically Yielding Hollow Interrupted or Intermittent.

■ Overwork during childhood. This pulse is Interrupted or Intermittent at an early age, between five and ten years, or Yielding Hollow Full-Overflowing and Slow between the ages of ten to fifteen years.

▪ Over-exercise early in life. This pulse is Yielding Hollow Full-Overflowing and Slow between the ages of ten to twenty years, especially if the exercise is suddenly and permanently suspended. It is then Empty and Slow between the ages of sixteen to twenty. The long-range effect is the diminishment of circulation that deleteriously affects the Heart (and mind).

▪ An insidious cause at any age is the attempt to slow the Heart rate through aerobic exercise, especially jogging, under the assumption that this will strengthen the heart muscle and because it temporarily relieves depression. Circulation increases because the Heart requires increased activity to push more blood through the system. This requires more Heart qi, which weakens the Heart, requiring more exercise to get the same circulatory result. The Heart weakens further, the rate becomes slower, and eventually the Heart cannot supply enough blood to the coronary arteries, leading to a variety of illnesses including coronary occlusion and arrhythmias.

▪ Protracted menorrhagia in pubescent and adolescent girls, often due to heavy exercise. This pulse is Empty Thread-like or Leather-like and Empty.

▪ Sudden cessation of extreme exercise. This pulse is Yielding Hollow Full-Overflowing and Rapid. Exercise causes the vascular system to expand and vessels to dilate in order to accommodate the increased volume of blood. When abruptly stopped, the blood volume decreases suddenly, but the vessels themselves remain expanded, leaving a gap reflected as a Hollow pulse quality. When the amount of circulating blood is rapidly diminished, the yang loses its grounding and moves out of control, disrupting the orderly circulation of yang to the channels and organs as well as disturbing the 'nervous system'.

▪ While a relatively uncommon finding, with sudden and very excessive lifting in a very deficient person, the pulse can also be Yielding Hollow Full-Overflowing Rapid.

▪ Extreme and prolonged emotional and physical abuse, as well as substance abuse, can be factors in producing 'qi wild' qualities and the associated, often cataclysmic, consequences.

'Qi wild' qualities with Regular rate

Empty Types of 'Qi Wild' Qualities

EMPTY The most serious is palpable only at the qi depth and no pulse quality is felt at the blood and organ depths. The least serious is Separating only at the organ depth (see Ch. 9, Fig. 9-3a-d). This pulse quality occurs in the yin stages of the six stages of disease, especially the lesser yin and terminal yin stages, and is usually a sign of advanced qi-yang deficiency and of potentially serious illness occurring within a few years.

The age at onset of this etiology is usually between fifteen and twenty. There may be severe neurosis and psychosis present. Rarely, this is a transient quality resulting from a sudden and very stressful life situation, representing an attempt to mobilize all energy at the surface to meet the emergency.

LEATHER-LIKE EMPTY   Similar to Empty, except much harder at the surface, representing a more serious deficiency of essence, yin, or blood.

EMPTY THREAD-LIKE (SOGGY, SOFT)   The Empty Thread-like (soggy or soft) pulse is "like a strand of cotton floating on the water"[7] at the qi depth, and disappears on pressure. It is a sign of extreme deficiency of blood, essence, and yang.

SCATTERED   When rolling the finger distal ↔ proximal, this quality feels as if the radial artery is broken into fragments; it signifies an extreme form of 'qi wild'. The damaging etiological events usually occur before the age of ten and often involve excessive deprivation. The prognosis is poor. It is seen in AIDS patients where it is referred to by some caretakers as the 'ceiling dripping' pulse. It is one of the traditional 'eight pulses of death'.

MINUTE   Resembling the Scattered quality in its lack of longitudinal continuity and found only at the blood depth, this quality is Thin and Feeble, showing little resistance to pressure. The Minute quality signifies extensive qi and yang deficiency in a seriously ill person in which there is not enough yang left to rise to the surface; it represents a more advanced 'qi wild' disorder than the Scattered quality, and can indicate impending death.

Yielding Hollow Types Of 'Qi Wild' Qualities

The Yielding Hollow Full-Overflowing and Rapid pulse quality results from the sudden cessation of extensive and prolonged exercise, usually practiced over a period of many years. Another similar 'qi wild' pulse quality is the Yielding Hollow Full-Overflowing and Slow quality that occurs in a very qi-yang deficient person who has exercised extensively since childhood.

These qualities represent slightly less serious conditions than the Yielding Hollow Intermittent or Yielding Hollow Interrupted pulses, which because of the abnormal rhythm also involve Heart function. The former can be caused by long-term environmental deprivation, overwork, and over-exercise between birth and age fifteen.

The Hollow quality is palpable at the qi depth, separating or missing in the blood depth, and again felt at the organ depth, whereas the Empty quality is felt only at the qi depth and is often Separating rather than Absent at the other depths. The Yielding Hollow Full-Overflowing quality informs us that the yin has even less control of the yang, and that the qi is even 'wilder' than with just the Empty quality.

YIELDING ROPY HOLLOW   This pulse quality is found after inordinately excessive exercise or very hard physical work beyond one's energy over an extended period of time, or in an environment characterized by significant deprivation of food, clothing, or shelter before the age of fifteen. As blood volume is diminished, by work or exercise beyond a person's energy, the yin blood and the more yang vessel wall become functionally dissociated from each other. Nutritional deprivation of the vessel wall increases as the blood volume decreases, causing the intima of the vessel walls to dry out and harden over time.

'Qi Wild' Qualities Characterized by Change

CHANGE IN QUALITIES   A Change in Qualities of the pulse is only slightly less serious than the Scattered pulse, the Yielding Hollow pulse, and pulses with rhythm disturbances such as the Yielding Hollow Interrupted or Yielding Hollow Intermittent. A Change in Qualities (Fig. 6-2) can occur over the entire pulse ('qi wild') or in one or more positions (loss of contact between yin and yang and significant organ disease). It can also indicate that the body or yin organ system is in a state of transition, either deteriorating or improving.[8]

CHANGE IN QUALITIES OVER THE ENTIRE PULSE: This represents an extreme imbalance and serious 'qi wild' condition where the patient is at great risk. It occurs in those who continually push themselves beyond capacity, use powerful chemical medications, have autoimmune diseases, or who live in geographic areas of chaotic energy.[9]

CHANGE IN QUALITIES IN ONE POSITION: This signifies extreme dysfunction and that the yin and yang have separated in a particular yin organ system.

Fig. 6-2 Change in Qualities

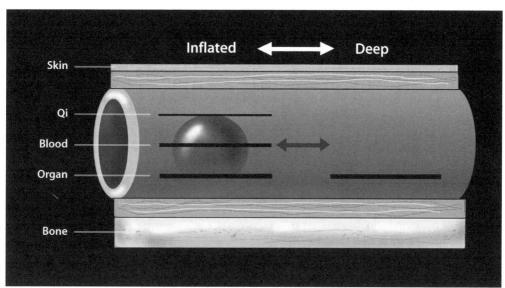

CHANGE IN QUALITIES BILATERALLY IN ONE BURNER: Assessing which of the organs within the burner has the primary deficiency (where the qualities are changing the most) may be required for successful treatment. This can reflect either a problem in the associated yin organ systems or a related area, that is, Change in Qualities in the upper burner positions can reflect a current or potential mediastinal tumor or breast cancer.

'Qi wild' qualities with Arrhythmic rate

The process leading to these qualities begins before the age of ten, and often before five. Unless very strong intervention is taken, these qualities are pathognomonic of a very short life due to severely compromised Kidney qi and essence and Heart qi-essence.

EMPTY OR YIELDING HOLLOW INTERRUPTED OR INTERMITTENT (CONSTANT)
This is a 'qi wild' pulse signifying the most serious life-threatening illness. The Interrupted (or Intermittent) quality alone (even without Hollow or Empty) signifies severe instability affecting the entire organism, especially of the Heart function. We refer to this as 'circulation out of control'. While this is not technically a 'qi wild' condition, it should be considered as such because it reflects advanced Heart qi and yang deficiency and exhaustion and has serious consequences for the entire organism. With the addition of the Hollow and Empty qualities, the seriousness is magnified many fold.

INSTABILITY RELATED TO HEART AND CIRCULATION, BUT UNRELATED TO RHYTHM AND RATE

Amplitude—the height to which the pulse is generated from organ to qi depth or beyond—represents the body's yang force. The seriousness of the instability grows with increased frequency and degree of the change (Figs. 6-3 and 6-4).

Entire pulse

CHANGE IN AMPLITUDE   Consistent Change in Amplitude (Fig. 6-3) over the entire pulse on first impression signifies Heart qi or yang deficiency, depending upon the accompanying qualities.

Change In Amplitude on first impression: Constant Over Time

ETIOLOGY: The etiologies are either the Heart affecting the circulation or the circulation affecting the Heart.

HEART AFFECTS CIRCULATION: A Change in Amplitude that is constant is a sign of Heart qi deficiency (smaller change) or yang deficiency (greater change). With Heart qi-yang deficiency the circulation of blood is diminished and is accompanied by cold hands and feet, migrating pain, and fibromyalgia.

Fig. 6-3 Change in Amplitude

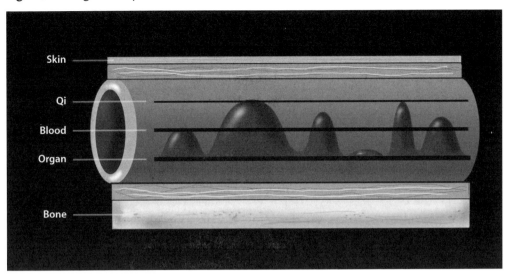

CIRCULATION AFFECTS THE HEART: The presentation of circulation affecting the Heart may be due to trauma and shock, emotional or physical.

Emotional shock drains Heart yin, thus the left distal position, especially the Pericardium at first, will be Tight. The Heart attempts to protect the other organs by shunting blood to them, including some of its own, resulting in yin deficiency (blood is yin). Shock also causes the Heart qi to contract ('close') so as to protect itself, leading to qi stagnation and accumulation of fluid that manifests as a Slippery pulse at the left distal position.

With regard to qi stagnation, if the physical condition is good, the left distal position may be Inflated; if poor, it may be Flat. There will be Change in Amplitude and Rough Vibration (a sign of shock to the Heart) over the entire pulse on first impression. In the beginning the rate is Rapid, however over a long period of time it decreases to very Slow (about 50-60 beats per minute) and the left distal position becomes Feeble.

Every physical trauma is also a shock to the Heart. The pulse becomes very Tight and Rapid. In the area affected by the trauma, the pulse will be Inflated in a person of relatively robust health, and Flat in a person with reduced qi. There will be Rough Vibration over the entire pulse, but little or no Change in Amplitude unless the Heart qi is diminished for some other reason. The left distal position will be as described just above. Over time, the rate will decrease to very Slow (50-60 beats per minute).

When the etiology is Heart affecting the circulation, the Heart qi is too deficient to move the circulation of blood sufficient to meet the needs of the body. Heart qi deficiency is often due to a constitutional deficit, disease (rheumatic), overwork, over-exercise, generally poor physical condition (Spleen qi or Kidney essence failing to produce blood), or a long-term mental and emotional drain (worry, obsession). The rate will be Slow (low 60s), and even Slower in those who exercise aerobically. The left distal position will show varying degrees of deficiency (Feeble-Absent) or separation of yin and yang, Change in Amplitude (mild), or Change in Qualities (severe). Eventually the left distal position becomes Slippery and shows Rough Vibration and a greater Change in Amplitude than the rest of the pulse.

Although it is unusual, the circulation can slow due to hypothermia. Here the pulse is Firm or Hidden and very Slow, too deep to show Change in Amplitude.

Change in Amplitude at First Impression: Inconstant over Time

When the Change in Amplitude does not occur each time the pulse is taken, the cause is usually stress affecting the Liver. When the Change in Amplitude involves the Liver, the sign appears with a significant increase of repressed feelings and disappears when the stress and the repression diminishes.

CHANGE IN AMPLITUDE UNDULATING FROM ONE POSITION TO ANOTHER

The amplitude waxes and wanes from one position to another, without pattern. This is a form of chaos, a 'qi wild' condition, especially the nervous innervation of the Heart. Clinically this pulse pattern has been found in people who have experienced early childhood sexual abuse.

CHANGE IN AMPLITUDE UNDULATING FROM ONE WRIST TO ANOTHER

Amplitude shifts from one wrist to another, usually at a constant level. This pulse is often associated with a current, powerful interpersonal conflict, and occasionally with a recent episode of exertion beyond one's normal strength.

CHANGE IN AMPLITUDE AFFECTING ONLY ONE SIDE   This is usually due to trauma to the side of the body on which it occurs. Without a history of trauma, Change of Amplitude only on the right side indicates pathology of the 'digestive system', and if only on the left, that the 'organ system' is impaired (see Glossary).

Individual Positions

Principal Individual Positions

A Change in Amplitude reflects a separation of yin and yang in the associated yin organ system, from mild [1-2] to moderately severe [4-5]. It is a less severe sign of separation of yin and yang than the other 'qi wild' qualities described above. The etiology is deficiency of qi, blood, and yang. A Change in Amplitude at any one position indicates a transition in function, usually from better to worse, although the opposite should also be considered.

Complementary Individual Positions

A Change in Amplitude is a sign of impaired function in the associated organ or area.

Distinguishing Change in Amplitude from Change in Qualities

With Change in Qualities, the change is sudden from one quality to another, whereas with Change in Amplitude, the change can be followed almost continuously as the pulse becomes more or less Robust.

Distinguishing Change in Amplitude from Arrhythmia

When the Change in Amplitude is considerable, the pulse may simulate a Change in Rate at Rest, or even an Interrupted quality. Careful and patient observation and experience are necessary to distinguish these. Hold the pulse for a few minutes with intense focus on the ends of your fingers.

Other Separation of Yin and Yang Qualities Found in Individual Positions

Other qualities that signify the separation of yin and yang and which appear only at individual positions, and never over the entire pulse, are the Unstable and Nonhomogeneous pulse qualities.

NONHOMOGENEOUS   This quality signifies extreme stagnation of all substances if the pulse is Robust, and extreme deficiency of an individual organ if it is Reduced. In both instances it represents separation of yin and yang and the resultant physiological anarchy of the organ associated with the pulse position where it is found. This is discussed in more detail in Ch. 11.

UNSTABLE   The Unstable quality has an irregular nature on smaller segments of the pulse, such as at one position or at one burner. It rebounds off the finger tremulously and erratically, like a pulsating point that moves from one part of the finger to another with a quick, jerky, and constantly changing movement. It is the sensation of chaos.[10] This quality is not the sign of a true arrhythmia, as that appears over the entire pulse at all positions.

This quality appears when there is severe injury to qi, blood, yang, and especially the parenchymal material of a yin solid organ. The condition is considered to be extremely serious unless further investigation proves otherwise (see Ch. 12 for specific discussion of pathologies of individual positions and areas[11]).

SPINNING BEAN   The Spinning Bean quality appears at an individual position with profound shock to the Heart at the left distal position, severe physical trauma to a specific organ at the position representing it, and sometimes with intractable pain (stomach ulcer) at the involved position (right middle with an ulcer) (see Ch. 11). It represents significantly impaired circulation.

'Blood Out Of Control' (Reckless Blood)

All of the qualities that indicate 'blood out of control' are under the Hollow category. Two of the three types of Hollow qualities signify 'blood out of control'—

Leather-like Hollow (most dangerous) and Tense-Tight Hollow Full-Overflowing—and the third, as we have already observed, is a sign of 'qi wild'—Yielding Hollow Full-Overflowing. (Further differentiation among the three Hollow qualities is found in Chs. 9 and 13.)

Hemorrhage, Rapid

LEATHER-HOLLOW   In this pulse, the qi depth is very Hard, the organ depth Tense, and the blood depth completely Absent. This quality signifies notable and even massive hemorrhage. This situation is life-threatening due to shock and typically appears in one position; it calls for emergency measures. If Rapid, the hemorrhage is imminent; if Slow, the hemorrhage has recently occurred, but could recur.

VERY TENSE-TIGHT HOLLOW FULL-OVERFLOWING   This quality rises above the qi depth, separates or is completely Absent at the blood depth, and is very Tense at the organ depth. If found over the entire pulse or on either side, it can signify hypertension with the potential for cerebral bleeding or thrombosis (stroke) always present. In insulin-dependent diabetes, it is usually more confined to the middle and (especially) proximal positions.

Hemorrhage, gradual

YIELDING PARTIALLY HOLLOW AND SLOW (FULL-OVERFLOWING WHEN VERY SERIOUS)   With these qualities, the qi depth is pliable, the blood depth separates, and the organ depth is Normal or slightly Diminished. It indicates more gradual bleeding, and can lead to a chronic severe drain of qi and a secondary 'qi wild' condition as well as 'blood out of control', as seen in heavy menstrual bleeding over time, repeated abortions, or deliveries with significant blood loss.

Fig. 6-4a Rhythm

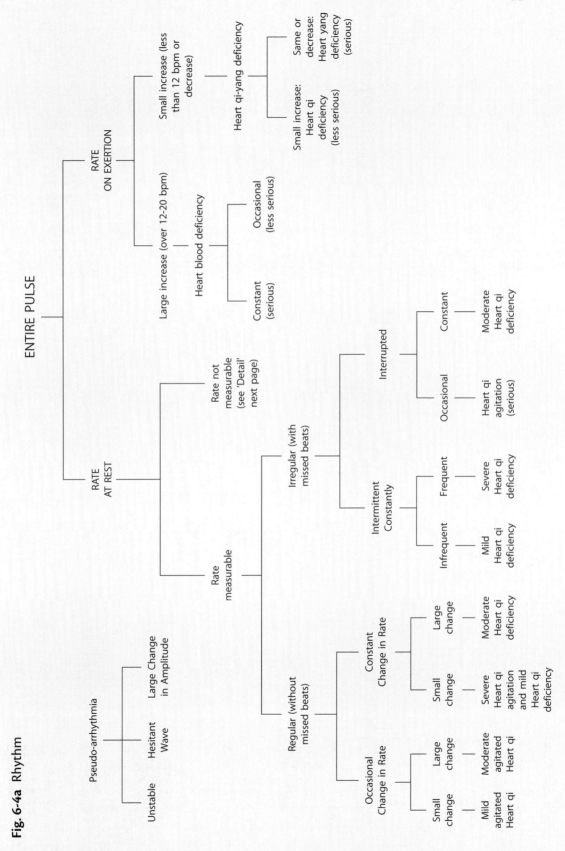

Fig. 6-4b Rhythm (detail)

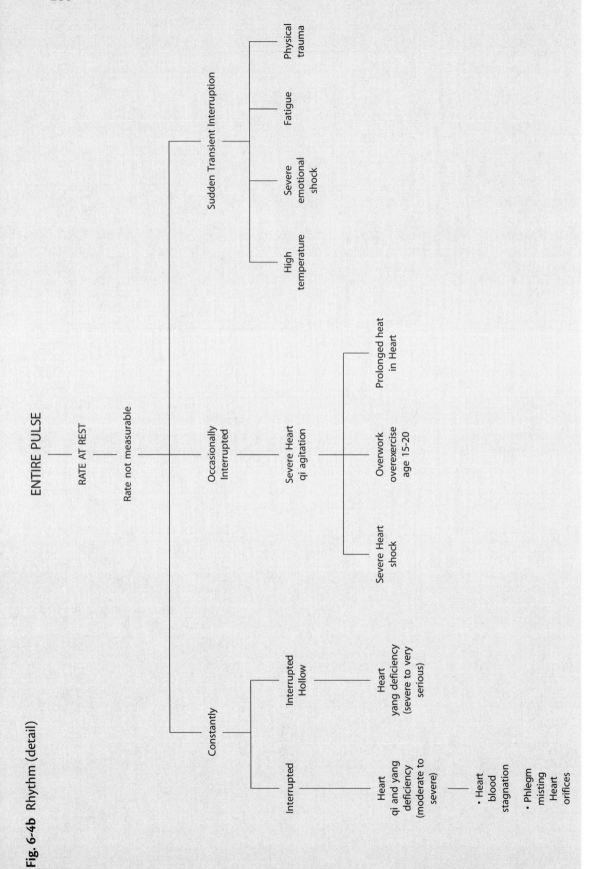

Fig. 6-5 Stability

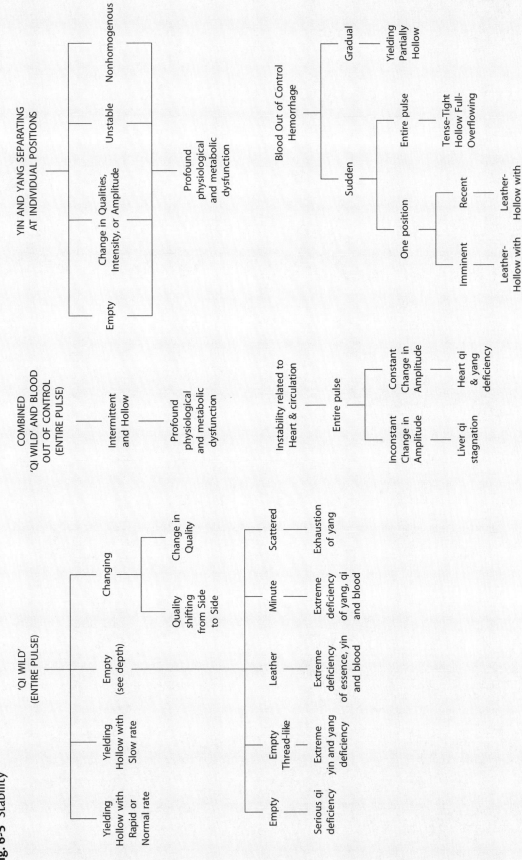

7

Rate

Hamilton Rotte, A.P.

TRADITIONALLY, THE RATE OF the pulse has been associated with conditions of either cold or heat.[1] However, according to Drs. Shen and Hammer, in our time, the rate more commonly involves factors that affect Heart function and circulation such as shock, over-exercise, and overwork. Since the Heart is the 'emperor', the rate and its regularity are the qualities that supersede all other considerations in the interpretation of the pulse and in choosing a therapeutic regimen.[2]

Rate always involves the entire pulse (all three positions on both wrists), and for reasons of accuracy should be measured for one minute with a nondigital watch rather than by the breath. (The changes discussed in this chapter are independent of, and easily distinguished from, the small changes in rate normally recorded with the breath, increasing with inhalation and decreasing with exhalation.)

In a few instances of toxicity to the Heart from powerful medications, we have found the rate in the upper burner to be more Rapid than that of the rest of the pulse, easily corrected by a change in medication. The subtleties of seasonal variations are of minor consequence in an era when environmental assaults on organisms are so profound.

THE NORMAL RATE ACCORDING TO AGE

Dr. Shen's view[3] of the Normal age-associated resting pulse rates in healthy individuals is shown in the following chart:

AGE	RATE
Birth to 4 years	84-90/min
4-10 years	78-84/min
10-15 years	78-80/min
16-40 years	72-78/min
40-50 years	72/min
50+ years	66-72/min

Normal children's pulses recorded by European neonatal nurses are the following rates:

AGE	RATE
Newborn	120-140/min
1 year old	100-120/min
5 year old	90-100/min
10 year old	~90/min
16 year old	~80/min

THE RAPID RATE

RAPID

A Rapid rate over any length of time weakens the qi, yin, and blood of the Heart and therefore it is a priority in treatment to return the rate to Normal as quickly as safety allows.

The Rapid pulse is traditionally associated with excess heat or yin deficiency. Empirical evidence, however, has revealed that a Rapid pulse more often involves the effects of shock and stress on the Heart and circulation and is often associated with severe anxiety. Although a very Slow rate is generally associated with conditions of severe deficiency, it is important to remember that the pulse can sometimes become very Rapid in circumstances of great deficiency of qi during the lesser yin and terminal yin stages of disease, when the yin is too weak to grasp the yang, which, as it slips out of control, causes the pulse rate to increase.[4]

BOUNDING

A Bounding quality is one in which the pulse feels as if it is running away faster than the actual rate (e.g., it feels like 120 beats/minute but is really only 100 beats/minute). This sensation is associated with severe anxiety and panic, high fever in a weak person, heat prostration and shock, and sometimes pain and trauma.

Rapid Pulses Due to External Etiology

External heat in the protective level (wind-heat)

In this pattern the pulse is slightly Rapid. It is Floating and more Yielding than with wind-cold. The increase in pulse rate is due to a rise in body temperature resulting from increased activity of the body's protective qi in defense of the organism.

Individuals affected by this pattern experience a sudden onset of the condition accompanied by a fever, headache, aversion to heat, and perspiration. Other symptoms include thirst, cough, sore throat, yellow and thick nasal discharge, yellow sputum, and generalized pain.

The tongue is slightly dry and moderately red, with raised red spots, and has a thin yellow coating. The eyes have red rims and the sclera are congested.

Heat stroke

The pulse is very Rapid (140-160 beats per minute), very Tense and Hollow Full-Overflowing, or collapses to Empty when 'shock' ensues. This pattern arises due to failure or inadequacy of heat loss, often associated with heat in the blood and dehydration after overexposure to the sun.

Associated symptoms are headache, weakness, sudden loss of consciousness, hot, red, and dry skin, and slight perspiration. The tongue is red and dry, and the pulse is Rapid, Tense, and Hollow Full-Overflowing.

Heat exhaustion

Heat exhaustion is due to excessive fluid loss with heavy perspiration. The pulse is Rapid and Feeble. Other symptoms include low blood pressure, cold, pale, and clammy skin, and in extreme cases, disorientation and sudden loss of consciousness. There may also be extreme fatigue, weakness, and anxiety.

Trauma

The pulse signs vary with the type (physical or emotional), size and extent of the trauma, as well as the passage of time elapsed and the location of the physical trauma. In general, the greater the trauma and the more deficient the body condition (terrain), the greater effect on the rate.

Physical trauma

Extensive physical trauma causes the entire pulse to be very Rapid, Bounding, Tight to Wiry (with pain), Inflated, or Flat. The tongue body has a purple hue; ecchymosis or a large purple blister is present on the area of the tongue corresponding to the trauma site on the body. On the side of the trauma, a horizontal blood vessel is evident on the inner mucosa of the lower eyelid separate from the vertical blood vessels. If a long time has passed since the trauma has occurred, the rate becomes Slower.

Emotional trauma

An emotional trauma leads to a Rapid, Bounding pulse with a Tight quality over the entire pulse that first appears at the left distal position. Rough Vibration over the entire pulse is another reliable sign of emotional trauma. The tongue and eyes are normal. If a long time has passed since an emotional trauma occurred, the rate becomes Slower as the Heart qi is drained by the effort of maintaining a state of urgency and an elevated rate for a prolonged period.

RAPID PULSES DUE TO INTERNAL-EXTERNAL CONDITIONS

Internal-external etiology refers to causes that are external, such as stress, which lead to an internal pathology.

The Heart

Here we are mentioning only those Heart conditions that involve a rate that deviates from normal.

Very mild Heart qi agitation

This pattern is characterized on the pulse by a Superficial Vibration with or without a slight elevation in rate (80-84 beats/min). The individual is worried about some current life event. As the vibration moves to all depths and positions, the person will find something to worry about even if there is nothing.

Mild excess heat in the Heart

An early sign of this condition is a Tight quality at the Pericardium position and a mild to moderate elevation of rate. The individual has been worrying for a relatively long period of time, such as several years.

Moderate to severe Heart qi agitation

As well as Changes in Rate at Rest, the rate is often moderately to severely elevated. This is equated with instability in the individual's life, usually with a history of shock. The individual feels that his life and emotions are on a roller coaster and finds it difficult to focus and ground himself.

Heart yin deficiency

The rate is relatively rapid (84-90 beats/min) with more severe symptoms of irritability and restlessness, including insomnia marked by waking and tossing and turning all night.

RAPID PULSES DUE TO INTERNAL CONDITIONS

Excess heat

With excess heat the pulse is usually very Tense.

Heat in the qi level

The pulse associated with this pattern is Rapid, Tense and Slippery, either at the organ depth or at all depths if chronic and severe, and in the more extreme cases with a Flooding Excess Wave.

The increase in pulse rate is due to a rise in body temperature resulting from increased activity of the protective and nutritive qi in defense of the organism. Infection or inflammation of an organ is usually the source, located by searching for a Flooding Excess Wave and/or the Tightest position on the pulse.

Individuals with this pattern are affected by acute high fever, sensation of heat, aversion to heat, thirst with a preference for cold beverages, profuse sweating, severe pain, cough with yellow sputum, either constipation with small hard feces or diarrhea with a burning sensation and tenesmus, bloody or purulent dysentery, abdominal pain, nausea and vomiting, dysuria, yellow and scanty urine, irritability and restlessness, and dizziness. In more serious cases, delirium or coma may ensue. Bleeding is more associated with the blood level of the four levels classification of warm diseases.

The tongue is red and dry with a thick yellow coating. The sclera are red and the face is flushed.

'Blood heat'

This heat syndrome, sometimes accompanied by a slightly Rapid rate, can be one of either excess or deficiency, depending on the etiology. The pulse of this pattern exhibits an expanded blood depth as finger pressure is released moving from the organ depth; it may also be Slippery. (See Chs. 10 and 13.)

'Blood thick'

With this pattern, the blood depth is greatly expanded to the qi depth as finger pressure is released from the organ depth. This syndrome is sometimes accompanied by Robust Pounding, a moderately Rapid and Bounding rate, and Slippery and/or Choppy qualities, and may later become Tense-Tight Hollow Full-Overflowing.

'Nervous system tense'

This condition may appear constitutionally in certain ethnic groups due to prolonged hypervigilance learned from generations of exposure to oppression and unexpected danger; in these cases, the rate is normal to slightly elevated. Or it may be the result of stress-induced tension, frustration, and anxiety in daily life. When the 'nervous system tense' is due to an individual's lifestyle, the pulse tends to be more moderately Rapid than the constitutional condition. All 'nervous system tense' conditions are identified by a uniformly Tense pulse and Thin and Tight qualities at the qi depth. We call this the 'vigilant pulse'. Over time, an individual who is living with nervous tension will show signs of yin depletion—as the heat from the tension depletes the yin—at which time the rate can become slightly elevated. (See Ch. 15.)

The principal symptom is a feeling of ongoing tension that may or may not be related to any particular life stress.

Yin-deficient heat

With deficient false heat the pulse is usually Tight (yin deficiency), Wiry (yin and essence deficiency), Leather-Hard (yin, blood, and essence deficiency), and is usually less Rapid than with excess heat.

Wind

This term is extensively used in Chinese medicine, but lacks a satisfactory explanation. It is used here as the consequence of the 'separation of yin and yang' in the Liver, in which the yang escapes from its bond with the yin and 'wanders' to the most vulnerable organ or area of the body where it interferes with the function of that organ or area. The pathogenesis of this condition, from repressed emotion through Liver qi stagnation, is described elsewhere in this book, dispelling the notion that the Liver 'attacks' and expounding its true physiology.

Entire pulse, without internal wind

If the condition has lasted for a short time the entire pulse is slightly Rapid; it is also somewhat Tight due to reduced yin-fluids, and sometimes slightly Thin if accompanied by blood deficiency. If the condition has lasted for a longer period due to prolonged tension in the 'nervous system', the pulse is slightly Rapid and Tighter to Wiry as well as Thinner.

Other causes are dehydration from illness and the overwork of one of the internal organs, such as the effect of alcohol on the Liver, tobacco on the Lungs, over-thinking on the Kidney and Heart (worry-obsessions), or long-term intake of spicy foods on the Spleen and Stomach. A new type of dehydration that is characterized by the Leather-Hard quality is due to environmental radiation (computers, cell-phones, microwave ovens, etc.).

Entire pulse, with internal wind

Mild internal wind (Liver wind) is characterized by a Floating Tight quality and mildly Rapid rate. Severe internal wind is signaled by a Very Tight Hollow Full-Overflowing quality that is associated with an impending major stroke, and a very Rapid rate.

Individual positions

Yin-deficient heat is manifested on the pulse as a hardening sensation that is called Tight when mild to moderately hard, Wiry when cutting, and Leather when very hard. Yin-deficient heat in a yin organ will therefore usually be accompanied by a Tight to Wiry or Leather-Hard quality in the position representing that organ.

Internal etiology other than heat

Imminent hemorrhage

The pulse of this pattern is Rapid and Leather-Hollow; the blood depth is totally absent and the qi depth is very hard.

Pain

Acute, severe pain causes a Rapid rate (90-106 beats/min) and Tight-Wiry Biting qualities. The pulse is less Rapid with chronic pain, and even Slow, with eventual qi depletion over a long period of time.

Acute phase of chronic illness

While chronic illness is associated with a Slow rate, the appearance of a Rapid rate in chronic disease may indicate an acute exacerbation of symptoms or, less often, that the organism is mobilizing and increasing circulation for the purposes of self-healing. This often accompanies a Flooding Excess Wave if the terrain is strong enough and Flooding Deficient if not. (See Ch. 8.)

Lesser yin heat pattern

A depletion of yin energies causes it to lose control of the yang, effectively separating yin and yang. The yang rises to the surface, resulting in a Rapid rate. This is a form of 'qi wild', resulting in a paradoxical drop in temperature.

Sudden cessation of exercise or heavy work

The pulse is Normal to Rapid Yielding Hollow Full-Overflowing.

Circulation, and ultimately the Heart, is impaired when one who has exercised a great deal suddenly stops. Consistent exercise causes blood volume to increase and the blood vessels to expand. With a precipitous cessation of exercise, blood volume decreases faster than blood vessel contraction, thus creating a break between yin (blood) and yang (qi).

Most of the symptoms of this condition fall into the category of 'qi wild' and commonly include profound anxiety, labile emotions, fatigue, 'spaced out' feeling, and depersonalization. There is also a sense of loss of control over body and mind, during which parts of the body no longer feel connected to the rest of the body, especially when lying down, resulting in a feeling of drifting away. Severe migrating joint pain is another common complaint, though the range of developing physical manifestations is unpredictable and often widespread.

The tongue and eyes are usually normal.

THE SLOW RATE

While a Slow pulse is ordinarily associated with conditions of severe deficiency, it is important to remember that deficiency can also cause a very Rapid pulse, especially upon exertion, due to the instability of the qi, particularly the qi of the Heart.

The Slow quality (see Fig. 7-2 at end of chapter) involves the entire pulse and reflects the functioning of the entire organism. According to Drs. Shen and Hammer, the most common cause of the Slow quality is circulatory deficiency due to either energy depletion, the long-term effects of shock, or over-exercise and overwork, all of which affect or are affected by the Heart and circulatory qi deficiency.

COMMON CAUSES IN CONTEMPORARY SOCIETY

External

Cold from external excess

Here the Slow pulse is due to stagnation of the protective and nutritive qi caused by a cold external pathogenic influence. The pulse is Floating, Tense, and Slow.

Internal

Cold from deficiency (qi and yang deficiency)

Longstanding internal disease, overwork, over-exercise, sex beyond one's energy, and protracted emotional strain can deplete qi and yang. Since the qi is the motivating force underlying the circulation, the lack of qi results in a diminished circulation and a Slow rate.

Heart qi and yang deficiency

A qi and yang deficient Heart is unable to circulate qi and blood, which leads to a slowing of the pulse.

Aerobic exercise

A Slow pulse associated with the depletion of Heart qi due to excessive aerobic exercise, including running, usually goes from somewhat Robust to Reduced Pounding as the Heart overworks to maintain function.

LESS COMMON CAUSES

Liver qi stagnation and deficiency

Liver qi stagnation and deficiency diminishes peripheral circulation and, while relatively rare, slows the pulse rate by depriving the circulation of the impetus that it normally supplies in moving the blood and qi through the vessels and channels. The pulse is Slow and Tense. More often the stagnation is experienced by diminished movement in another organ such as the Stomach, with the slowing of peristalsis for which Liver qi is partially responsible.

Internal excess heat: late-stage 'blood thick' (middle-stage arteriosclerosis)

The circulation is slowed and the pulse is Ropy and Tense, all due to increased viscosity of the blood from the accumulation of lipids, plaque formation, and heat in the blood over a long period of time. By this stage the slowing process due to the viscosity outweighs the accelerating process associated with the initial etiology of excess heat.

Yin deficiency (late-stage arteriosclerosis)

In advanced yin deficiency the pulse can be very Ropy and Slow. When the vessels lose their elasticity, the rate may initially increase as the Heart attempts to overcome this resistance to circulation; but later, when the Heart becomes exhausted from this losing battle, the pulse slows even more than in the 'blood thick' pattern.

Toxicity

Over a long period of time, poisoning gives rise to a very Slow and Deep pulse. The rate is usually under fifty. This has been observed in artists and welders after many years of exposure to toxic solvents. Frequently, they also show a 'blood unclear' pulse.

Medications

The beta-blocker and calcium channel blocker classes of medications cause the pulse to become very Slow and suppress the wave. With the ever-increasing prescription of these drugs within our society, this etiology is increasing.

Shock

Unresolved physical or emotional shock (trauma) initially inhibits the circulation of qi and blood, causing the Heart to work harder and the rate to increase. Over a long period of time, in the attempt to open circulation of qi and blood, the organism becomes depleted and the pulse becomes Slow.

UNCOMMON CAUSES

Cold from internal excess

Internal cold arises when cold foods and beverages are consumed excessively from an early age; from excessive use of cold applications in the treatment of pain; or from frequent bathing in very cold water. Extremely inadequate wintertime heating and attire because of poverty unfortunately are still more common than one cares to believe, both here and in Third World countries, and leave their mark on children for their entire lives. The pulse associated with this pattern is Slow and Tight. Internal cold can lead to blood stagnation, which is reflected as a Choppy quality in deficient areas of the body, such as the Pelvis/Lower Body position and proximal positions.

Please refer to the source text for a more detailed discussion of the classification of conditions according to the degree of Slowness.

WIDE VARIATION IN RATE OVER TIME

When the rate is very different when taken at different times over the course of a pulse examination, the condition is Heart qi deficiency. Heart qi is too deficient to maintain rate stability over the course of approximately one hour that it takes for the initial assessment. It may sometimes be Slower and sometimes more Rapid.

Fig. 7-1a Rapid rate

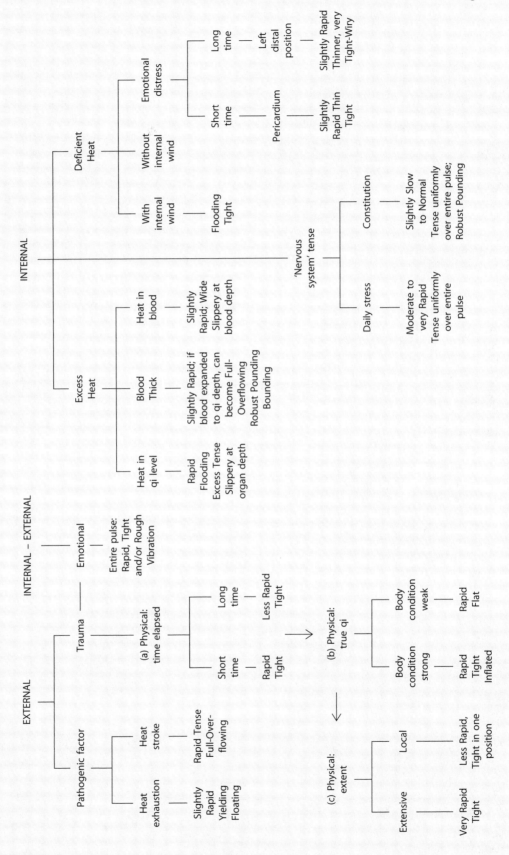

114

Fig. 7-1b Rapid rate (detail)

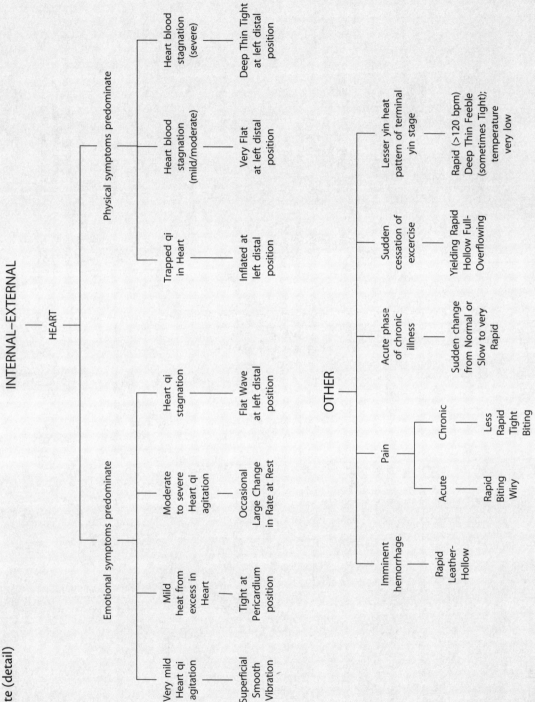

Fig. 7-2 Slow rate

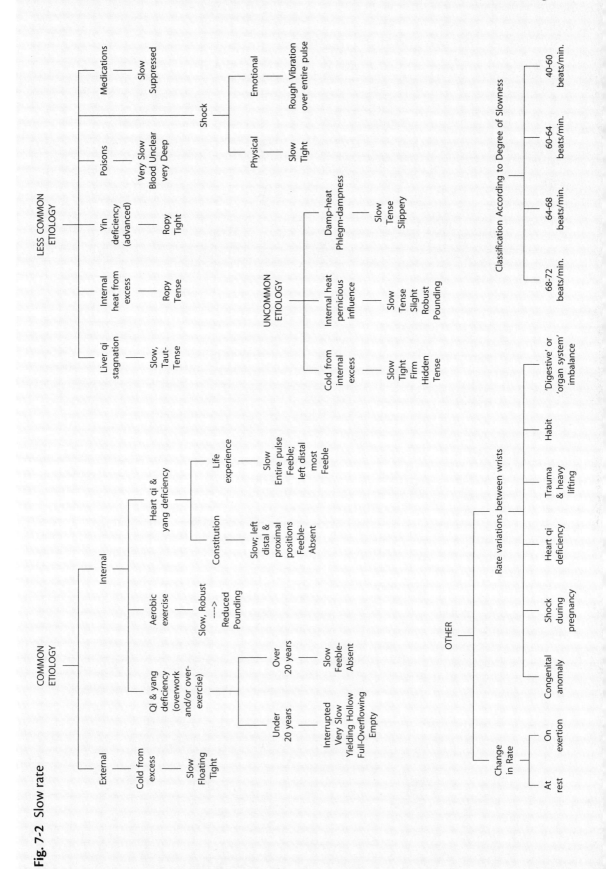

8

Volume

Brandt Stickley, A.P.

THE VOLUME OF THE pulse is expressed largely through the amplitude of the waveband and partially through the intensity or the width. Amplitude is defined as the height to which the pulse is generated from the organ depth to the qi depth and beyond. As a reflection of the functional basal metabolic yang energy, high amplitude suggests a robust yang force and low amplitude suggests diminished yang. The qualities are divided into Robust and Reduced categories.[1] Volume is also determined by the substance of the pulse, that is, the amount of the pulse as measured by its width.

ROBUST QUALITIES

HOLLOW FULL-OVERFLOWING

CATEGORY: The Hollow Full-Overflowing quality is categorized with various indicators of 'yang excess energy' as a pulse rising forcefully above the qi depth. Distinct from other classifications of this quality as Full or Overflowing is the Hollow sensation that accompanies this quality.

SENSATION: The Hollow Full-Overflowing wave form (Fig. 8-1) has a normal sine wave that begins between the organ and blood depths and rises above the qi depth. The Hollow Full-Overflowing wave often feels as if it is coming from the blood-organ depth, but it can be distinguished from the Normal wave form in that it clearly rises above the qi depth. The Hollow Full-Overflowing separates under pressure at or around the blood depth, and then regains its substance as one moves toward the organ depth. However, because it seems to begin higher and rises above the qi depth, the position of the blood depth is also a little higher than with the Normal pulse. The interpretation of the Hollow Full-Overflowing depends upon the other qualities present.

Fig. 8-1 Hollow Full-Overflowing quality

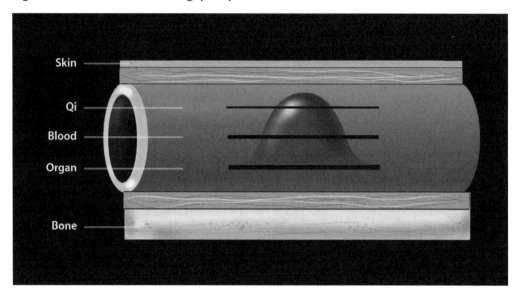

PATHOGENESIS: The process begins with stagnation due, for example, to repressed emotion in the Liver. Metabolic heat is brought to the organ in question to overcome the stagnation. If the metabolic heat is unable to overcome the stagnation, it accumulates and becomes toxic excess heat. The body attempts to neutralize the destructive excess heat with fluid (yin), gradually depleting the yin sufficiently to create a separation of yin and yang and a 'wandering' or 'aimless' Liver yang. In an effort to spare the Liver, the excess heat goes into the blood as a retained pathogen, leading to all of the conditions described in the Hollow Full-Overflowing section of this chapter.

With regard to the 'separation of yin and yang', since yang is function, Liver function in this instance will be impaired and the 'wandering' yang will go to the most vulnerable organ and interfere with its function, for example, the Spleen-Stomach, Heart, Lung, or one of the vulnerable areas of the chest, breast, diaphragm, or lower burner.

Types

There are three types of Hollow Full-Overflowing pulse: Tense Hollow Full-Overflowing, Yielding Hollow Full-Overflowing, and Tight or Wiry Hollow Full-Overflowing. Their differences are evident in both sensation and interpretation.

TENSE HOLLOW FULL-OVERFLOWING   The Tense Hollow Full-Overflowing quality feels forceful, especially as it surges from between the organ and blood depths to beyond the qi depth. This accords with historical descriptions comparing it to the "roaring waves of the sea." The term Tense is used to reflect the width and expansiveness of the quality.

YIELDING HOLLOW FULL-OVERFLOWING   The Yielding Hollow Full-Overflowing quality is characterized by the same forceful surge above the qi depth, but it separates more easily under pressure at the qi depth.

TIGHT-WIRY HOLLOW FULL-OVERFLOWING   The Tight to Wiry Hollow Full-Overflowing has two determining factors. Above the qi depth at the surface of the pulse it is harder, less resilient, less yielding and diminished in diameter. It also may lose the Hollow quality associated with the Tense and Yielding Full-Overflowing qualities.

Etiology

Historically, the etiology of the Hollow Full-Overflowing quality was limited to excess heat patterns; however, our discussion includes excess heat, yin deficient heat , and 'qi wild'. Whatever the etiology, it is our basic premise that only a susceptible, vulnerable circulatory system will be involved in the pathologic process which leads to the creation of a Full-Overflowing pulse quality.[2] 'Circulatory system' is what Dr. Shen generally thought of as the peripheral circulation—the integrity of the muscular structure of arteries, veins, arterioles, and capillaries.

■ Tense Hollow Full-Overflowing quality (excess heat)

In the Tense Hollow Full-Overflowing quality, the excess heat is located in the 'circulatory system', in the blood vessels, where it is less immediately damaging to the vital organs whence it came. This quality is a sign that the organism is trying, perhaps with only partial success, to eliminate the heat from overworking organs into the blood, and from the blood and the body, by expanding the circulatory system and by a general acceleration in function. (See Ch. 10.)

Ultimately, the heat in the vessels damages the intima and media of the vessel wall, weakening the wall, which expands so that the blood has less immediate contact with the vessel wall. This produces the Hollow quality.

Its etiology includes dietary indiscretions, including excessive sugars, fats, and alcohol, and emotional stress that can contribute to the production of heat, especially in the Liver. The Liver can transmit heat to the blood via its blood storing function, so that conditions that give rise to Liver stagnation and heat can also be associated with the development of this quality. According to Dr. Shen, physical overwork, including excessive exercise, can also produce heat in the Liver. When present over the entire pulse, this quality is associated with the early and middle stages of the biomedical condition of severe hypertension, and ultimately, of a dangerous stroke. Severe, persistent acne in adolescence is an early sign of heat in the blood, usually associated with poor nutrition, that can later develop into hypertension (Hollow Full-Overflowing, Ropy) later in life.

■ Yielding Hollow Full-Overflowing quality ('qi wild')

The Yielding Hollow Full-Overflowing quality develops from overwork or over-exercise for a very long period of time when a weak or vulnerable organism is striving to muster compensatory energy to meet the demands of life.

The factors giving rise to this type of debility are manifold including consti-tutional weakness in which the rate is Slow; the sudden cessation of overwork or of excessive exercise, in which the rate is Rapid; and serious illness with extreme loss of qi, blood, and fluids. The Yielding Hollow Full-Overflowing is a 'qi wild' pulse that is encountered with increasing frequency as massive qi defi-ciency is seen in younger and younger people.

■ Tight to Wiry Hollow Full-Overflowing quality (heat from yin deficiency)

The Tight to Wiry Hollow Full-Overflowing pulse is produced by the body's response to the excess heat patterns described previously. The body demands fluids to counteract the heat generated by repressed emotions that ultimately drains and damages yin. Eventually we have a deficient (yin-deficient) rather than excessive disorder that primarily affects the Heart, Liver, and later the Kidneys. Yin-deficient false heat damages the blood vessels by causing the mus-cular walls to become dry, brittle, and fragile. This quality is associated with hypertension, atherosclerosis, and ultimately stroke.

FLOODING EXCESS

CATEGORY: The Flooding Excess pulse can be confused with the Hollow Full-Overflowing quality because both are found above the qi depth, are often as-sociated with the Rapid and Robust Pounding qualities, and involve excess heat. However, it is actually different in both sensation and interpretation. The Flooding Excess wave lacks the full sine wave seen in the Hollow Full-Overflowing quality. It also represents acute heat in the yin organs rather than chronic (deficient or excess) heat in the blood. Flooding Excess qualities that appear in the literature are associated with patterns of heat (see Ch. 10).

SENSATION: The Flooding Excess wave form (Fig. 8-2) is felt as the first part of a strong sine curve wave originating at the organ depth, surging over the qi depth, and then dropping off precipitously at its apogee. It can be found over the entire pulse or in an individual position.

INTERPRETATION: The Flooding Excess wave form primarily indicates acute excess heat, usually associated with a significant infection when found over the entire pulse. When it is found in one position it indicates intense heat or fire and infection in that organ. The Flooding Excess wave form is found in acute hepatitis, the yang brightness phase of the six stages, the manic phase of bipolar disease, and acute fulminating infection. In these conditions, other signs of heat are present such as the Robust Pounding quality and Rapid rate.[3, 4]

The Flooding Excess wave is also found in chronic infections, especially at the left middle position, where it is associated with such conditions as chronic hepatitis and mononucleosis, in which case there is less Robust Pounding and a Slower rate.

Fig. 8-2 Flooding Excess quality

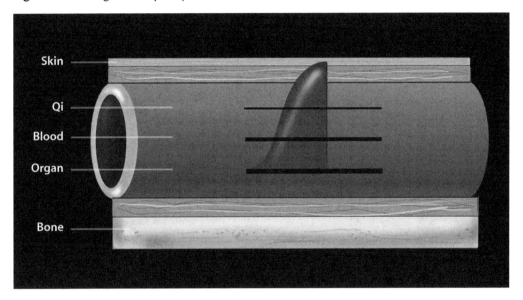

INFLATED

CATEGORY: This pulse has been identified with the term 'Full' in some sources, including Dr. Shen. We use the term Inflated to prevent confusion and to join the quality firmly with its sensation.

SENSATION: The Inflated quality (Fig. 8-3) feels like an inflated balloon; the sensation doesn't give way under pressure but follows the finger as it is lifted. It has a constant level of tension within the three depths and is equal at all of them.

INTERPRETATION: The Inflated quality reflects qi trapped in an organ or area. It can be due to physical or emotional trauma having occurred when the body condition or qi is robust, in contradistinction to the Flat quality created by a similar etiology in a deficient person, where the qi cannot enter an organ or area. If found in the left distal position, an Inflated pulse often suggests a history of breech birth, although for this reason it may also appear bilaterally at the distal positions. An Inflated Tense quality can appear with trauma, repressed anger, respiratory diseases, emphysema, chest surgery, and a single major episode of lifting far beyond one's energy.

TYPES: Three types of Inflated qualities may be distinguished: Inflated Yielding, Inflated Tense, and Inflated Very Tense. In terms of etiology, all derive from events that produce trapped qi and varying degrees of heat. The Inflated Yielding quality is, while still balloon-like, characterized by a more yielding sensation. It is associated with mild trauma, incorrect breathing techniques, trapped wind-cold, sudden lifting beyond one's energy, and mild yet repressed anger. The Tense Inflated quality of similar but more severe etiology is defined by an increasing resistance to pressure. The Inflated Very Tense quality has the most resistant sensation of all the Inflated qualities, and indicates a potentially serious complication of trauma or extraordinarily heavy lifting that has ruptured vessels and given rise to extravasated blood.

Fig. 8-3 Inflated quality

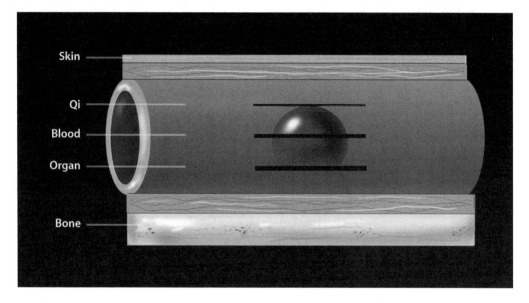

ROBUST POUNDING

CATEGORY: Nowhere in the literature is there a pulse described that reflects this quality (see Table 1-1). Surging and Flooding include aspects of Robust Pounding, but also involve a wave form that is not part of this quality.

SENSATION: The pulse hits the finger with great force, the amount of which depending upon the degree [1-5].

INTERPRETATION: Robust Pounding is the most common sign of excess heat on the pulse; it also accompanies, for example, the Tense and Tight Hollow Full-Overflowing and Flooding Excess qualities. Excess heat is considered toxic to tissue wherever it is found. Covered under the reduced qualities as Reduced Pounding, there are times when even Robust Pounding is a sign that a depleted organism or organ is mobilizing as much qi, blood, and body fluids as it can to continue functioning. It is usually short lived, except in the aged.

SUPPRESSED

CATEGORY: This represents an entirely new category that has come into existence with the physiological burden of potent synthetic chemical medications.

SENSATION: In the Suppressed quality (Fig. 8-4), the sine wave of the Normal pulse is cut off at the apex.

INTERPRETATION: Antihypertensive and antidepressant medications have been most closely associated with this finding. It may also be associated with suppressed feelings of resentment and with the linked pattern of indirect venting of frustrations through the use of humor or inference. Unlike the unconscious repression reflected in the deeper Flat quality, patients with the Suppressed quality demonstrate at least veiled awareness of their difficult feelings. Over time, and actually more often, this manifests as a Cotton quality (see Ch. 9).

Fig. 8-4 Suppressed quality

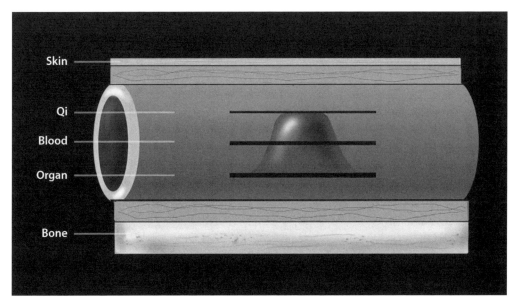

REDUCED QUALITIES

The classification of the Reduced qualities has typically involved some confusion. The difficulties of classification and interpretation are resolved by closely allying the terminology with perceived sensations, and by focusing interpretation on modern clinical realities. Additionally, some of the qualities described below represent additions to the traditional categories. Generally speaking, in terms of sensation, the Reduced qualities are those whose impulse and pulse wave lack force, amplitude, and substance.

YIELDING AT QI DEPTH

CATEGORY: This is a new category representing a subtle but significant deviation from the Normal pulse.

SENSATION: The qi depth is more pliable, or yielding, on gentle pressure (Fig. 8-5).

INTERPRETATION: This is the earliest sign of qi depletion. It indicates deficiency of protective qi *(wèi qì)* and deficiency at the qi level of energy. Inadequate sleep and rest, minor illness, incomplete recovery from pregnancy or delivery, and other failures to conserve or recover energy can give rise to this quality. Rest is indicated to prevent more serious illness.

Fig. 8-5 Yielding at Qi Depth quality

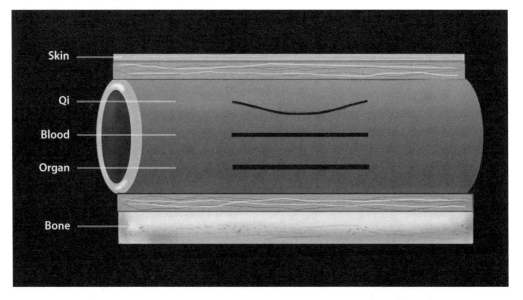

DIMINISHED OR ABSENT AT QI DEPTH

CATEGORY: This is another new category that indicates the subtle progression of mild qi deficiency.

SENSATION: The pulse at the qi depth is either diminished or absent (Figs. 8-6 and 8-7).

INTERPRETATION: In the hierarchy of deficient qualities this represents the second stage of qi deficiency. It is associated with overwork, and requires stronger tonification and circulation of qi.

SPREADING AT BLOOD DEPTH

CATEGORY: This is also a new category and shows a larger degree of deficiency than the Yielding and Absent at Qi Depth qualities.

Fig. 8-6 Diminished at Qi Depth quality

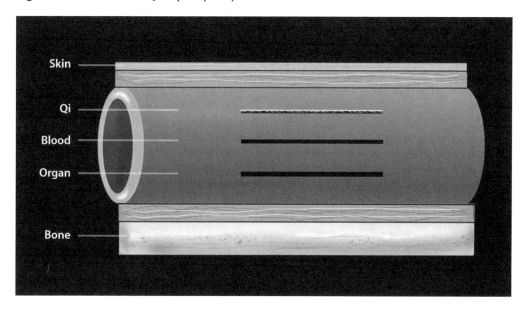

Fig. 8-7 Absent at Qi Depth quality

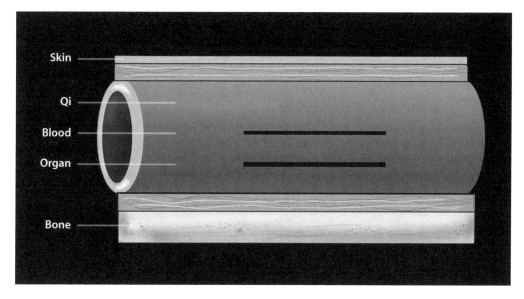

SENSATION: The pulse at the qi depth is Yielding or Absent, and at the blood depth separates on pressure (Fig. 8-8).

INTERPRETATION: While this quality represents the third stage in the progression of qi deficiency, it also indicates that this process has progressed to include both qi and blood deficiency, thus indicating either a condition of longer duration or some other reason for the depletion of both vital substances.

Fig. 8-8 Spreading quality

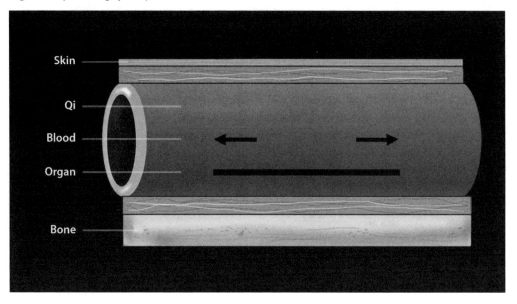

FLOODING DEFICIENT WAVE

CATEGORY: The Flooding Deficient Wave quality is categorized as a 'push pulse' in Dr. Shen's terminology.

SENSATION: The front part of the sine wave is similar to the Flooding Excess quality but it has less force, as it only reaches or almost reaches the qi depth and then falls or precipitously drops out from beneath the fingers (Fig. 8-9).

Fig. 8-9 Flooding Deficient Wave quality

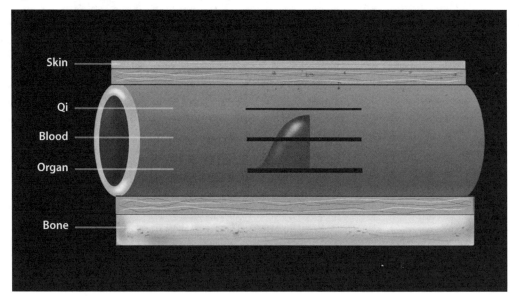

INTERPRETATION: The Flooding Deficient quality is a sign of qi deficiency in the yin-solid organs. It denotes physical overwork or work beyond one's energy coupled with an effort to push oneself obsessively day and night. It is also a sign of the fourth stage of mild to moderate qi deficiency. Individuals with this pulse tend to collapse suddenly for short periods and usually recover with rest.

REDUCED POUNDING

CATEGORY:　There is no category in the traditional literature identified as Pounding.

SENSATION:　The Reduced Pounding quality beats against the finger without force, energy, or vigor. It may at first give the impression of force and power, but it does not retain this strength. Reduced Pounding is found either over the entire pulse or at a single position.

INTERPRETATION:　As a sign of the fifth stage in the progression of qi deficiency, this quality represents the body's attempt, but compromised ability, to maintain function. Over the entire pulse it infers a 'true qi' deficiency and at individual positions is a sign of moderate qi deficiency in the organ associated with that position.

SUBSTANCE

Substance refers to the strength, elasticity, buoyancy, and resilience of a pulse quality. Traditionally, aspects of substance have been included in the category of Stomach qi (see Ch. 11).

REDUCED SUBSTANCE

CATEGORY: Substance refers to the strength, elasticity, buoyancy, and resilience of a pulse quality, so this term is used to modify the description of other qualities. Traditionally, aspects of substance have been included in the category of Stomach qi as a measure of the true qi of the organism.

SENSATION: The Reduced Substance quality (Fig. 8-10) lacks form, substance, strength, elasticity, buoyancy, and resilience when compared to the Normal pulse. It is a sensation somewhere between Normal and Feeble. It feels like a cigarette from which some tobacco has been removed, and, having less resistance, spreads out on pressure. Another analogy is that it feels like a threadbare sweater. Reduced Substance can be found over the entire pulse, at an individual position, or at different depths.

There has been some confusion between the sensations of Reduced Substance and Separation (Empty). With reduced substance there is less resistance side to side. With Separation and the Empty pulse, the reduced resistance is from distal-proximal and there is no pounding under the finger in the middle of the position.

Fig. 8-10 Reduced Substance quality

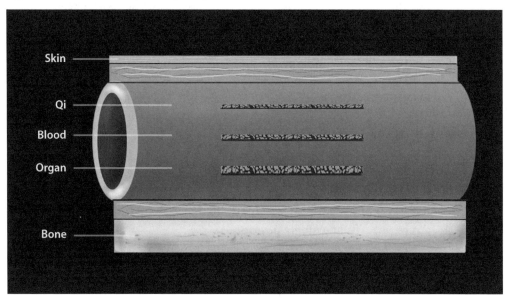

It is important to keep this distinction in mind since Reduced Substance is a sign of qi-blood deficiency, whereas the Empty quality reflects the more serious 'separation of yin and yang' and points in the direction of the much more serious 'qi wild' disorder.

INTERPRETATION: Reduced Substance suggests the sixth stage of advancing qi deficiency, but also includes some deficiency of blood and yin. It represents a slightly less qi deficient quality than the Feeble quality.

DIFFUSE

CATEGORY: There is no other system of classification that describes this quality.

SENSATION: The sensation of the Diffuse quality (Fig. 8-11) lacks clearly defined borders and boundaries with the surrounding tissue and pulse qualities. It is most often coupled with Reduced Substance, though other sensations, such as Tense, Thin, or Tight, may appear in the center of the position.

INTERPRETATION: The Diffuse quality is a sign of moderate qi deficiency. Combined with the Thin Tight quality, it is a sign of combined qi, blood, and yin deficiency. It represents the seventh stage of qi deficiency. Although it seems counterintuitive, this is another example of a Wide deficient quality.

FLAT

CATEGORY: By its sensation the Flat quality can be classified under two categories: Submerged, due to its deep position, and Shape, due to its lack of a wave form. It is also catalogued with Reduced volume, and thus represents a form of deficient and stagnant qi.

Fig. 8-11 Diffuse quality (longitudinal cross section of radial artery)

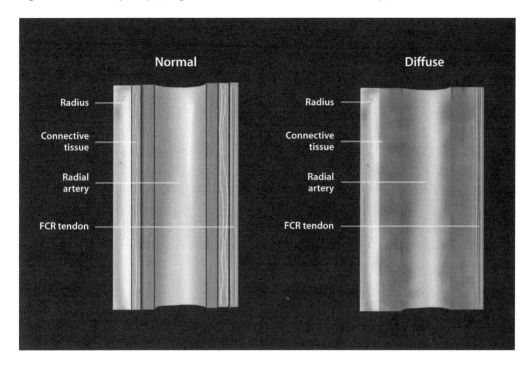

SENSATION: The Flat quality (Fig. 8-12) is usually found at the organ depth. It is stifled and compressed, with a very small or even no wave. In Dr. Hammer's experience, it is found only at individual positions, most often at the distal positions, especially the left.

Fig. 8-12 Flat quality

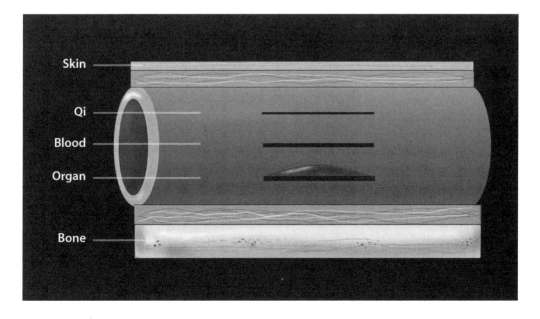

INTERPRETATION: The Flat quality reflects an energetic situation in which qi cannot penetrate into an already deficient organ. These conditions usually occur if the patient is already weak when receiving a significant insult to physiological function. Due to the vulnerability of organs in a weakened state, this results in a diminishment of the yin organs' storing capacity. The Flat pulse quality is found most commonly in the upper burner, especially at the left distal position, where it suggests emotional trauma (shock to the Heart) early in life (exemplified by a young person losing a loved one while their energy is immature), birth trauma (as in having the umbilical cord wrapped around the neck), or physical trauma, especially to the chest when the body condition is weak (see Ch. 12).

DEEP

The Deep quality is briefly mentioned here to demonstrate its place in the hierarchy of increasing qi deficiency. It is more properly classified under the rubric of Depth in Ch. 9.

FEEBLE-ABSENT

CATEGORY: The terminology of Contemporary Chinese Pulse Diagnosis uses Feeble to suggest an insubstantial sensation and Absent to suggest the complete absence of any impulse. The clinical significance of this distinction differs only to a slight degree, and thus, although distinct perceptually, the qualities are discussed in tandem.

SENSATION: The Feeble-Absent quality is usually applicable to the organ depth. However, we have already seen the hierarchy Yielding and Diminished at the qi and Spreading at the blood depth. The Feeble (Deep) pulse is barely palpable at the organ depth and the Absent (Deep) pulse is missing altogether. When present, it may be Thin or Wide, depending on the relative deficiency of blood or qi, respectively.

INTERPRETATION: There are a few salient features of the Feeble-Absent pulse. When the organ depth is Feeble-Absent, it indicates a deficiency of both blood and qi *(zhèng qì)*.

According to Dr. Shen, the Feeble-Absent pulse indicates a state of vulnerability to serious disease. In the absence of symptoms, it was his opinion that the individual would become ill within one year without intervention. (Dr. Hammer estimates this period more conservatively as being one to three years.) The Feeble-Absent pulse suggests a history of some chronic, prolonged, or serious drain to the organism.

Otherwise, in a young person, this pulse may indicate a serious illness or constitutional vulnerability. In the elderly, it is associated with natural decline.

Fig. 8-13a Feeble quality (early stage)

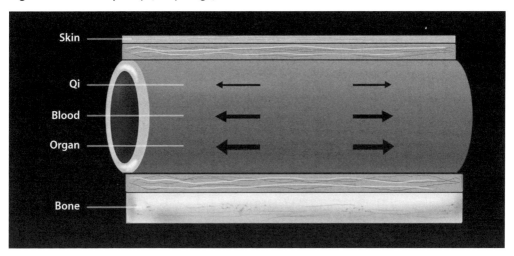

Fig. 8-13b Feeble quality (later stage)

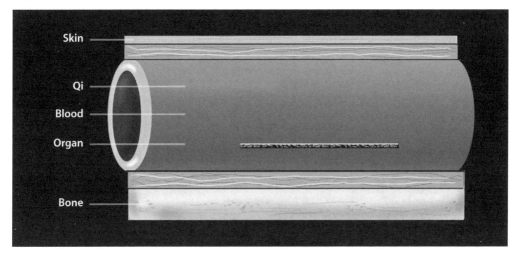

Fig. 8-14 Absent quality

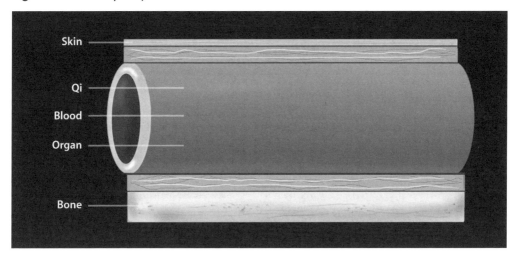

MUFFLED

CATEGORY: The Muffled quality does not appear in the literature. It has been most fully described through Dr. Hammer's clinical observation. Dr. Shen corroborated the seriousness of the sign and described it as an example of a 'stagnant' pulse quality.

SENSATION: The Muffled quality feels obscured, as if the other qualities are being felt through layers of cloth (Fig. 8-15). The sensation is muted and unclear.

INTERPRETATION: The Muffled quality indicates neoplastic activity, or breakdown of cellular function. A minor degree of the Muffled quality found over the entire pulse is sometimes associated with emotional depression. Heavier degrees of this quality are associated with potential or current serious disease.

At the left distal position, it is indicative of the Heart type of depression, characterized by a lack of joy. In the Pelvis/Lower Body position, it suggests extreme qi and blood stagnation and has been associated with uterine and ovarian tumors. The Muffled pulse quality has also been reported following surgery and is typically found in the pulse positions most closely reflecting the anatomical location of the procedure.

Fig. 8-15 Muffled quality

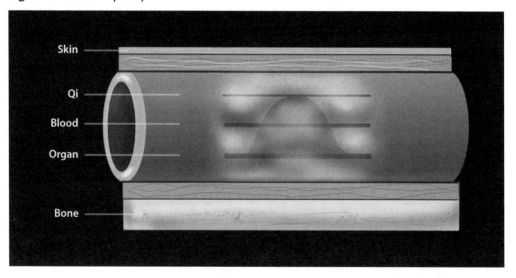

DEAD

CATEGORY: No category exists for this quality. Dr. Shen described the Dead quality only in personal communication, but omitted it from his lectures.

SENSATION: There is a sensation of a presence and substance that is lacking in movement. It is literally like touching a dead animal.

INTERPRETATION: Although not frequently identified, the Dead quality has always been clearly associated with advanced malignancy.

9

Depth

Hamilton Rotte, A.P.

DEPTH GIVES US INFORMATION ABOUT the location and stage of a disease. Generally, the superficial pulses are associated with acute diseases involving the surface protective qi and the deeper pulses are a sign of more profound, chronic illness of the yin organs. Exceptions to this are mentioned in the discussion of individual qualities; as a general exception, heavier people normally have slightly deeper pulses. This discussion of pulse depth is organized by superficial and submerged (deep) qualities.

EXCESS AND DEFICIENCY
....

Pulses that are Deep are associated with internal conditions. Theoretically, they could be due to excess, but most commonly in modern times, they reflect deficiency.

SUPERFICIAL PULSE QUALITIES
....

COTTON

CATEGORY: This quality, demonstrated clinically by Dr. Shen, is not discussed elsewhere in the literature. It is a commonly identified quality with a reliable clinical meaning. The Cotton quality is felt only above the qi depth and to the depth at which other qualities are first accessed; therefore it is classified as a superficial pulse.

SENSATION: The Cotton quality (Fig. 9-1) usually manifests over the entire pulse and less often at individual positions. It is spongy, amorphous, structureless (connective tissue) and has a resistance that increases as gentle pressure is exerted from the surface down to whichever depth other qualities can be first accessed. If the qi depth is absent, the Cotton quality is felt down to the blood depth, or to the organ-qi depth if the blood depth is absent, and even down to the organ-blood (O-B) and organ-substance (O-S) depths if the pulse is Feeble-Absent. Neither individual beats nor the wave are palpable with the Cotton quality. Obese individuals have a thickening of the connective tissue that is distinguished from the Cotton quality by its sensation of hardness.

Where the wave of the radial pulse is above the qi depth or the structure of the artery protrudes above the surrounding tissue, the Cotton quality is palpated to the side of the artery.

INTERPRETATION: The Cotton quality is a sign of superficial qi stagnation with several etiologies. Over time, the body's efforts to overcome the stagnation will cause depletion, and eventually the blood circulation will be affected. The Cotton quality is usually caused by suppression of emotions and less commonly by physical trauma.

Fig. 9-1 Cotton quality

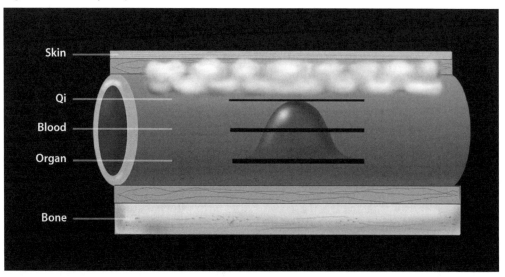

Emotional Suppression and Resignation

The Cotton quality reflects feelings of oppression, resignation, sadness, and hopelessness due to the perception that one cannot change adverse conditions in one's life. One example of this is an unhappy marriage in which the individual cannot leave even though the commitment to make it work is clearly not present. Individuals with a pronounced Cotton quality tend to blame others for their predicament, thereby suppressing awareness of the cause of their feelings, although it is close to the surface of consciousness. The conditions that create the Cotton quality are often present in a person's daily life, and are more likely to be consciously accessible to them than other causes of emotional problems. Treatment of Kidney yang-essence deficiency and concomitant diminished will power have been found to diminish the Cotton quality.

Trauma

A major physical trauma obstructs qi circulation in the channels and at the surface of the body and may give rise to the Cotton quality. The Cotton quality can reflect this stagnation when pain is present; and the qualities at the qi, blood, and organ depths of the pulse are Tight. The facial color is darker, and there may be a horizontal line at the back of the inside of the lower eyelid and a purple blister on the tongue at the side of the body affected by the trauma.

FLOATING

CATEGORY: The Floating quality is a superficial pulse found above the qi depth just under the skin. The qi depth is located using a very specific amount of finger pressure, but almost no pressure is required to access the Floating quality.

SENSATION: The Floating quality (Fig. 9-2) is accessed by gently laying the fingers on the skin with almost no pressure; it does not have a wave form. The Floating quality is not connected to other qualities found deeper in the pulse, even if those other qualities at times rise above the qi depth. The Floating pulse sensation can be Tense, Tight, Slippery, or Yielding.[1]

Fig. 9-2 Floating quality

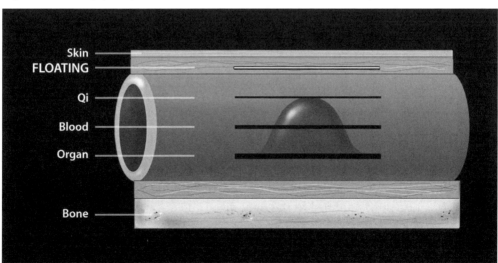

DIFFERENTIATING FLOATING FROM OTHER QUALITIES

In the literature, expansive qualities, chiefly the Empty, Hollow Full-Overflowing and Flooding Excess pulses, are classified as Floating. We differentiate these qualities as follows.

Floating and Empty, Hollow Full-Overflowing, and Flooding Excess

When the body mounts a response to an external pathogen, energy is brought to the surface to expel the pathogen. When a Floating pulse manifests, some of the substance of the pulse within the three depths may be diminished, but essentially it remains intact. The Empty quality, with which the Floating quality is sometimes confused in the literature, is the result of a profound separation of yin and yang energies. It is felt clearly at the qi depth but not above it, and the blood and organ depths are separating or absent. When the blood and organ depth are finally absent and only the qi depth remains, observers in the past have classified this as Floating, although the qi depth is well below the skin. The Hollow-Full Overflowing and Flooding Excess qualities are described in Ch. 8.

ETIOLOGY, PATHOGENESIS, AND INTERPRETATION OF THE FLOATING PULSE

External disharmony

Usually the Floating quality is a sign of increased activity of the superficial, fast-moving protective energies of the body.

The entire pulse, or the right distal position alone, will be Floating in the early stages of an external pathogenic factor invasion, such as an attack of wind-cold or wind-heat. Later, when an external pathogenic factor invades the Lungs and reaches the deeper qi level (four levels)—as seen with allergies, asthma, bronchitis, and pneumonia—the right distal position can still be slightly Floating, and there may also be signs of internal heat in the Lungs, such as the Robust Pounding quality. In such instances, the Special Lung position is usually Floating and may also have Robust Pounding and Slippery qualities.

Wind-cold

The pulse is Floating Tense and slightly Slow. The Floating quality usually affects the entire pulse, but in mild conditions it may be confined to the right distal and to the Special Lung positions.

Wind-heat

The pulse is Floating Yielding and slightly Rapid; this may include the entire pulse or be confined to the right distal and Special Lung positions.

Wind-water (phlegm with wind-cold or wind-heat)

When dampness (and the resultant phlegm) accompanies a wind-cold or wind-heat pattern, the Floating quality is attended by the Slippery quality. This quality, also known as wind-water, is a sign of stagnation of qi (wind-cold) or agitation of qi (wind-heat), which interferes with the movement of fluids at the surface of the body. The Floating Slippery quality is also sometimes associated with hives.

Internal disharmony

FLOATING TIGHT   The Floating Tight quality is a sign of Liver 'wind'. Initially it is found at the left middle position and, as the condition becomes more serious, the Floating Tight quality appears over the entire pulse. This quality may be a precursor to stroke, preceded or accompanied by wind in the channels, and characterized by transient neurological symptoms such as numbness, tingling, other parasthesias and transient ischemic attacks (TIA). Prior to a major stroke, the Floating Tight quality may accompany the very Tight Full-Overflowing quality that is most pathognomonic of an impending stroke.

EMPTY

CATEGORY: The Empty quality is categorized as superficial because it is most clearly felt at the qi depth.

SENSATION: With the Empty quality (Figs. 9-3a-c) the qi depth is fully intact. With greater pressure, the blood and organ depths separate or disappear entirely. The ability to discern the separating movement at the blood and organ depths is essential to identifying the Empty quality. When the pulse is Empty, we may find the qi depth to be Tight, Tense, Leather, or Yielding depending on the associated disorder.

There has been some confusion between the sensations of Reduced Substance and Separation (Empty). With Reduced Substance there is less resistance side to side. With the Empty pulse the reduced resistance is from distal-proximal and there is no pounding under the finger in the middle of the position.

It is important to keep this distinction since Reduced Substance is a sign of qi-blood deficiency while the Empty quality is a sign of the more serious 'separation of yin and yang' and suggests a much more serious 'qi wild' disorder.

ETIOLOGY: The Empty quality found in a single position is a sign of profound deficiency of yin or yang that will induce a functional alienation between yin and yang ('separation of yin and yang'). When found over large parts of the pulse, we have the extreme physiological chaos known as 'qi wild'.

Yang, or functional qi, is expansive and is held in place by the centripetal, sinking, and heavy aspects of yin, or nourishing qi. If the yin energies are not strong enough to hold the yang, the yang energies will float aimlessly away to the surface and functionality will be lost. If the yang is not strong enough to move the yin, a similar process of separation and consequence occurs.

INTERPRETATION: The Empty quality, when found over the entire pulse, is a sign of a 'qi wild' disorder. The 'qi wild' condition is characterized by chaos. It is the most serious disruption and disorganization of normal physiology and is associated with illnesses such as cancer, autoimmune and mental illness. If found over the entire pulse, the presence of an Empty quality demonstrates that a person is in the early stages of a 'qi wild' condition, and without corrective

Fig. 9-3a Empty (early stage)

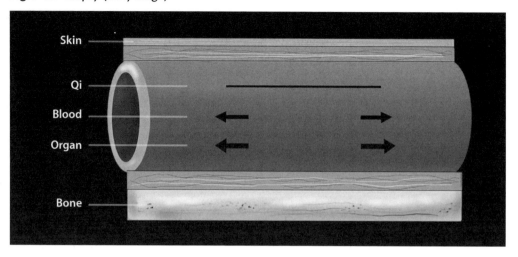

Fig. 9-3b Empty (middle stage)

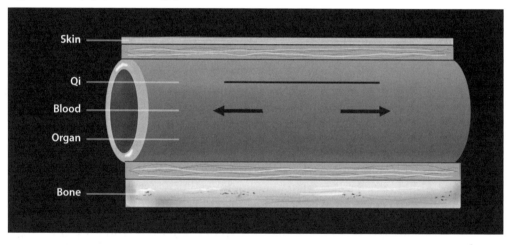

Fig. 9-3c Empty (later stage)

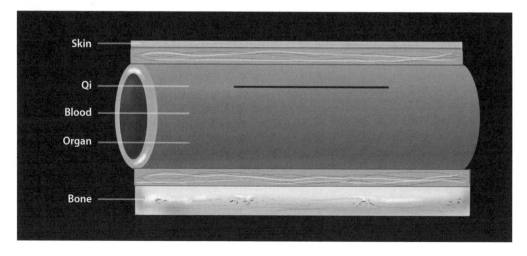

measures will suffer a major illness within six months to three years. Severe early malnourishment, overwork, or over-exercise beyond one's energy, significant fetal distress, as well as long use of the cold-natured recreational drugs are common etiologies, the latter accessed primarily at the left distal position. Found in the course of a serious illness, it denotes a poor prognosis and is one of the eight pulses of death.[2]

The Empty quality over the entire pulse for a short period of, say, a few weeks, may also manifest acutely in an individual who is in acute emotional distress and whose energy comes to the surface to cope with the circumstances. This should be interpreted and treated as a post-traumatic stress disorder rather than a 'qi wild' condition. Treating it as a 'qi wild' disorder could make the person's condition worse.

Another condition in which the Empty quality can appear for a short time, days to weeks, is with an invading common cold where the qi rises to eliminate it. It is important to inquire when finding the Empty quality whether or not the person may have a cold because, again, treating the invading cold as if there is a deficient condition associated with 'qi wild' might make the condition worse.

YIELDING EMPTY THREAD-LIKE

CATEGORY: Although this quality can be classified with the reduced-volume pulses, it has been placed with the superficial pulses because it is only at the depth at which the Yielding Empty Thread-like quality is felt.[3]

SENSATION: The Yielding Empty Thread-like quality (Figs. 9-4a and 9-4b) feels like a thread floating on water at the qi depth. Like the Empty quality, the Yielding Empty Thread-like quality separates or disappears under pressure.[4]

Fig. 9-4a Yielding Empty Thread-like (early stage)

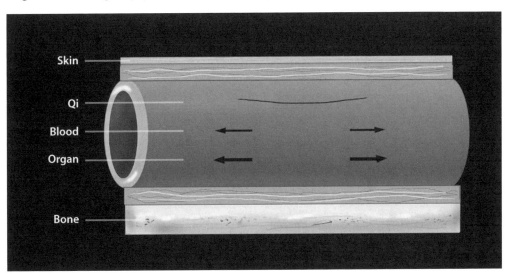

Fig. 9-4b Yielding Empty Thread-like (later stage)

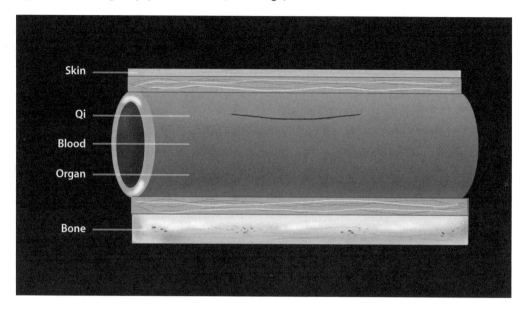

INTERPRETATION: Yielding Empty Thread-like is a rare pulse quality that indicates extreme deficiency of yin and yang. It is found primarily in persons who are in the terminal stages of disease, and is a more severe sign of a 'qi wild' disorder than the Empty pulse.[5]

LEATHER-EMPTY

CATEGORY: The Leather quality is classified as a superficial pulse because it is accessed at the qi depth.

Fig. 9-5a Leather (early stage)

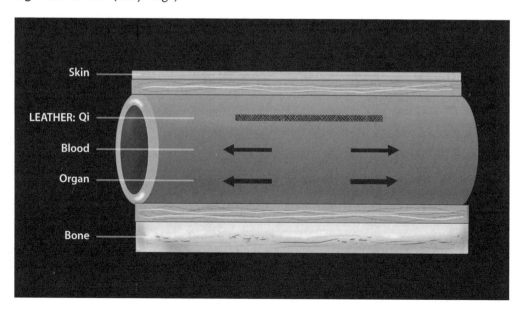

Fig. 9-5b Leather (later stage)

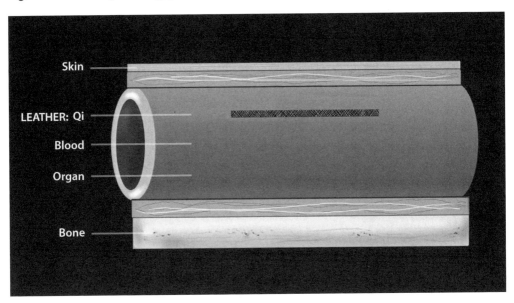

SENSATION: Found at the qi depth, the Leather quality (Figs. 9-5a and 9-5b) feels hard, like the surface of a drum, and separating at the blood and organ depths, especially in the later stages of the Leather-Empty quality.

INTERPRETATION: The Leather-Empty quality is a sign of extreme yin, blood, and especially essence depletion. It is similar in meaning to the Empty quality in terms of its association with the separation of yin and yang in a 'qi wild' disorder. The hardness that is accessed at the qi depth communicates the profound depletion of the yin-essence energies of the body associated with prolonged chronic disease and damage to the bone marrow.

SCATTERED

CATEGORY: The Scattered quality is one of the most serious Empty qualities, falling into the category of extreme 'qi wild'.[6]

SENSATION: The Scattered quality (Fig. 9-6) is felt at the qi depth. Instead of feeling continuous, as one rolls one's finger longitudinally, it disperses into separate pieces, as if divided. A very apt classical metaphor describes the sensation as a "superficial pulse, like willow flowers scattering in the wind."[7]

INTERPRETATION: The Scattered quality occurs with profound deficiency of qi, blood, and yang (especially Kidney yang) and is a sign of extreme 'qi wild'. Attendants to late stage AIDs patients have described it as the 'dripping ceiling' pulse.

Fig. 9-6 Scattered quality

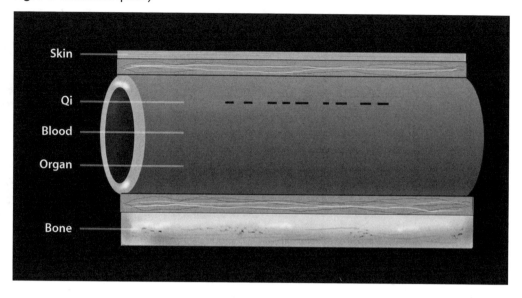

MINUTE

CATEGORY: The Minute pulse, like the Empty and Scattered qualities, is absent or markedly diminished at the organ depth and has a similar meaning to the Empty and Scattered 'qi wild' qualities, except more serious.

SENSATION: The Minute quality (Fig. 9-7) is found only at the blood depth. It is Thin but ill-defined ('blurry'), gives way under pressure like the Empty quality, and, like the Scattered quality, is not continuous as the fingers are rolled from the proximal to distal positions.

Fig. 9-7 Minute quality

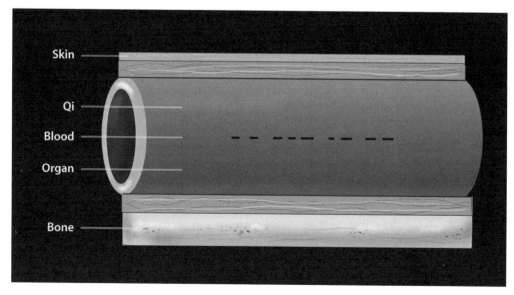

INTERPRETATION: The Minute pulse signifies an extreme deficiency of qi and yang and is a 'qi wild' quality that represents a more advanced pathology than even the Empty or Scattered qualities. The presence of the Minute quality indicates that there is not enough yang left to rise to the surface. The Minute quality is uncommon but has been found in AIDS patients and in the terminal stages of other illness.[8]

HOLLOW

CATEGORY: The Hollow quality is classified as a superficial pulse because it is primarily accessed at the qi and organ depths.

SENSATION: The Hollow pulse is felt clearly at the qi depth. As pressure is increased to the blood depth, the pulse separates (moves to the sides) and diminishes or altogether disappears until the organ depth is reached, where the pulse returns. The Leather-Hollow pulse has no sensation at the blood depth, but all other Hollow qualities have the separating quality at the blood depth. It is important to distinguish the Hollow pulses from the Empty quality. Both can be palpated at the qi depth, both can separate or are absent at the blood depth, but unlike the Empty quality, the Hollow pulse feels as though it has a bottom when pressure is applied from the qi through the blood and to the organ depths.

The Hollow quality is sometimes mistaken for the Slippery quality because the pulse separates at the blood depth, and to some this separating movement of the substance of the pulse feels like Slipperiness. However, a Slippery quality moves on its own in only one direction, while a Hollow quality separates and moves both proximally and distally only under pressure.[9]

The Hollow quality is also often confused with the Inflated Yielding quality. The Inflated quality is like a compressible balloon and sometimes gives the impression of hollowness. However, unlike the Hollow quality, it does not separate at the blood depth with pressure, and when pressure is released, the Inflated quality fills out and follows one's finger up to the qi depth. Though it does not expand beyond the qi depth, it feels as if it will. The Hollow quality separates, diminishes, or disappears at the blood depth and has much less sense of filling out with the release of pressure.

INTERPRETATION: There are multiple types of Hollow qualities and the interpretation varies according to each type. Almost every Hollow quality is an indication that the blood vessel wall and the blood itself are sufficiently out of contact and that there is a notable functional disengagement of yin and yang in the blood vessels.

Types of Hollow qualities[10]

Tense Hollow Types

TENSE HOLLOW FULL-OVERFLOWING The Tense Hollow Full-Overflowing quality, described fully in Ch. 8, is associated with excess heat in the blood due to any of its varied causes.

Yielding Hollow types

YIELDING PARTIALLY HOLLOW   The Yielding Partially Hollow quality (Fig. 9-8) is a sign of mild general blood deficiency, less so than with a Thin quality, but more than with a Spreading quality.

Fig. 9-8 Yielding Partially Hollow quality

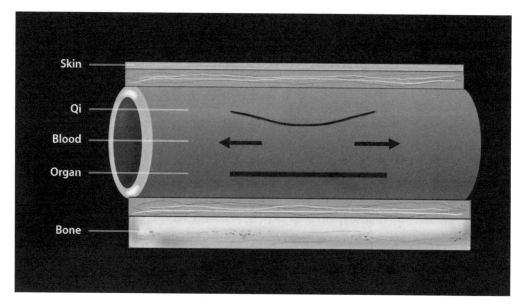

YIELDING HOLLOW FULL-OVERFLOWING   When found over the entire pulse, the Yielding Hollow Full-Overflowing quality signifies one of the most severe types of the 'qi wild' disorder, considerably more of a 'qi wild' condition than is signified by the Empty quality.

The Yielding Hollow Full-Overflowing quality with a Slow rate is caused by inordinately excessive exercise or labor, especially in childhood; significant deprivation of food, clothing, or shelter in childhood or prolonged, severe menorrhagia can also lead to this quality.

The slightly Yielding Hollow-Full Overflowing quality with a Normal or slightly Rapid rate occur together when an individual who has been exercising beyond his or her energy capacity for a prolonged period of time suddenly stops exercising. When the exercise is stopped suddenly, the blood volume contracts more quickly than the blood vessels and the yin (blood) and yang (vessels) lose contact. The symptoms—which develop quickly—include severe fatigue, severe anxiety, panic, dissociation and depersonalization, explosive anger, cold extremities, migrating joint pain, and many other seemingly bizarre symptoms.

The Yielding Hollow Full-Overflowing quality with the Intermittent or

Interrupted rate is a sign of a severe form of 'qi wild' where the instability is already in the yin organs, especially the Heart (the 'emperor'). Here we have the combination of general yin organ and circulatory chaos. The presence or imminence of serious disease and death is great.

YIELDING HOLLOW ROPY   The Yielding Hollow Ropy quality is caused by excessive exercise over a long period of time beyond one's energy, especially in an individual who is still maturing, though I have found it in the moderately elderly. The blood volume is gradually reduced due to its overconsumption by this excessive activity; when it is unable to nourish the vessel walls, they eventually become harder.

SUBMERGED PULSE QUALITIES

DEEP

SENSATION: The Deep quality (Fig. 9-9) is only accessed at the organ depth; the qi and blood depths are absent.

INTERPRETATION: Traditionally, a Deep quality over the entire pulse is associated with depletion of the true qi and blood from chronic or serious internal disease that is difficult to cure. True qi is strongly linked with the yang basal metabolic heat that drives the body and is based on the integrity of Kidney yang. The pulse will become deeper as this energetic heat is used up through either physical or mental work beyond a person's energy, or from poor eating habits like anorexia and bulimia, lack of sleep, excessive sex, or chronic illness.

Fig. 9-9 Deep quality

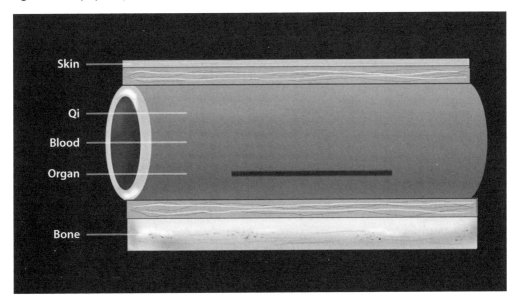

A rare cause of the Deep quality in our time, in developed countries with central heating, is stagnation of qi due to excess cold that prevents the yang qi from rising. Usually this occurs with an external pathogenic factor when the yang qi is already deficient.

In an obese person, a relatively Deeper pulse in all positions may be normal. In a healthy person the entire pulse will be slightly Deeper in the winter, but this is barely discernible. A transient Deep quality can be found in very introverted people whose initial response to new social contact is to energetically withdraw; this quality will, on repeated examination, revert to the enduring and valid pulse picture.

On the positive side, although the presence of the Deep quality implies that the true qi is depleted, the yin organ energies are still more or less intact and functioning. The Deep quality is less serious than the Feeble-Absent quality or the 'qi wild' condition associated with the Empty qualities.

THE ORGAN-BLOOD AND ORGAN-SUBSTANCE DEPTHS

According to Dr. Shen, there are three divisions of the organ depth (Fig. 9-10), which have been identified as the organ-qi, organ-blood (O-B), and the more material organ-substance (O-S) depths. These names replace what has previously been called the organ depth, blood subdivision of the organ depth, and the deepest part of the organ depth. Thus, for example, we find at the Liver organ depth, the Liver organ-qi, Liver organ-blood, and Liver organ-substance depths.

Recent investigation into these three levels of the organ depth indicate that the organ-blood and organ-substance levels tell us about the hidden pathogens

Fig. 9-10 The nine depths

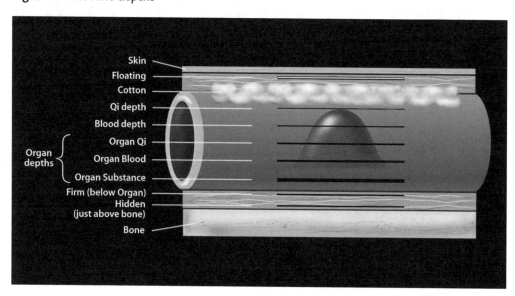

in the body, especially damp-heat of diverse etiologies, since the Slippery quality and increased Robust Pounding can be found here when not found at the organ-qi level. Increasingly, the Choppy quality also appears at these depths, informing us about the burgeoning problem of retained toxicity.

FIRM

SENSATION: The rarely found Firm quality (Fig. 9-11) is slightly deeper than the Deep quality (below the divisions of the organ depth) and slightly more superficial than the Hidden quality. It feels hard and unyielding to the touch, and, as Wu Shui-Wan says, it "does not respond to the finger."[11] This aspect clearly differentiates it from the organ-blood and organ-substance positions described above.

Fig. 9-11 Firm quality

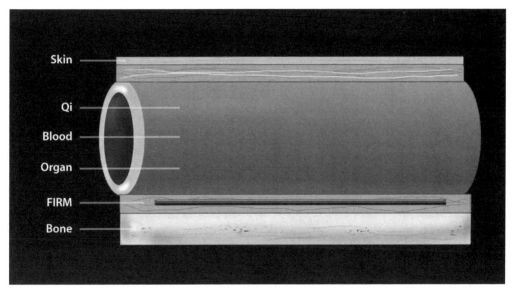

INTERPRETATION: In the literature,[12] stagnation and serious interference with qi, blood, and fluid circulation by internal cold are associated with this quality. This factor was more significant in times and places of the distant past when people were subjected to extreme cold and had limited sources of heat. Currently it could occur with hypothermia in winter mountain climbers. Found in any position, it must be viewed as a sign of serious illness until proven otherwise.[13]

HIDDEN

SENSATION: The Hidden quality (Figs. 9-12a and 9-12b) is felt only with extreme pressure below the organ depth, on or just above the radius bone. (NB: In learning this quality, there is a danger that students will mistakenly learn to exert excessive pressure when taking the pulse. In fact, the most common mistake in pulse-taking is the tendency to press too deeply, beyond the fine parameters of this model and beyond the realm of its interpretive function.)

INTERPRETATION: With the Hidden Deficient quality, the yang qi is severely deficient and unable to bring the pulse wave to the surface. It is a sign of serious illness in which the disease process has entered profoundly into the yin organ system. With the Hidden Excess quality (like the Firm quality), cold may be a factor, as described above. It is very rare, though it is reported in the literature. It may be due to internal cold that has transformed into heat, or even more rarely, to stagnation of food, phlegm, or blood, or to extreme heat transforming into internal wind.

Fig. 9-12a Hidden Excess quality

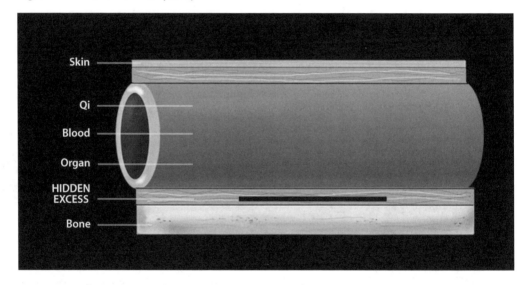

Fig. 9-12b Hidden Deficient quality

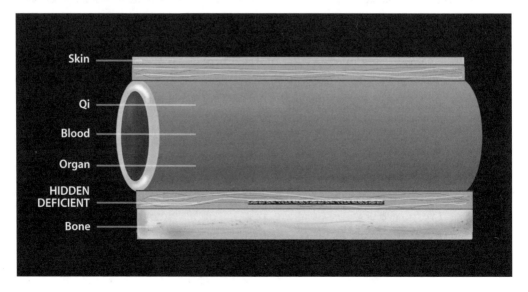

Fig. 9-13 Depth

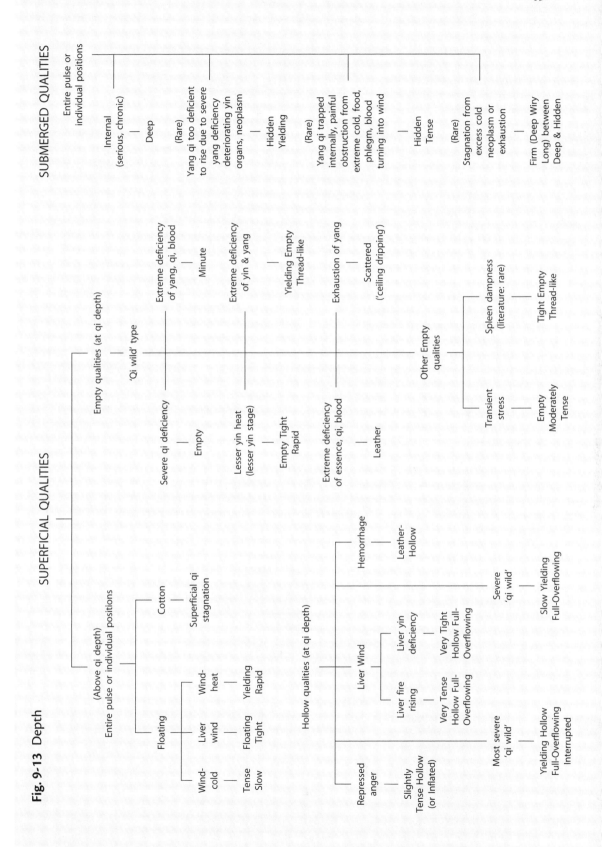

10

Size: Width & Length

Brandt Stickley, A.P.

WIDTH

The width of the pulse primarily describes the condition of the blood in terms of excess, toxicity, heat, viscosity, plasticity, and deficiency. By contrast, amplitude, or the depth and height of the pulse, conveys the condition of the qi and yang, and hardness informs us of the condition of the yin. Wide pulses are broadly associated with excess conditions[1] while Narrow qualities generally reflect deficiency. Divergences from this general scheme are noted.

WIDE PULSE GROUP

There are three categories within the group of Wide pulses: Wide Excess, Wide Moderate, and Wide Deficient.

Wide excess qualities

CATEGORY: The Wide Excess category includes pulses that are wider than normal. These have been described in the literature as 'big' and 'large'.

SENSATION: The Wide Excess pulse is broader than the Normal pulse and also exhibits strength and substance. The depth and extent of the wider sensation informs its interpretation. For example, at the organ depth the Flooding Excess quality is particularly wide and strong. The Tense Hollow Full-Overflowing quality usually begins wider and stronger somewhat higher, between the organ and blood depth, and the Hollow therefore appears a little higher than with the Normal pulse. The width of the Blood Unclear quality is more moderately wide than the Blood Heat or Blood Thick qualities.

INTERPRETATION: In general, Wide Excess qualities pertain to excess heat. A major contribution to the interpretation of conditions affecting the blood is found in the elaboration of the Blood Unclear, Blood Heat, and Blood Thick qualities. To assess these qualities, one would palpate the organ depth and then gradually release pressure through the blood and qi depths. A barely perceptible increase in width at the blood depth suggests the Blood Unclear quality. If the pulse significantly widens and fills out at the blood depth and narrows at the qi depth, it is the Blood Heat quality. If the pulse continues to widen as one releases pressure through the qi depth, then the Blood Thick quality is present. These qualities are described more fully in Ch. 13.

BLOOD HEAT

SENSATION: With the Blood Heat quality (Fig. 10-1) the blood depth fills out significantly as one releases pressure from the organ depth, and then the pulse diminishes on further release of pressure to the qi depth.

INTERPRETATION: The etiology of this excess heat in the blood is due to repressed emotional stress causing Liver qi stagnation; rapid eating or excessive eating of spicy foods, shellfish, coffee, chocolate, and sugar; consuming alcohol; shock that causes Heart qi agitation; exercise beyond one's energy; and stimulating drugs such as cocaine.

Fig. 10-1 Blood Heat quality

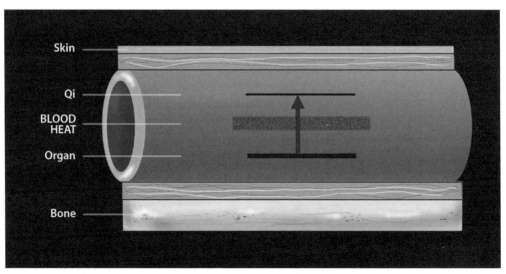

BLOOD THICK

CATEGORY: Blood Thick (Fig. 10-2) is classified with the Wide Excess qualities due to both its extremely excessive width and strength.

SENSATION: The blood depth is extremely Wide and continues to expand up to the qi depth as one releases pressure from the organ depth.

INTERPRETATION: Blood Thick involves a greater degree of heat in the blood (or inflammation), increased deterioration of the blood vessel walls, and the presence of excessive destructive lipids. Its etiology includes all the factors that cause Blood Heat, as well as excessive intake of fatty and rich foods and prolonged emotional stress.

Fig.10-2 Blood Thick quality

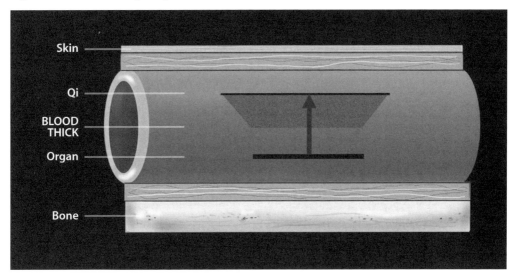

TENSE HOLLOW FULL-OVERFLOWING

SENSATION: The pulse is Wide at the blood depth and expands to above the qi depth with a full sine wave. It feels slightly Hollow to pressure around or just below the qi depth.

INTERPRETATION: The Tense Hollow Full-Overflowing quality (Fig. 10-3) is a sign that the body is unsuccessful in attempting to discharge excess heat. This is normally accomplished through the urine, bowel movements, and perspiration. Unreleased heat may accumulate in and dilate the vessels. An overworking 'nervous system', dietary indiscretions (including excessive ingestion of sugar, fats, and alcohol), and emotional stress can all contribute to the production of heat. This quality may occur in conjunction with the progression from Blood Heat to Blood Thick, and may be associated with headache, epistaxis, hematemesis, hypertension, and ultimately stroke (see Ch. 8).

FLOODING EXCESS

CATEGORY: The Flooding Excess quality is categorized among the 'big' pulses in

Fig. 10-3 Tense Hollow Full-Overflowing quality

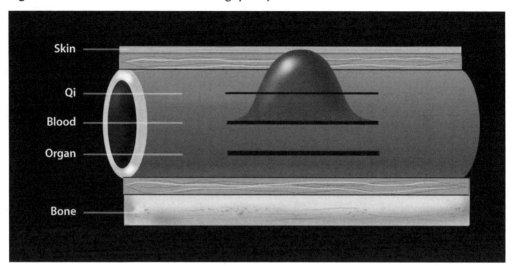

the literature. Unlike the Tense Hollow Full-Overflowing quality, the Flooding Excess wave lacks the full sine curve. It also represents heat in the yin organs rather than heat (deficient or excess) in the blood. Flooding Excess qualities are associated with patterns of heat in the literature.

SENSATION: The Flooding Excess quality is Wide at the organ depth. It is felt as a strong sine wave originating at the organ depth, surging over the qi depth, and then dropping off precipitously at its apogee.

INTERPRETATION: The Flooding Excess wave form primarily indicates extreme excess heat, usually associated with a significant infection. When it is found in one position, it indicates intense heat or fire and infection in that organ. The Flooding Excess wave form is found in acute hepatitis, the yang brightness stage of the six stages, the manic phase of bipolar disease, and acute fulminating infection. In these conditions, other signs of heat, such as the Robust Pounding quality, can be found. The Flooding Excess wave is also found with less Robust Pounding and a Slower rate in chronic infections and subliminal chronic hepatitis (see Ch. 8).

Wide moderate qualities

BLOOD UNCLEAR

SENSATION: The pulse exhibits a barely perceptible increase in size, rather than a decrease, at the blood depth as the finger is raised from the organ depth. As pressure is released from the blood to the qi depth, the size diminishes. Sometimes the pulse is also Slippery.

INTERPRETATION: The Blood Unclear quality indicates toxicity in the blood due to environmental toxins (especially solvents), inadequate metabolism of toxins in the Liver, or inadequate digestion, particularly of proteins. Especially in the context of toxicity, the symptoms associated with the Blood Unclear quality include fatigue, joint pain, and skin conditions like eczema and psoriasis. Dr. Shen compares this condition to a glass of water in which dirt is suspended.

LEATHER-HOLLOW

SENSATION: The pulse is Leather-Hard at the qi depth, becomes completely Hollow at the blood depth, and reappears at the organ depth.

INTERPRETATION: The Leather-Hollow pulse is always a serious sign. It is associated with hemorrhage. If the rate is Rapid, then bleeding is imminent. If the rate is Slow, it suggests past hemorrhage. It is worth noting that this pulse may presage a life-threatening condition due to the potential for shock associated with sudden blood loss. When found in a single position, it appears as the result of the associated organ losing control of its blood, as in the case of bleeding stomach ulcers.

TENSE ROPY

SENSATION: The Tense Ropy quality feels like a cord, with the edges clearly delineated, sometimes straight and sometimes twisted. It feels as though one could lift the Ropy pulse away from the surrounding tissues. It is usually found over the whole pulse, and rarely, only in the left middle position. It may vary in both hardness and size.

INTERPRETATION: The Tense Ropy quality indicates hardening of the vessel walls due to chronic heat in the blood that has vulcanized the vessel walls. It is associated with developing atherosclerosis or arteriosclerosis, sometimes preceded or accompanied by hypertension. It may also be associated with a history of a protracted 'nervous system tense' disorder or a diet of excessively rich foods.

Wide deficient qualities

WIDE YIELDING HOLLOW FULL-OVERFLOWING WITH NORMAL OR SLIGHTLY RAPID RATE   The Yielding Hollow Full-Overflowing pulse is discussed under the rubrics of Rhythm and Stability, and Volume (Chs. 6 and 8).[2] With the Rapid rate, it is associated with a 'qi wild' disorder with symptoms of depersonalization, severe panic and anxiety, irritability, and extreme fatigue. It often results from sudden cessation of prolonged periods of excessive exercise, or, with the Slower rate, prolonged overwork and/or over-exercise in a vulnerable person, especially since childhood. These conditions, in which yin and yang have lost functional contact, are very serious.

REDUCED SUBSTANCE

SENSATION: Reduced Substance pulse lacks density and feels like a threadbare sweater. Reduced Substance can be found over the entire pulse, at an individual position, or at different depths. It is a sensation somewhere between Normal and Feeble.

INTERPRETATION: Reduced Substance suggests advancing qi, blood, and yin deficiency. It represents a slightly less qi-deficient quality than the Feeble quality.

DIFFUSE

SENSATION: The boundary of the vessel is partially or completely obliterated. Diffuse is usually found with other qualities, chiefly Reduced Substance and Reduced Pounding.

INTERPRETATION: Diffuse suggests a state of more advanced qi deficiency.

YIELDING ROPY

SENSATION: The Yielding Ropy quality is cord-like, big, and distinct from the surrounding tissue, but without the hardness of the Tense Ropy quality. Rather it is like a soft tube, with a slightly hollow and pliable surface.

INTERPRETATION: This quality is associated with very long periods of physical activity (thirty or more years) beyond one's energy. In this case, the drying of the intima of the vessels is derived from yin-blood deficiency rather than chronic heat. Yin and yang in the blood vessels have lost contact and the yin cannot adequately nourish the vessel walls.

NARROW PULSE GROUP

THIN

CATEGORY: The terms Thin, Fine, Thready, and even Small are all frequently encountered in the literature as terms for this quality. We use the word Thin because it is unambiguous and clearly contrasts with the term Wide.

SENSATION: The Thin quality (Fig. 10-4) is narrower than the Normal pulse. There are two types, Thin and Pliable and Thin and Hard (usually Tight).

INTERPRETATION: The Thin quality is associated with blood deficiency. The Thin and Pliable qualities are a combination of blood and qi deficiency. The Thin and Tight qualities are signs of blood and yin deficiency.

The Thin pulse, demonstrating blood deficiency, is more common in women due to the demands of menstruation and childbirth. It is less common in men.

If found in a young man it is a sign of severe qi deficiency and has been associated with chronic disease. There is a hierarchy of seriousness depending on the depths and positions at which it is located.

The Thin quality found over the entire pulse at first impression means that the entire organism is depleted of blood. In individual positions it is a sign of blood deficiency in that organ. At the left distal position it is a sign of Heart blood deficiency and indicates that the Heart cannot circulate the blood and nourish it's own muscle. At the right distal position it means that the Lungs cannot provide the blood with sufficient oxygen; at the left middle position it means that the Liver cannot store the blood; at the right middle position it means that the Spleen is not sufficiently making blood from food; at the left and right proximal positions it means that the Kidney essence is not producing sufficient blood from the marrow (bone).

Fig. 10-4 Thin quality

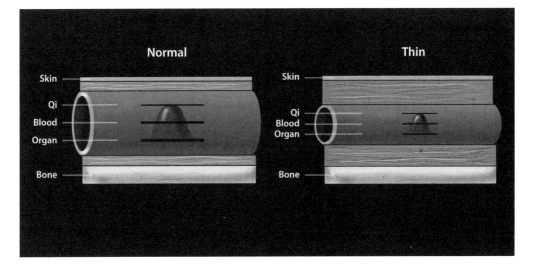

LENGTH

The significance of the length of the pulse is not emphasized in Contemporary Chinese Pulse Diagnosis. Restriction in the length, however, does have some clinical significance.

Extended Length

LONG

CATEGORY: The Long pulse is regarded as being one of the 28 traditional pulse qualities.

SENSATION: The Long quality (Fig. 10-5) feels elongated through the three principal positions.

Fig. 10-5 Long quality

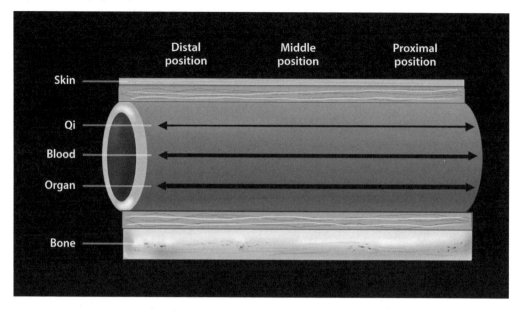

INTERPRETATION: With other qualities that define the Normal pulse, it is a sign of a robust body condition unless it is very Tense or has substantial Robust Pounding, which implies excess heat.[3]

DIMINISHED LENGTH

SHORT

CATEGORY: The Short quality is described in terms of its diminished length. The discussion below will be elaborated in terms of Contemporary Chinese Pulse Diagnosis.

SENSATION: A Short pulse is one whose position feels disconnected from its contiguous position; its sensation feels isolated from those around it. In practice, the Short pulse appears most often in the middle burner, especially the left, and the position has very robust qualities such as Tense and Robust Pounding. Frequently with this pulse pattern, the distal and proximal positions are simultaneously Feeble/Absent (Fig. 10-6).

INTERPRETATION: The configuration described above suggests deficiency in the upper and lower burners and stagnation in the middle burner. The issue is whether the upper and lower burner are truly deficient or simply appear that way due to stagnant qi, blood, dampness, or food in the middle burner that is interfering with the circulation of energy and substance between above and below. If treatment using the Girdle vessel releases the stagnation in the middle burner, and the apparent deficiencies in the upper and lower burner disappear, we know that the cause was one of excess in the middle.

Fig. 10-6 Short quality

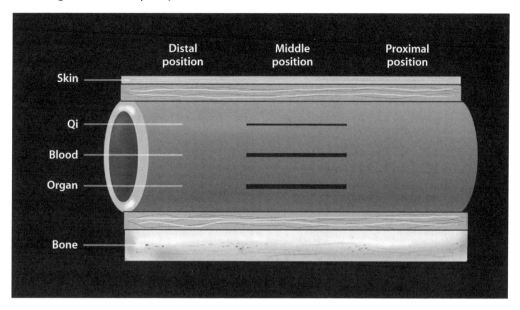

If on the other hand the upper and lower deficiencies persist, then the Short pulse in the middle is due to severe upper and lower burner deficiency that is unable to move the vital substances through the middle burner. This may sometimes be a Kidney-Heart disharmony.

RESTRICTED (LENGTH)

SENSATION: The Restricted pulse, found only in the Special Lung Position, is very short and feels constricted. It occupies a very small area.

INTERPRETATION: The Restricted quality is associated with severe Lung qi stagnation. Conditions in which this pulse has been found include chronic pulmonary obstructive disease and cancers of the lung, chest, and breast.

Fig. 10-7 Width

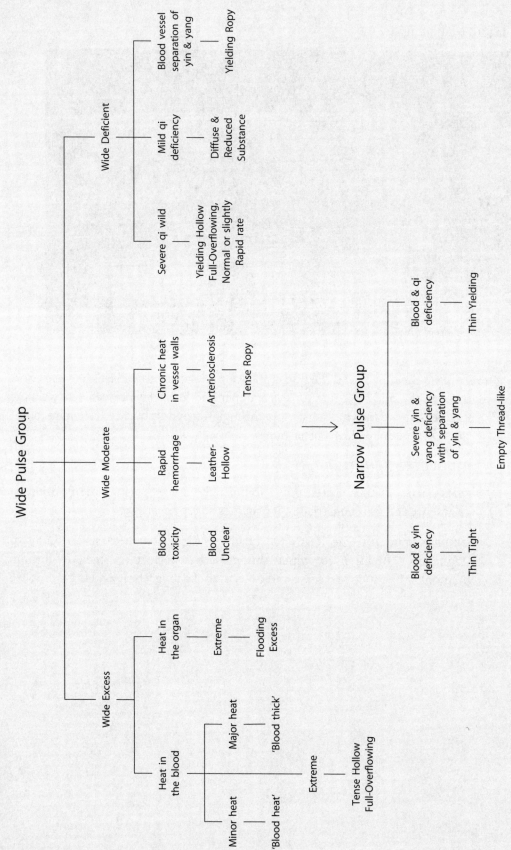

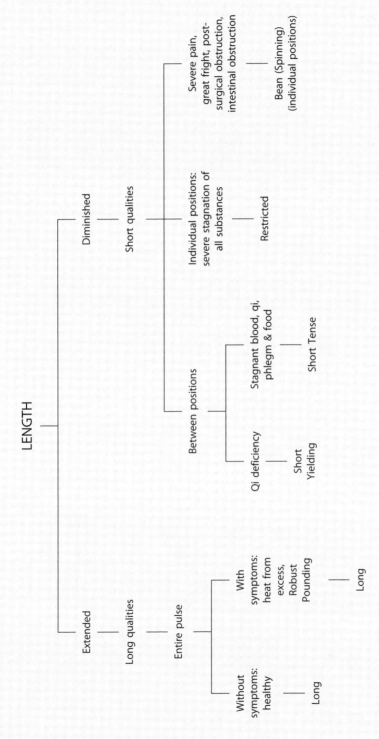

Fig. 10-8 Depth

11

Shape

Oliver Nash, L.Ac., M.B.Ac.C.

Karen Bilton, L.Ac.

Classification by shape implies that the pulse quality is recognized more by its shape than by other descriptive parameters such as depth, width, volume, length, rate, and rhythm. Shape may be subdivided into qualities with sensations that are relatively unyielding and lack fluidity, such as the Taut, Tense, Tight, Wiry, Ropy, Leather-Hard, Choppy, and Vibrations; and those that are fluid and more yielding, of which there is only one quality, Slippery. The clinical value of classifying the harder qualities in this way is discussed below.

FLUID QUALITIES

SLIPPERY

CATEGORY: The Slippery quality is classified under the category of shape and represents a form of stagnation that is due to a wide variety of causes.

SENSATION: With the Slippery quality (Fig. 11-1) the pulse slides rapidly under the fingers in one direction. The movement is independent of finger pressure.

This feeling of movement makes the Slippery quality easy to confuse with other qualities: the Robust Pounding quality at the organ depth, the separating sensation of the Spreading quality, and the Empty (stage one and two) and Hollow qualities; each of these qualities has a sensation of movement that is similar to that of the Slippery quality.

The wide and forceful nature of the Robust Pounding quality at the organ depth can add an expansive character to the sensation, causing the organ depth to seem to move in both directions.

The movement associated with the Separating quality is felt to occur in two directions, distally and proximally, but is not felt directly under the center of the finger. The sensation of separation grows with an increase in finger pressure. Dr. Hammer refers to this as the Pseudo-Slippery quality.

The Slippery quality is different in sensation to both the Robust Pounding and Separating qualities as its movement flows in one direction only, is felt clearly under the center of the finger, and does not alter with a change in finger pressure.

INTERPRETATION: Except in pregnancy, Dr. Shen regarded the Slippery quality as always indicating a damp condition. Perhaps the principal source of a damp condition is when the body brings fluid (yin) to cool and balance excess heat in an organ or area of the body. If the attempt fails, the dampness accumulates and will impair function in that area or organ, and will be perceived on the pulse as Slippery. While in the literature the Slippery quality is also often associated with excessive fluid, closer examination reveals a much more complex situation.

Fig. 11-1 Slippery quality

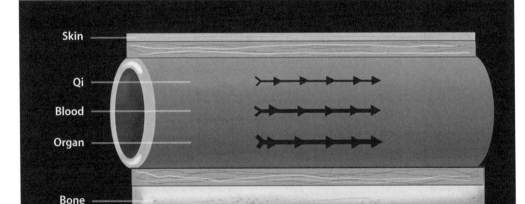

ENTIRE PULSE AT ALL DEPTHS

The interpretation of the Slippery quality over the entire pulse depends on the depth where it is found.

Pregnancy

The appearance of Slipperiness at all depths over the entire pulse may be a very early sign of pregnancy, sometimes lasting the entire first trimester. It is interpreted as an excess of fluid in the form of blood necessary to sustain the fetus.

Elevated blood lipids and glucose

With elevated lipids, the Slippery quality is most often found only at the blood depth. However, Slipperiness over the entire pulse at all three depths can also be a sign of increased blood viscosity as a result of increased serum lipids (cholesterol and triglycerides) and glucose. In this case the Slipperiness usually appears in conjunction with the Tense quality, indicating blood turbulence. If the blood vessel walls are damaged, a Tight Rough Vibration will be felt at the blood depth.

Blood Infection

If the pulse rate is also very Rapid, the overall quality Tight-Tense, and the color under the eyelids is very red, we are dealing with a serious condition of heat or fire known in biomedicine as septicemia (systemic blood infection). Also, the temperature is often elevated.

Heart qi deficiency

Diminished circulation can result from severe Heart qi deficiency, shock, or trauma directly to the circulation; these can lead to turbulence in the blood causing a Slippery and Slow quality over the entire pulse at all three depths. With Heart qi deficiency the left distal position will have deficient qualities such as Reduced Substance, Deep, and Feeble.

Iatrogenic

Steroids and corticosteroids can cause water retention and are another major etiology of the Slippery quality when it presents with the Feeble and Slow qualities at all depths.

Hypertension

Slipperiness found with Tight Hollow Full-Overflowing and a Rapid rate indicates impending stroke as an expression of a Spleen dampness condition. The excess fluid revealed by the Slippery quality arises as compensation for heat in the blood. Sometimes the phlegm created by the heat and dampness can cloud the orifices of the Heart.

Blood dyscrasia and autoimmune disease

Slipperiness found with the Feeble and Slow qualities over the entire pulse at all depths can indicate blood dyscrasia such as sickle cell anemia and hemochromatosis, or autoimmune diseases such as lupus.

Floating

A Floating Slippery quality can be a sign of dampness in the protective level due to an attack of wind, an allergic response often accompanied by hives.

QI DEPTH

If the pulse rate is Slow, the Slippery quality at the qi depth alone indicates that the qi is deficient and less able to move fluids in the connective tissue. When the pulse rate is elevated and the Slippery quality is found at the qi depth, it is often a sign of elevated blood glucose.

BLOOD DEPTH

When found at the blood depth, Slippery is a sign of turbulence in the blood flow and an indication that the conditions for the laying down of arterial plaque (atherosclerosis) already exist.

Slippery at the blood depth often accompanies pulse qualities described by Dr. Shen as 'blood unclear' (toxicity), 'blood heat,' or 'blood thick'. In Western medical terms, the latter would be perceived as increasing blood viscosity.

ORGAN DEPTH

Slippery at the organ depth alone over the entire pulse is associated with severe systemic infection. This includes parasites, especially as they release their off-spring (larvae).[1]

INDIVIDUAL POSITIONS

When the Slippery quality is found at an individual position it generally implies that there is dampness in the organ represented by that position, usually in response to excess heat in that organ. The combination of heat and dampness creates phlegm.

Slipperiness is often found at the right distal position and Special Lung positions associated with acute or chronic lung infection. At the left distal position it indicates phlegm misting the Heart with a propensity to neurotic behavior, some emotional disturbance, and even psychosis. When found at the Mitral Valve position, Slipperiness may imply mitral valve prolapse, panic attacks, and phobias.

In the Gallbladder position the Slippery quality is a sign of a damp-heat inflammatory condition, and, depending on the depth, in the Liver position it can be a sign of chronic infection (hepatitis). Somewhat less obviously, in the Esophagus position it can mean inflammation and stagnation, and in the Stomach-Pylorus position it can be a sign of increased gastric acidity, ulcer, and damp food stagnation.

NONFLUID QUALITIES

Over the years the Chinese terms that describe the hard nonfluid qualities have been variously and confusingly translated. Therefore, in order to present a clear analysis of these qualities, new classifications have been created based on sensation and interpretation, interrelated with specific clinical signs and symptoms.

OLD CLASSIFICATION OF NONFLUID QUALITIES

The descriptive terms tight, wiry, bow-string, string-taut, threadlike, and stringy are found in many of the standard texts on pulse diagnosis. Although these terms are all used to refer to the hard, nonfluid qualities, their descriptions often lack clarity either in terms of sensation or interpretation.

Furthermore, some of the traditional interpretations of the hard, nonfluid qualities do not reflect current clinical experience. While in older texts the Tight pulse is almost always associated with stagnation due to internal cold, in our time it is much more often found with deficient heat. This reflects the different states we encounter now compared with those found in ancient China. Modern practitioners do not commonly see the acute medical problems (such as malaria and internal cold obstruction) that were mentioned by traditional writers.

In developed countries present-day practitioners are primarily engaged in treating chronic disease largely due to responses to stress. Basing treatment on interpretations of pulse qualities from a time so different from our contemporary environment—that is, treating a Tight pulse as if there were cold stagnation when in fact there is yin-deficient heat—is obviously not in the best interest of the patient. What follows is a new, more structured and integrated classification system.

NEW CLASSIFICATION OF NONFLUID QUALITIES

There are at least five categories of increasing hardness included in the range of nonfluid pulse qualities. At one end of the spectrum is Taut, the least hard, followed by Tense, Tight, Wiry, and finally Leather-Hard. Clinically, we find there is a gradual progression from Taut through Tense and Tight to Wiry and Leather-Hard. Perhaps the most common error in pulse diagnosis is mistaking the hard qualities for excess, when in fact the Tight, Wiry, and Leather-Hard qualities signify a very important deficiency of yin and yin-essence. With this arrangement of the hard nonfluid pulse qualities, their interpretation and treatment becomes more logical and rational.

Pathogenesis

The hard nonfluid qualities progress pathologically along a continuum. The sequence of increasing hardness from Taut through Tense to Tight and then to Wiry and Leather-Hard reflects both growing degrees of qi stagnation and the development of excess heat generated by the body's attempt to overcome the stagnation. The body supplies yin to balance the excess heat; the yin is thus consumed over time, leading to deficiency of yin. A progression to the Leather-Hard quality reveals deficiency of yin, blood, and especially essence, the etiology of which is discussed below.

Sensation

These five nonfluid qualities are characterized by their sensation of decreasing diameter and increasing tension and hardness. The Taut, Tense, Tight, and Wiry pulses are on this continuum. The Wiry quality is the thinnest and hardest, feeling almost cutting, and the Leather-Hard quality is as hard as the Wiry but as wide as the Tense quality.

These qualities can also be likened to the strings of a violin (Fig. 11-2): the most flexible G string would be likened to the Taut pulse, the slightly less flexible D string to the Tense pulse, the even less flexible A string to the Tight pulse, and the thinnest, least flexible and most rigid E string to the Wiry pulse.

Fig. 11-2 Violin strings (nonfluid qualities: Taut, Tense, Tight, Wiry)

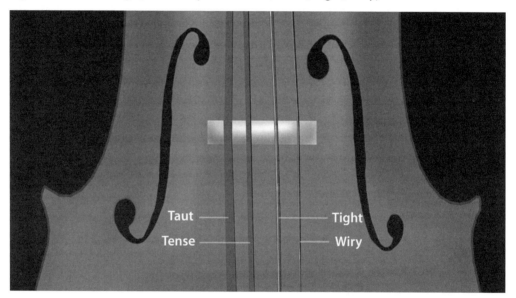

Clinical significance

To put these qualities in perspective, consider the following sequence of herbal formulas that might be prescribed for progressive Liver qi stagnation. Each of the formulas is appropriate for the pulse quality associated with a particular stage in the development of the disorder. (*Warning*: These formulas are chosen only for the purpose of illustration and should not be prescribed without a complete diagnostic assessment.)

The Taut quality represents mild qi stagnation and only minimal excess heat. This would call for herbs that primarily move stagnation rather than remove excess heat. Frigid Extremities Powder *(sì nì sǎn)* would be appropriate for this purpose.

The Tense quality is associated with greater qi stagnation, increasing excess heat, and also some yin-deficient heat; the pulse is becoming harder. A blend of herbs that have stronger qi-moving and excess-heat-removing properties is indicated. Here, a formula like Minor Bupleurum Decoction *(xiǎo chái hú tāng)* would be appropriate.

With the Tight quality we must still deal with some qi stagnation, but now the thrust is more toward building yin and blood. Six Flavor Pill with Rehmannia *(lìu wèi dì huáng wán)* might be considered at this stage.

Once the pulse becomes Wiry our focus is almost entirely on building yin-essence as quickly as possible. Formulas such as Lycium Fruit, Chrysanthemum, and Rehmannia Pill *(qǐ jú dì huáng wán)* or Restore the Left [Kidney] Decoction *(zǔo guī yǐn)* would be appropriate.

The above examples illustrate the importance of making diagnostic distinctions, a process indispensable to proper treatment.

EVEN NONFLUID QUALITIES

TAUT

SENSATION: This quality has the resilience and flexibility of a very wide rubber band that has been moderately stretched, but has considerable give on pressure. It may be likened, as already noted, to the widest and most supple of violin strings, the G string.

INTERPRETATION: This quality represents the earliest sign and first stage of qi stagnation from causes other than shock. It is the mildest form of qi stagnation perceptible by pulse diagnosis in a person with a relatively good level of energy and of average to good constitution. By itself, it is the closest quality to Normal that any of us will probably ever feel.

ETIOLOGY: The most common cause is moderate repression of emotion on a daily basis. Taut is commonly found in the left middle position, which represents the Liver. This organ contains the emotions associated with daily stress, including those associated with the 'nervous system tense' vigilant condition. Other common etiologies include physical labor beyond one's energy over a very long time, generalized but relatively mild chronic pain, and chemical stress from environmental pollution and stimulants (e.g., coffee and early-stage use of drugs such as cocaine and amphetamines).

Found in individual positions, the Taut quality may have other causes. Taut in the right middle position can indicate mild food stagnation or excess cold due to overindulgence in cold food and drink, both of which may be accompanied by mild abdominal pain. Taut may also appear in the right distal position where it represents mild invading cold from excess, associated with external pathogenic influences.

TENSE

CATEGORY: The Tense pulse is a Taut pulse which has advanced further along the path of qi stagnation and is now developing signs of excess heat as the body tries to overcome the stagnation.

SENSATION: The Tense quality has a somewhat more narrow sensation to that of the Taut quality. It also has less flexibility and resilience and thus feels harder against one's fingers, though still more elastic than the Tight or Wiry qualities. It corresponds to the thinner, though still relatively wide, second (D) string on the violin.

INTERPRETATION: The slight narrowing and hardening of the pulse (relative to the Taut quality) signifies increasing qi stagnation with the development of mild to moderate excess heat.

ETIOLOGY: The etiologies of the Tense and Taut qualities are similar, but with the Tense pulse the condition is either more severe or has persisted for a longer time. As with the Taut quality, the qi stagnation is most often due to stress, primarily in the form of repressed emotion. For example, there may be slowly growing unexpressed anger and resentment. When Liver qi, the irresistible force of the body's energy, meets the immovable object of repression, these two opposing forces create a stalemate.

When found uniformly over the entire pulse this quality is referred to as the 'vigilance' pulse and reflects a 'nervous system tense' condition. It can be found constitutionally in ethnic groups whose survival through the centuries has required extraordinary vigilance. This pulse may now also be found in anyone living in a large city or dangerous environment. If the 'nervous system tense' condition is constitutional, the pulse rate will be slower than if the condition is due to modern living.

Other etiologies include physical stress from prolonged working beyond one's energy, generalized but relatively mild chronic pain, chemical stress from exposure to pollution, and the moderate use of stimulants, including coffee, cocaine, and amphetamines. This pulse quality can also be felt where infection or toxicity creates acute internal heat. In individual positions such as the right middle, the Tense quality could be a sign of excess heat from food stagnation.

LEATHER-HARD

CATEGORY: This quality is a variation of the Tense quality with a very different interpretation. It is placed here because of its physical similarity in terms of width. The term Leather is inherently confusing because there are three known variants, all of which feel similar at the qi depth but vary considerably at other depths. They are the Leather-Hard quality described here, the Leather-Empty quality (floating drumskin, tympanic; see Ch. 9) associated with a 'qi wild' condition, and the Leather-like Hollow quality associated with severe hemorrhage (Ch. 10).

SENSATION: The distinguishing aspect of the Leather-Hard quality is its extreme hardness, especially at the qi depth; it has the same relative width as the Tense quality, less width than the Taut quality, and greater width than the Tight. Because the other depths are present, it is distinguished from the Leather-Empty and Leather-Hollow qualities mentioned above.

INTERPRETATION: The Leather-Hard quality is a sign of extreme yin, blood, and especially essence deficiency. Once a rare quality, it is now quite common due to our increasing exposure to electromagnetic fields.

ETIOLOGY: This quality was initially observed primarily in people who had received radiation therapy for cancer. Now it is found with alarming, and ever increasing, frequency among the general population. This is perhaps due to escalating levels of radiation in our environment. Over the past fifty years the prevalence of electronic devices such as portable telephones, cell phones, computers (found even in cars and other machines), microwave ovens, wireless internet, mp3 players and so forth has increased dramatically. Our homes, offices, schools, and even streets are filled with wires carrying electricity. Given that everything electrical radiates an electromagnetic field, we are gradually increasing our exposure to these forms of radiation.

Leather-Hard can also result from other factors: an extreme loss of blood over time, the premature cutting of the umbilical cord, the 'nervous system tense'[2] condition, the so-called exercise revolution, and cocaine abuse.

In the case of 'nervous system tense,' the body is seriously depleted of Kidney yin and essence by its attempt to balance excess heat generated in the Liver as a response to Liver qi stagnation; this leads to a drying and hardening of the vessel walls.

The modern propensity for excessive exercise has led to people over-exerting themselves[3,4] and sweating too much, thereby depleting yin and blood. This in turn stresses the Heart, and ultimately drains the Kidney storehouse of yin and essence.

TIGHT

CATEGORY: As a matter of interpretation, the Tight quality described here is a totally new category which most clearly corresponds with descriptions of the Wiry quality in the traditional literature.

SENSATION: In relation to the Tense quality, the Tight quality is harder, less resilient, less flexible, and thinner. It may best be identified as feeling like the A string on a violin: the next to thinnest string. With pain, the Tight quality often has a sharper, biting sensation.[5]

INTERPRETATION: In today's world the Tight quality is associated primarily with false heat due to yin deficiency. There are, however, other possible interpretations. These include pain, trauma, infection, inflammation, hyperactivity, and external cold. To recognize which of these interpretations may be more appropriate, it is helpful to understand how the Tight quality can arise in the first place.

Etiology and pathogenesis of heat from deficiency

When the Tight quality reveals yin-deficient heat it is due mainly to stagnation from a long-term condition of 'nervous system tense'. The shift in sensation from Tense to Tight reflects the shift in the body from a predominance of stagnation and excess heat to that of a consumption of yin mobilized to balance the excess heat, and the consequent development of yin-deficient heat. With extreme yin deficiency, the yin can no longer hold onto the yang, resulting in a 'separation of yin and yang' and a wandering yang that usually rises and interferes with function of the most vulnerable organ, Spleen-Stomach, Lung, or Heart.

When the Tight quality is found in an individual position it is usually the result of the organ related to that position overworking for a long period of time: when found at the left middle position a common cause could be emotional stress; when at the left distal position it may be the result of excessive thinking, worry, or emotional shock; at the right distal position it may be caused by smoking; at the right middle, eating too rapidly; and at the proximal positions, excessive thinking over a period of years.

Yin and blood deficiency

Since the description of a Tight quality suggests a degree of Thinness, concurrent blood deficiency inevitably comes to mind. However, although yin and blood deficiency often occur simultaneously in clinical practice, it is important to remember that while a blood deficient pulse may be as Thin as the Tight quality, it will not be as hard. It is the hardness of the pulse quality that signals the yin deficiency. It is possible to have a Thin blood-deficient pulse that is not hard.

Pain, trauma, infection, inflammation

The Tight quality can also appear with pain due to stagnation of qi, blood, or fluids, especially from trauma and with cold, or food stagnation. With abdominal pain, the Tight quality can have a sharp, biting sensation in the Small and Large Intestine positions, and represents bowel irritability as well as abdominal discomfort.

If the Tightness is a sign of inflammation and infection (fire toxin), the pulse position that is most Tight is the location of the organ or area where the infection originated or is currently most active.

On rare occasions the Tight quality may be due to invading external cold; in this situation it will appear in that part of the body or burner exposed to the cold. For example, one might encounter a very Tight quality at the proximal and/or Pelvis/Lower Body positions in a person who has been walking in the snow with inadequate protection on his feet.

ALTERNATING FROM TIGHT TO YIELDING

There are occasions when the pulse can be felt to alternate from Tight to Yielding. Although apparently contradictory, this combination of qualities can be a sign of combined yin and qi or yang deficiency. This is a situation in which the 'nervous system' has been tense for a long time and the patient has also worked physically beyond his energy with insufficient rest. These are two different, simultaneously existing, conditions being revealed by the alternating qualities of the pulse.

WIRY

CATEGORY: The term 'wiry' is perhaps the one most misapplied term in the vocabulary of Chinese pulse diagnosis. In the current literature and practice, the term is misused, being closest to the Taut or Tense sensations described above. The Wiry pulse as described here is therefore a new quality, in sensation and interpretation, once relatively rare and now more common.

SENSATION: In our system the Wiry quality literally feels like a metal wire. With the slightest pressure it feels thin, hard, and cutting to the touch. It is long and continuous, and does not move away with an increase in finger pressure. Consider the sensation of palpating the E string, the narrowest violin string. Anything less than the thinnest, hardest, and most rigid cutting sensation does not justify the term Wiry.

INTERPRETATION AND ETIOLOGY: While there is considerable overlap with the Tight quality, the Wiry quality represents extreme yin and essence deficiency. (The Leather-Hard quality is likewise a sign of yin and essence deficiency, but also of blood deficiency.)

The Wiry quality in the proximal positions, and sometimes in the left middle position, is a sign of impending or present diabetes, a disease associated in Chinese medicine with Kidney essence deficiency. In the left middle and distal positions, it is a sign of cocaine use.

When combined with elevated blood pressure, the Wiry quality felt over the entire pulse is a sign of a potentially very severe and widespread stroke, the final sequelae of prolonged nervous tension. The pulse at this stage is usually Wiry Hollow Full-Overflowing, and often Slippery if a Spleen damp condition is also involved.

The Wiry quality at one position may be a sign of intractable pain in the associated area of the body, usually accompanied by muscular spasm and inflamed nerves. On rare occasions the Wiry quality may be due to invading external cold throughout the body. In such instances it will appear over the entire pulse, and be found especially in young people with prolonged exposure to cold. This cold obstructs the circulation of qi and blood in the muscles and also in the nervous system.

A Wiry Robust Pounding quality in one position with a Rapid pulse rate, accompanied by a high fever, can indicate localized infection. For example, when found in the left middle position (Liver) this combination of qualities can indicate acute hepatitis. Found in a stronger person, this etiology is often accompanied by the Flooding Excess quality.

Chemicals such as ethyl alcohol have a drying effect, especially on the Liver. The long-term effect of exposure to these is hepatic cirrhosis. The resulting depletion of yin and essence leaves the pulse with a Wiry quality, especially in the left middle position. Cocaine use causes Liver and Heart fire, leading eventually to the very severe depletion of yin and essence manifested by the Wiry quality in the left distal and middle positions.

UNEVEN NONFLUID QUALITIES

ROPY

CATEGORY: The Ropy quality has been placed under the general category of Shape, where there is a progression in the continuum of the pulses that ranges from stagnation (Taut) to excess heat (Tense) to yin-deficient heat (Tight, Wiry) in the blood vessels. It is found only over the entire pulse in all positions simultaneously, though sometimes it appears first at the middle position due to the Liver's function of storing the blood (see Fig. 11-3).

There are two types of Ropy pulse, one that is Tense and one that is Yielding and Hollow. They are discussed separately.

TENSE ROPY

SENSATION: The vessel is cord-like, big, hard and round, and is distinct from the surrounding anatomical structures. It varies in degree of hardness and in size, is sometimes straight and other times somewhat twisted, and is always continuous through all positions unless confined to the left middle in the beginning of the process.

Fig. 11-3 Ropy quality

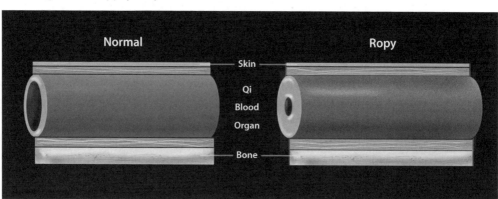

INTERPRETATION: The Tense Ropy quality is specifically a sign of chronic excess heat in the blood. The heat vulcanizes the intima of the vessel walls, causing them to lose all flexibility and elasticity (yin deficiency). This pulse represents a generalized arteriosclerotic process, often accompanied by hypertension.

This quality is generally encountered in older individuals with a lifelong 'nervous system tense' condition and/or a history of excessive ingestion of rich, difficult to digest foods and consequent excess Stomach heat that goes to the blood.

ROPY YIELDING HOLLOW FULL-OVERFLOWING

SENSATION: The vessel is cord-like, big, and round, but Yielding and Hollow rather than hard. It is also distinct from the surrounding anatomical structures, giving the same impression as Tense Ropy that the vessel could be grasped, lifted, and moved, yet more like a soft flexible tube than a hard rope.

INTERPRETATION: Dr. Shen attributed this pulse to long-term participation in vigorous sports, especially when one has exercised or worked beyond one's energy for a very long period of time. (This 'qi wild' condition is discussed in the section on the Hollow and Hollow Full-Overflowing qualities in Ch. 8.) The drying out of the intima and media of the vessels in this case is due to lack of nourishment rather than heat.

There are two types, one with a Slow rate that indicates that the person was gradually depleted, and the other with a more Rapid rate that is a sign that the person stopped suddenly (see Ch. 9). The latter is more serious.

CHOPPY

CATEGORY: The Choppy quality (Fig. 11-4) is categorized by its unique serrated

Fig. 11-4 Choppy quality

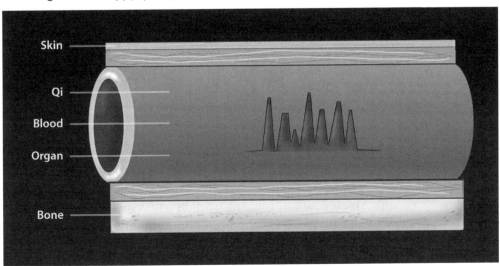

shape and was described as 'scraping bamboo' in the eighth century by Sun Si-Miao.

SENSATION: The Choppy quality is rough to the touch and if one rolls the finger distal to proximal across the position, the sensation is uneven and grating, like rubbing it across a washboard. The degree of roughness varies with the position and the degree of associated pathology. In discussing the Choppy quality it is necessary to mention the quality with which it is most often confused, Rough Vibration.

Choppy and Rough Vibration

The sensation of the Choppy quality is sometimes confused with the Rough Vibration quality. The Choppy quality is a rougher sensation and feels 'grating', whereas the Vibration quality is finer and feels more like a rough 'buzzing' sensation. The Choppy quality specifically lacks the buzzing sensation of the Vibration quality. They are sometimes found together, indicating simultaneous but separate disharmonies.

The Choppy quality, once rare, is now commonly found. Previously palpated principally at the proximal and the Pelvis/Lower Body positions, and associated with blood stagnation in the lower burner, it is found more recently during the First Impression phase of pulse diagnosis and at many positions associated with toxicity.

INTERPRETATION: Depending upon the degree, the Choppy quality is usually a sign of a serious pathology.[6] The interpretation depends upon the position where it is found. The three possible causes—blood stagnation, toxicity, and inflammation—are discussed separately.

Blood stagnation

Blood stagnation can be classified according to location. The Choppy quality signifies the presence of blood stagnation in the tissues. The cause of the blood stagnation can be excess heat, qi stagnation, qi deficiency, blood deficiency, excess cold, neoplasm, or trauma.

Blood stagnation in the blood itself is signified by the Blood Heat, Blood Thick, Hollow Full-Overflowing, Ropy, and Liver Engorgement (of the portal system) qualities. When accompanied by the Choppy quality, these qualities are even more serious.

The Choppy quality is a sign of Heart blood stagnation (coronary artery disease) when palpated at the left distal position; with inhaled toxins at the right distal and Special Lung positions; with chemical toxins at the left middle position; with microbleeding from inflammation at the right middle, Gallbladder, Stomach-Pylorus, and Intestine positions; and with dysmenorrhea, fibroids, endometriosis, and ovarian cysts at the proximal and Pelvis/Lower Body positions.

When found in the lower burner during pregnancy, the Choppy quality can indicate imminent miscarriage. This is theoretically due to the fetus not being properly nourished, and the practitioner should check the patient's tongue for lengthwise black lines.

Toxicity

Recently, the Choppy quality has been associated with toxicity which, in its terminal stages, creates blood coagulation.

When the organism is unable to excrete toxins they are conveyed away from the vital organs and retained as pathogens in the blood, joints, and vulnerable areas of the body where they may be destructive but not life-threatening.

This may be represented on the pulse by a Choppy quality over the entire pulse and particularly at the O-Q (organ-qi), O-B (organ-blood), and O-S (organ-substance) depths. The more extensively the Choppy quality is found and the greater its degree [1-5], the more severe is the retained toxic pathogen. The association between this quality and toxicity has been clearly established in the clinic, and was first seen with our veterans from the first Gulf War. There are many reports from a variety of sources relating toxicity and blood coagulation.[7]

Inflammation

The Choppy quality is sometimes found at the Gallbladder, Stomach-Pylorus Extension, and Intestine positions in conditions of extreme inflammation and consequent ulceration, necrosis, and microbleeding.

Differentiating the Vibration qualities

The sensory distinction between the Choppy and Vibration qualities has already been explained. In terms of interpretation, depending upon where it is found, the Choppy quality is a sign of blood stagnation, toxicity, and microbleeding. The Rough Vibration quality, also discussed in this chapter, is often a sign of parenchymal damage and severe physiological disorganization of the organ in which it is found, or severe Heart shock when found over the entire pulse.

VIBRATION

CATEGORY: The Vibration quality doesn't appear in the literature of pulse diagnosis. It is a quality that was first described by Dr. Shen and recognized consistently ever since.

SENSATION: The Vibration quality is a more delicate 'buzzing' sensation while the coarser Choppy quality is closer to the sensation of 'grating' ('scraping bamboo'). There are broadly two types of Vibration, Smooth and Rough. Another important distinction between the two is that one sometimes has to roll one's finger along the position in order to access the Choppy quality; by contrast the movement of the Vibration quality is felt while one's fingers are stationary on the position.

Fig. 11-5 Smooth and Rough Vibration qualities

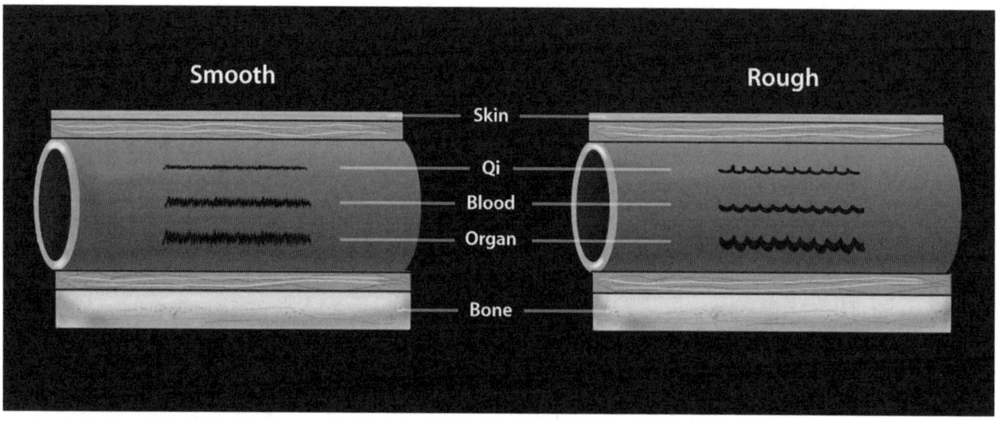

SMOOTH VIBRATION   Smooth Vibration is a fine buzzing sensation under the finger. Useful synonyms are shaking, trembling, tingling, reverberating, palpitating, shivering, wavering, quivering, vacillating, and oscillating. Students have described it with the words 'seltzer bubbles' and 'sparkles'. This sensation varies from very smooth to slightly less smooth, the different meanings of which will be explained below.

ROUGH VIBRATION   With Rough Vibration the sensation under one's fingers is that of a very coarse buzzing.

INTERPRETATION AND ETIOLOGY: Vibration is a quality whose interpretation varies depending on the degree of its smoothness, consistency, position, depth, and response to treatment as well as the length of time it has existed.

Smooth Vibration over the entire pulse is a sign of Heart qi agitation, current worry or a tendency to worry, or mild emotional shock. Rough Vibration over the entire pulse is either a sign of severe emotional shock, or it indicates a physical shock with a strong emotional component. In the latter case there will sometimes also be fear, terror and guilt, especially when there is already Heart qi deficiency. When Smooth Vibration is found at one position only, it is most often at the left distal, the Mitral Valve, or the Neuro-psychological position, and is also a sign of Heart qi agitation.

Rough Vibration at any individual position is a sign of parenchymal damage and physiological dysfunction, depending upon the degree [1-5]. As a sign, the deeper, rougher, more consistent the Vibration, and ubiquitous its appearance, and the longer it has persisted, the more serious the condition.

If the Rough Vibration in an individual position persists as it was after a week of rest or after one or two treatments, it is an indication that the parenchymal damage to the organ associated with that position is more serious. If, after rest and a few treatments, the Vibration is present at fewer positions, becomes less consistent and more superficial, and is less rough, the condition is less serious.

MISCELLANEOUS SHAPE QUALITIES

NARROW   The Narrow quality is found only at the Special Lung positions (SLP) and describes a thin position that is a sign of moderate Lung qi stagnation. The term Narrow is used here to avoid confusion with the Thin quality found elsewhere on the pulse, which is a sign of blood deficiency.

RESTRICTED   The Restricted quality is also found only in the Special Lung positions as a sign of more serious Lung qi stagnation. The position is shorter than normal.

NONHOMOGENEOUS

CATEGORY: There is no other system of classification that we have reviewed that describes this quality.

SENSATION: The sensation is not accessed uniformly within the domain of a particular position. In some parts of the position there is consistently more substance to the pulse than in other parts, as if one's finger is passing over a smooth topographical surface with elevations and depressions.

INTERPRETATION: This quality is a sign that yin and yang have separated and that physiological function of the associated organ is very seriously impaired. If the position is Robust it is a sign of stagnation of all substances. If the position is Reduced it is a sign of deficiency of all substances. This quality can be found at any position, although we find it most often in the left distal position when it is Robust, and in the left proximal position when it is Reduced.

BEAN (SPINNING)

CATEGORY: This quality is problematic in terms of the disparity between our experience and the descriptions in the literature. We find the 'bean' aspect to be far more prominent in our experience than the 'spinning'. Dr. Hammer has emphasized the Bean component but retains the term Spinning in parentheses so that it will be recognizable to those more familiar with the original terminology.

SENSATION: This quality is relatively rare and is usually found to be very Tight to Wiry, hard, short, without a wave, with a sense of urgency, and sticks out on the pulse in unpredictable shapes, but always dramatic. Sometimes it has been accessed as a hard object such as a splinter sticking out from and counter to the longitudinal flow of the rest of the pulse. In any position in which a quality is present but devoid of any recognizable shape and lacks a wave, Bean (Spinning) should be considered. The experience is spectacular and not easily missed.

INTERPRETATION: Clinically this quality is associated with profound emergencies and traumatic events. Shock, a major life-threatening physical trauma, severe fright or terror, and very severe, intractable pain are the life experiences and conditions with which this quality is most commonly identified. It always involves a profound disturbance to the physiology.

DOUGHY

CATEGORY: The Doughy quality is not described in any other system of classification.

SENSATION: This is the most common quality found in the Neuro-psychological positions. It is an ill-defined, undifferentiated impulse that is perhaps best described as an amorphous glob of clay, whose shape is never the same and whose volume varies from very faint to moderately robust.

INTERPRETATION: Dr. Shen associated the Doughy quality with chronic neurological disease, especially multiple sclerosis. Due to the role of Kidney essence in controlling the central nervous system (marrow), the Doughy quality has been identified as a sign of Kidney yang-essence deficiency. In this connection, Dr. Shen theorized that since yang is associated with the faster moving energies of the body, it is functionally associated with the myelin sheath where the central nervous system's most rapid electrical impulses occur, and where the lesions of multiple sclerosis occur.

It should also be noted that the Doughy quality has been found frequently at this position with no clinical signs of such serious disease. There has been no consistent medical condition associated with the Doughy quality. Though rarely, intractable headaches and a history of electro-shock therapy have been noted in some case histories. The entire position is currently the subject of a database study to better correlate the findings of Chinese and biomedical diagnoses. Recent evidence suggests that signs in one of the Neuro-psychological positions are associated with pathology in the opposite side of the brain.

COLLAPSING

CATEGORY: The Collapsing quality is not described in any other system of classification that we have reviewed. Clinically it presents with increasing frequency in both the old and young.

SENSATION: With this quality there is a tendency for the pulse and all qualities to completely disappear suddenly under the fingers. It usually occurs on one side and less often over the entire pulse or in one burner. It differs from Change in Qualities, which reflects a gradual process.

INTERPRETATION: This quality has been interpreted and treated as a 'qi wild' condition in which there is physiological chaos. It occurs when one's physiology is no longer able to maintain stable functioning and may be expressed by the person as an experience of near total physical and/or emotional-mental collapse. At other times it has been observed, as with the Amorphous pulse, when the blood in an anomalous artery and in the radial artery shift and the radial artery empties.

AMORPHOUS

CATEGORY: The Amorphous quality is not described in any other system of classification that we have reviewed.

SENSATION: There is a total lack of definition to the pulse and no distinct qualities from the first moment of access throughout the examination. The sensation is one of palpating very loose cotton through the radial pulse, and occurs only over the entire pulse.

INTERPRETATION: The Amorphous quality is associated with the Three Yin *(sān yīn mài)* and Transposed *(fǎn quán mài)* pulses. As with the Collapsed quality, we find this sensation to sometimes alternate with a full set of qualities, at which time the anomaly *(fǎn quán)* could not be felt. It has been postulated that somehow the blood was shunted back and forth from the anomaly to the radial artery.

ELECTRICAL

CATEGORY: The Electrical quality is not described in any other system of classi-fication that we have reviewed.

SENSATION: It feels akin to that of holding a live wire, and though it is not as powerful or continuous, it is very distinct.

INTERPRETATION: Clinically, the Electrical quality represents some form of neurological or neuro-propagation problem. It seems to occur more frequently at the Neuro-psychological position than at any other and indicates epilepsy in any of its forms, including grand mal, petit mal, or psychomotor. Other positions and interpretations include the left distal (petit mal epilepsy), left middle (grand mal epilepsy), and Mitral Valve position (bundle branch block).

LEISURELY (LANGUID *[huǎn]*)

CATEGORY: Demonstrated by Hamilton Rotte, A.P., at a Pulse Intensive seminar, this quality is also referred to as Moderate and Slowed-Down in the principal literature. Some have mistakenly referred to it as Soggy (or Soft), though the latter term is identical in sensation to the Yielding Empty Thread-like quality of our system, and to Weak-Floating elsewhere in the literature.

SENSATION: The amplitude comes and goes at a very slow pace and is indepen-dent of the rate or the amount of change. This quality can be found over the entire pulse or at any position.

INTERPRETATION: This quality is identified with a damp condition, especially, though not necessarily, if accompanied by a Slippery quality.

QUALIFYING TERMS

BITING

The 'biting' sensation is a form of the Tight and Wiry qualities and involves a nipping sensation at the finger pad. It is found almost exclusively at the Intestine positions and is a sign of abdominal discomfort and pain.

ROUGH

CATEGORY: The term 'rough' is used to modify the description of other qualities. The term is most often used to modify the depiction of the Vibration quality.

SENSATION: Rough is partially defined by its opposite, smooth. It feels grating and uneven.

INTERPRETATION: With regard to Vibration, the rougher the sensation, the more serious the implications of the Vibration.

SMOOTH

CATEGORY AND SENSATION: 'Smooth' is a term used to modify the description of other qualities. A smooth sensation has no roughness and feels more level, regular, uniform, unvarying, and homogenous than the rough sensation.

INTERPRETATION: Smooth is associated with a less serious condition than is indicated by the rough sensation. For example, the Rough Vibration quality is a sign of parenchymal damage if found at principal positions, and of shock if found over the entire pulse; Smooth Vibration is a sign of worry and Heart agitation.

SUBTLE (VAGUE)

CATEGORY: The term 'subtle' is an adjective that further defines other qualities. We have not found it in the literature.

SENSATION: Subtle means that the pulse it qualifies is more elusive, and its access requires a finer palpatory distinction.

INTERPRETATION: A subtle sensation is generally associated with less pathology than a quality that is not subtle.

EPHEMERAL (TRANSIENT)

CATEGORY: We have not found the term 'ephemeral' in the literature.

SENSATION: This is a characteristic that is transient and fleeting, appearing and then disappearing at a particular position throughout the examination.

INTERPRETATION: The ephemeral sensation modifies the meaning of the principal quality in the direction of a less disharmonious condition than when the same quality is more enduring at that position.

ROBUST OR REDUCED FORCE

CATEGORY: Pounding, Hollow Full-Overflowing, and Flooding are the qualities in the literature that are most commonly associated with a pulse that has force and is 'robust'. The term 'reduced' indicates less force. ('Without strength' is an expression used by Li Shi-Zhen with regard to the Soft,[8] Scattered,[9] and Thin[10] qualities.)

SENSATION: In reference to pulse diagnosis, 'force', usually with regard to qi, can be defined as strength, energy, vigor, and power. A pulse quality can be robust (with force or power) or reduced (without force or power). The strength of the impulse is the measure of how robust or reduced it is. This modifying quality can be accessed at any position or over the entire pulse.

INTERPRETATION: These terms are most commonly used to modify the depiction of the Pounding, Substance, and Full-Overflowing qualities. A Reduced Pounding pulse begins strongly but loses momentum and hits the finger without the follow-through or impact of a pulse that has Robust Pounding. It is a sign that a depleted body is attempting, but failing, to function normally. A Robust Pounding quality is usually a sign that the body is attempting to rid itself of excess heat. Sometimes it can be a sign that the attempt to maintain function in the presence of deficiency is succeeding, for the moment.

ROBUST (WITH) SUBSTANCE AND REDUCED (WITHOUT) SUBSTANCE

Reduced Substance is a sign of qi deficiency and feels like pressing a cigarette from which some tobacco has been removed, in contrast to when it is fully packed. (See the discussion of this topic in Ch. 8.)

SEPARATING

CATEGORY: This characteristic is not described in the literature. Separating is a modifying term, not a true quality, since it has no interpretation apart from in relation to other qualities.

SENSATION: On pressure, the pulse moves in two directions, distally and proximally, at the same time. Simultaneously there is no sensation felt directly under the pad of the finger.

INTERPRETATION: This modifier helps define a sensation of the Empty, Hollow, and Spreading qualities in one or more positions or over the entire pulse.

CONDITIONS (QUALITIES) RELATED TO ABNORMALITIES IN RADIAL ARTERIES

ANOMALOUS QUALITIES

A rule of biomedicine, confirmed by clinical experience, is that if there is one anomaly, one should expect to find the existence of at least one other. Finding one of the following anomalous vessels at the wrists means that the pulse qualities there are clinically unreliable. However, such a discovery should lead the practitioner to consider the possibility that there may be other anomalies elsewhere in the arterial system.

Three Yin pulse *(sān yīn mài)* [11]

This is a congenitally anomalous artery on the dorsal side of the left arm that, if found, renders the left radial artery unavailable to the diagnostic process. The entire pulse on the left side is Amorphous. This is thought to be a congenital anomaly and both this characteristic and the qualities that can be discerned are of no clinical significance. We have found that this can occur alone on the right side as well. (Further discussion is found above under the Amorphous and Collapsed qualities.)

Transposed pulse *(fǎn quán mài)*

This is a congenitally anomalous artery on the dorsal side of both arms that, if found, renders the entire pulse unavailable to the diagnostic process.

We find the Transposed and Three Yin pulse qualities to be present more frequently than is indicated in the literature. With the Transposed pulse there are degrees of clinical significance with regard to any qualities found at the wrist.The level of significance depends on how much of this anomaly is detected on the ventral surfaces of the arms above the wrist. The absence of familiar qualities, or the presence of the Amorphous and Collapsed qualities at the radial position with the simultaneous existence of this anomaly, diminishes the reliability of the radial qualities. Usually the greater the presence of blood in this anomalous artery, the less reliable the radial artery is as a source of diagnostic information in our system. As noted above, we increasingly find that the radial and anomalous vessels may alternate in blood volume, creating a shift in strength between the real qualities at the wrist and the Amorphous vessel further up the arm.

Ganglion

A ganglion is a small synovial cyst that can form at any time over the radial artery for no clear reason, perhaps trauma, that again renders the pulse at that position useless as a diagnostic tool.

Trauma

The radial artery can be traumatized by intra-arterial tubes inserted for the emergency delivery of blood as well as by the 'cutting' compulsion. This damage can interfere with the transmission of the impulse.

ANOMALOUS RADIAL ARTERIES

Multiple radial arteries

In rare instances more than one radial artery can be palpated at the wrist. This can be the result of a bifurcation of the vessel in its passage through the forearm. Clinically, the deeper of the vessels transmits the more valid information, if it transmits any at all.

Split vessels

Split vessels are rare and mostly found at the middle positions and, occasionally, at the proximal positions. Clinically, they have been encountered where there is a preoccupation with death. Most importantly, discovery of a Split vessel has proved to be an opportunity to help many patients open up and discuss their thoughts of suicide, thoughts that they managed to keep hidden from even their closest friends. Sometimes such discussion has saved lives. Split pulses have appeared with concerns about one's own potentially fatal disease and significant losses among one's friends and family.

Fig. 11-6 Shape

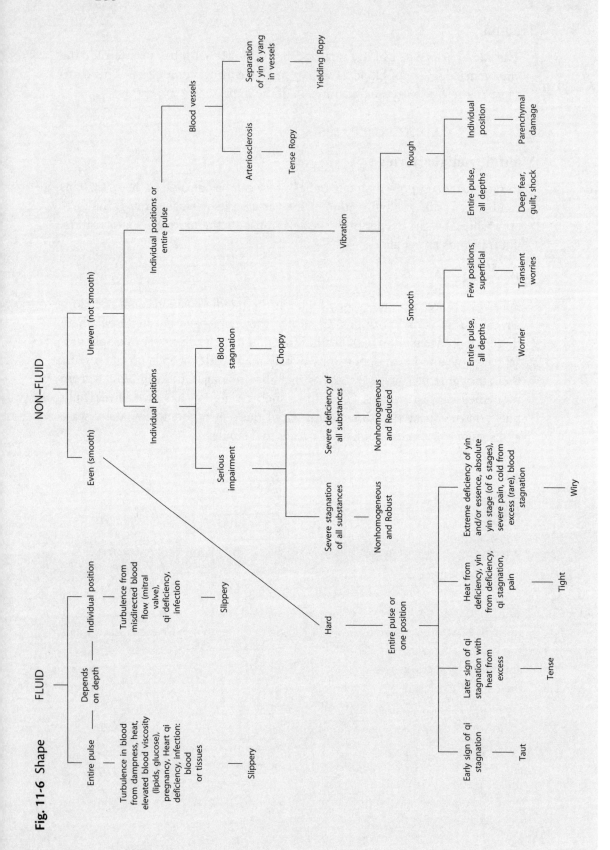

12

Individual Positions

Oliver Nash, L.Ac., M.B.Ac.C.

I N ORDER TO AVOID unnecessary repetition, the reader is referred to other chapters for further discussion of specific qualities relevant to each position. Information regarding the left distal position, which represents the Heart, is discussed at some length in this chapter due to its physiological importance as the 'emperor'. For the physical descriptions of the individual pulse positions, see Ch. 4.

LOCATION OF THE PRINCIPAL IMPULSE AND AMPLITUDE

The first vital step in taking the pulse is to accurately find the principal impulse. The vessel must be palpated directly in the center of its path, as the qualities just to the side of the center of the artery can be considerably different from those of the principal impulse. In our experience, when different practitioners feel different things on the same pulse, it is most frequently due to their not having located the center of the artery for each position. Likewise, qualities are recorded only as they appear at the height of the amplitude.

When locating the principal impulse, it is worth keeping in mind that the anomalous qualities (*sān yīn mài* and *fǎn quán mài*), as well as ganglia and local vessel trauma (discussed in Ch. 11), can, if present, obscure or obliterate the pulse. We should also remember and compensate for the tendency of the middle position qualities to overflow into other positions, particularly into the distal ones (see Ch. 2).

The distal positions are anatomically different from the other principal positions. When we feel the pulse in the middle or proximal positions, we are palpating the radial artery longitudinally (along the vessel). However, when we feel the distal positions we are not accessing the radial artery as such; rather, we are feeling a wave transverse to the vessel. This is created by fluid dynamics as the blood meets the trifurcation of the radial artery at the wrist. This wave informs us about the physiological integrity of the Heart and Lungs.

Due to the diminished space the distal positions occupy on the wrists, the three depths are not easily accessed there. Superficial and Deep qualities are easily recognized, as are those qualities which rise above the qi depth: Hollow Full-Overflowing, the Inflated quality (which seems to expand from the position), and the Empty quality (felt only at the superficial aspect and absent from the deeper aspects).

For ease of use, in this chapter we have listed qualities in order from the most common to the least commonly encountered for each position.

LEFT DISTAL POSITION

The descriptions below are of qualities associated with energy patterns and not with parenchymal damage to the Heart (unless otherwise stated). However, if a pattern remains uncorrected, some parenchymal damage can be a likely outcome.

LOCATION

To locate the left distal position, the right index finger and entire arm of the examiner must be rolled distally toward and slightly under the left scaphoid bone. The position is accessed horizontally, along a radial-ulnar, medial-lateral axis with the radial side of the index finger rather than its flat pad. Once in position, it is important to lighten up the pressure slightly to avoid obliterating the impulse.

COMMON QUALITIES

TENSE   Excess heat and qi stagnation in the Heart, both mild, usually accompany this quality. Insomnia with difficulty in falling asleep could be a symptom.

TIGHT   Over entire position with a slightly Rapid rate, this is a sign of Heart yin deficiency. Symptoms could include some agitation and a restless sleep pattern with frequent waking, and tossing and turning during the night. Occasionally the Tight quality is a sign of pain due to cardiac ischemia (angina).

THIN   This is a sign of Heart blood deficiency. Symptoms could include waking after four or five hours of sleep with little difficulty in getting back to sleep, dizziness (postural hypotension), becoming easily fatigued on exertion, and diminished memory and concentration. Originally, according to Dr. Shen, the pulse rate sign of Heart blood deficiency was an increase on exertion of between 8-12 beats per minute. However, further experience has shown that it is actually closer to an increase of more than 20 beats/minute.

FEEBLE-ABSENT   Usually this is a sign of Heart qi and yang deficiency. More rarely this quality can appear in combination with a Feeble-Absent quality at the left proximal position and a high diastolic blood pressure reading, in which case it may indicate advanced essential hypertension, with or without the presence of Heart qi and yang deficiency.

SLIPPERY   At the left distal position, the Slippery quality is a sign of phlegm 'misting the orifices' of the Heart and is associated with emotional disturbances that fall under the category of neurosis and psychosis. Epilepsy is also mentioned in the texbooks. The phlegm aspect of stroke, when the rate is very Rapid and the right side Deficient, is an extreme presentation of the condition in very obese persons.

MUFFLED   The Muffled quality at the left distal position indicates a repression of joy and pleasure and a form of depression usually associated with some loss involving a strong emotional bond, even to money and objects, though more often to people. It has less often been reported with a thickening of the pericardium or occlusion of the coronary arteries.

SUPERFICIAL, SMOOTH VIBRATION   This is a sign of mild Heart qi agitation marked by transient worry or mild emotional shock.

TIGHT IN THE PERICARDIUM POSITION AND MODERATELY RAPID   The Tight quality in the Pericardium position feels like a pencil point sticking into the finger from the middle of the left distal position, and indicates excess heat and qi stagnation. It is also often accompanied by difficulty in falling asleep.

CHANGE IN AMPLITUDE, CHANGE IN QUALITIES   Extreme deficiency of Heart qi and yang, with probable mild 'separation of yin and yang' within the Heart.

CHOPPY   Though increasingly commonly found at this position, this is a very serious sign of blood stagnation in the coronary arteries.

ROUGH VIBRATION, CONSTANT AT ALL DEPTHS OR DEEP   Increasingly common, this is a sign of parenchymal damage to the heart muscle itself and consequently possible Heart qi-yang deficiency.

LESS COMMON QUALITIES

DEEP, THIN, FEEBLE-ABSENT AND VERY SLOW   According to Dr. Shen, this pulse is associated with severe Heart qi deficiency that has existed for a very long period of time and has caused deterioration of peripheral circulation.

INFLATED, YIELDING TENSE, AND SLIGHTLY RAPID   Qi, or excess heat, is trapped in the Heart and cannot escape. This is often birth-related and can occur when the head is engaged in the birth canal for a prolonged period of time (as in breech birth), or can be due to unresolved grief (in such cases the Inflated quality is more often also found at the right distal position). Less common causes of this quality may be violent anger that is repressed while being physically active, or an episode of lifting an extraordinarily heavy weight.

FLAT WAVE   This pattern of Heart qi stagnation is usually either the result of efforts to repress emotional pain early in life or from the umbilical cord having been wrapped around the newborn's neck at delivery. The Flat Wave, in contrast to the Inflated quality, is a sign that the Heart qi was immature or deficient at the time of the incident, and is interpreted to mean that qi is unable to enter the Heart.

This quality is also found in the early stages or mild transient cases of Heart blood stagnation, when the coronary arteries are in spasm but not yet blocked; in Dr. Shen's terms, the Heart is "suffocating." If uncorrected, this will ultimately lead to occlusion of the coronary arteries (heart attack).

The Flat wave in the left distal position is a sign of Heart qi stagnation and/or Heart blood stagnation. The Heart is 'closed' to tender feelings towards and from others and is associated with a vengeful, jealous character. Chronic Heart blood stagnation is associated with lifelong fear. With Heart blood stagnation the Choppy quality is often felt here, though it is more difficult to feel when the wave is Flat.

SLIPPERY AND RAPID   This signifies phlegm-fire disturbing the orifices of the Heart. If the patient does not have a high fever then this sign is usually accompanied by agitated depression, manic-type mental disorder, or schizophrenia.

UNCOMMON QUALITIES

WIRY   This quality is found at the left distal position in patients with a history of long-term cocaine abuse, chronic mania, or who are in the later stages of Grave's disease. The yin-essence of the Heart is extremely deficient. More rarely, the Wiry quality is found here with severe angina.

RARE QUALITIES (USUALLY ASSOCIATED WITH EXTREME ILLNESS)

EMPTY   Extreme deficiency of Heart qi and yang with possible separation of yin and yang within the Heart is indicated by this quality.

SLIPPERY AND VERY RAPID   When accompanied by a very Tight Hollow Full-Overflowing quality, this is a sign of impending stroke with a phlegm-fire aspect.

VERY TENSE HOLLOW FULL-OVERFLOWING   This is a rare sign of excess heat in the blood vessels of the heart and is pathognomonic of the elevated diastolic blood pressure type of hypertension.

LEATHER-HOLLOW   This feels like an Empty quality except that the surface is very hard. Bleeding from the heart into the pericardium (cardiac tamponade) is either imminent (with Rapid rate) or recent (with Slow rate).

UNSTABLE AND NONHOMOGENEOUS   These are serious signs of extreme physical deterioration of the heart, such as an infarction and failure.

BEAN (SPINNING)   This quality has been found at the left distal position with profound emotional shock accompanied by great terror.

VERY TENSE INFLATED   Observed rarely in patients using cocaine and amphetamines (usually Wiry) and concomitant 'phlegm misting the orifices'. The Very Tense Inflated quality is associated with trapped blood in other positions.

COMPLEMENTARY POSITIONS ASSOCIATED WITH THE LEFT DISTAL POSITION

Pericardium Position

The Pericardium occupies the center of the left distal position and is accessed by rolling the radial side of one's right index finger medially to laterally so as to scan the whole width of the position. It has a quality that stands out as distinct from the rest of the position only with the pathologies discussed below. However, if the Heart is 'closed' and the majority of its qi is in defensive mode, then the Pericardium qualities may be the only ones present at the left distal position.

Common quality

TIGHT-TENSE   This quality is felt at the center of the left distal position and feels like a pencil point sticking into one's finger. As a sign of qi stagnation and excess heat in the Pericardium, it is an early indicator of potential excess heat in the Heart and is often accompanied by difficulty in falling asleep. By contrast, at most other positions, the Tight quality indicates deficient heat. It can also be a sign of pain due to transient ischemia of the heart (angina).

Uncommon qualities

SLIPPERY   While still confined to the center of the left distal position, it occupies space beyond the pin-point mentioned above. This is a sign of phlegm in the Pericardium that was preceded by excess heat that had an oppressive and suffocating effect on the Heart. Usually this situation is accompanied by symptoms such as mania, depression, chest discomfort, or epilepsy. If the left distal position is also Pounding Robust and Tense, and there is a high fever, this quality can be a sign of myocarditis.

INFLATED   Inflated only at the center of the left distal position is difficult to distinguish from an Inflated quality over the entire left distal position. Dr. Shen viewed this as a specific sign of phlegm misting the orifices of the Heart.

Mitral Valve position

Location

The Mitral Valve position is located on or around the tendon of the abductor pollicis brevis muscle as it passes over the styloid process to the scaphoid bone. Some of the qualities found here tend to be accessed very superficially, while others can be found slightly deeper.

Qualities

SLIPPERY   This is a definitive sign of a defective and incompetent prolapsed mitral valve (seriousness depending on degree of Slipperiness) and of Heart qi deficiency with greater signs of anxiety, panic, and fatigue than normally associated with Heart qi deficiency.

SMOOTH VIBRATION   Here Smooth Vibration is a sign of Heart qi agitation.

ROUGH VIBRATION   This is a more questionable sign of an incompetent mitral valve and of mild Heart qi deficiency.

CHANGE OF AMPLITUDE   It has been observed by a number of practitioners that when the Change of Amplitude is more obvious as one's finger moves from deep to superficial, it can indicate mitral valve defect. When the change is more obvious moving from superficial to deep, it can indicate atrial septal defect.

Large Vessel position

Location

This position is accessed by rolling the index finger medially and distally toward the ulna. At the intersection of the tendon of flexor carpi radialis and the scaphoid bone is a 'hole' or cave-like place that is palpated by the radial distal edge of the index finger. This 'hole' normally lacks any pulse quality. Be aware that many strong impulses originating from other directions can appear to be coming from this cave. It is important to distinguish where any impulse originates.

Qualities

TENSE INFLATED   This combination reliably represents an aneurysm in the vital large vessels, most often the aorta and less often the cerebral arteries. It has been found once as a sign of a disruption of cerebrospinal fluid due to an Arnold-Chiari malformation, indicating its significance as representing any disturbance in the circulation of body fluids.

HOLLOW FULL-OVERFLOWING   (Very rare.) This is associated with true hypertension, and expansion of veins and arteries due to heat in the blood.

Heart Enlarged position

This position is the distal portion of the left Diaphragm position, which is between the left distal and middle positions. The presence of a 'Heart enlarged' condition is discernible when the distal aspect of the left Diaphragm position is more Inflated and/or Rougher than the proximal aspect.

A positive finding here indicates that the Heart is enlarged, at least energetically. This will create discomfort in the chest, especially when lying on the left side. The greater the degree of Inflation or Roughness, the more likely the enlargement will be morphological as well as energetic. A chest x-ray and referral to a cardiologist are indicated to differentiate between the two.

Left distal and left proximal position (Kidney-Heart disharmony)

For a full discussion of this topic, please consult pp. 405-6 in *Chinese Pulse Diagnosis: A Contemporary Approach.* This includes Tight in both positions, Feeble in both positions, left distal position Feeble/Absent and left proximal position Tight, and left distal position Tight and left proximal position Feeble-Absent.

Neuro-psychological position

This position is found just above both distal positions, in and around a slight depression in the trapezium bone. This position, delineated by Dr. Shen, is not mentioned in the literature and the meaning of the qualities found here is the subject of on-going research. Thus far, findings at the Neuro-psychological position on one wrist reveal pathology on the opposite side of the brain and skull.

Qualities

DOUGHY   Described best as an ill-defined and amorphous small glob of soft clay, this is the most common quality found in this position. Dr. Shen associated this quality with Kidney yang-essence deficiency, primarily in patients with multiple sclerosis. Dr. Hammer has not found this association.

SMOOTH VIBRATION   In this position it is associated with Heart qi agitation, anxiety, and sometimes extreme fear. Dr. Shen said that such Heart qi agitation can either affect the 'nervous system', or that the 'nervous system' can affect the Heart qi.

ROUGH VIBRATION   More physical in nature than Smooth Vibration, this quality indicates that there is damage to the yin-essence (marrow) rather than to the psyche. It seems to reveal severe qi stagnation, possibly from head trauma, even that which occurred during the birth process. Symptoms can include severe intractable headaches that are somewhat related to the changing strength and circulation of qi. This quality has also been found with current deep fear and terror, multiple sclerosis, and even a history of electroshock therapy.

CHOPPY   This quality is associated with multiple past head traumas and chronic intractable headache, probably involving manifold micro loci of intracranial blood stagnation. Endocrine dysfunction has also been noted with this quality.

MUFFLED   In this position, Muffled has been linked with heavy use of LSD, but also with cerebral palsy, epilepsy, ADD, and dissociative mental states.

VERY TIGHT   This quality, though rarely reported, has indicated Arnold-Chiarri syndrome, glioblastoma, and in one person very severe head trauma.

RIGHT DISTAL, SPECIAL LUNG, AND PLEURAL POSITIONS

Right distal position

The right distal position represents the current function of the Lungs. Together with the left distal position, it also tells us about the energy of the chest and upper burner. While the right distal position can be used to access the different lobes of the material lung, this information is found more readily and accurately using the Special Lung positions.

Location

The right distal position, like the left, is accessed horizontally, along a radial-ulnar, medial-lateral axis just under the right scaphoid bone. The left index finger and entire arm of the examiner must be rolled distally toward and slightly under the right scaphoid bone, where the qualities are accessed with the distal phalange of the radial side of the index finger rather than the flat pad. Once in position it is important to lighten up the finger pressure slightly to avoid obliterating the impulse.

Due to the diminished space of this position, the three separate depths are not easily accessed, but superficial and deep qualities can be easily recognized.

Qualities

FLOATING   This is a sign of an attack by an external pathogenic factor in an early stage. Floating Tense with a slightly Slow rate is a sign of wind-cold; Floating Yielding with a slightly Rapid rate is a sign of wind-heat. If the tongue has a thin white coating, the illness is very recent; if the coating is no longer thin and white, the illness has existed for a longer time.

TENSE   This is a sign of mild Lung qi stagnation with mild excess heat, usually due to an unresolved cold external pathogenic factor.

The sudden appearance of a very Tense quality in this position can be due to recent mild chest trauma or an episode of lifting beyond one's energy. A feeling of chest oppression with inability to expand the chest can be a symptom of this temporary impairment of Lung function.

TIGHT   This is a sign of Lung yin deficiency that may be due to a drying out of the Lungs from tobacco, nasal sprays, bronchial anti-spasmodics, frequent wind-heat invasions, high fevers, dry climates, tuberculosis, or general systemic yin deficiency. The Tight quality may also be a sign of chest pain from chest trauma.

Alternatively, with 'separation of yin and yang' of the Liver and escaping Liver qi going to a vulnerable qi-deficient Lung, the resulting spasm of the bronchioles may result in asthma. The right distal position might be Tight as a sign of the spasm. (The Liver controls the autonomic nervous system.)

Having spent any amount of time in a neonatal incubator will often lead to a severe Lung yin-deficient condition and a very Tight-Wiry quality at the right distal position, often leading to intractable asthma.

WIRY   A rare sign of advanced Lung yin deficiency, perhaps with severe yin-deficient asthma (sometimes with a history of incubator confinement), tuberculosis, severe chest pain due to trauma or bronchial spasm, use of bronchial anti-spasmodics, or excessive use of tobacco or cocaine. This sign could also be an indicator of an early neoplastic process.

INFLATED   The Inflated quality is a sign that qi cannot easily leave the Lungs and is often associated with a breech birth and Inflated quality at the left distal position. The Inflated quality appears with the same associated etiologies as the Flat quality in relatively stronger subjects.

YIELDING INFLATED   When found at this position (and often at the left distal position) it is associated with 'trapped qi' due to repressed emotion (probably grief). Found only at this position it may reflect overworking Lungs (singing or talking), poor breathing techniques, or chronic lifting.

TENSE INFLATED   A sign of 'trapped qi and heat' in the Lungs that has accumulated over a long period of time. This is primarily associated with the excessive use of tobacco or other toxic inhalants leading ultimately to emphysema.

It is also found in adults who had inhalant allergies or frequent upper respiratory infections as children. These infections may have been resolved by medication, but the invading cold pathogen remained to create qi stagnation. Metabolic heat is generated by attempts to remove the stagnation and accumulates if the attempts fail, leading to the Tense Inflated quality.

SLIPPERY   A sign of damp-phlegm stagnation in the Lungs, the Slippery quality readily occurs when the accumulation of excess heat, described in the etiology of the Tense Inflated quality, has been balanced by fluids (yin).

It appears frequently when the Lungs fail to disseminate and make the fluids descend. With Lung qi deficiency, the fluids that the Lungs would normally cause to descend and disseminate instead stagnate in the upper burner and exit through the nose, often resulting in allergies and asthma with difficulty exhaling.

This may be compounded if the Heart cannot maintain blood circulation in the Lungs (edema); if the Kidneys fail to adequately anchor the descending Lung qi; if escaping stagnant Liver qi interferes with Lung function; if deficient Spleen qi results in accumulation of fluids; or if the Triple Burner and internal ducts fail to control food and water metabolism.

FLAT   A form of stagnation in which qi cannot enter the Lungs, it appears primarily in a deficient or physiologically immature person or yin organ, and may be the result of the same etiologies that would create an Inflated quality in someone stronger.

When feelings are repressed early in life and close off the flow of Heart and Lung qi, or if a person suffers birth trauma involving the cord wrapped around the neck, then the Flat quality is usually felt in both the left and right distal positions, sometimes for life.

This is also the case in qi-deficient individuals who suffer chest trauma or have lifted weight far beyond their capacity. A Flat quality in the right distal position may also be an early sign of lung tumors.

REDUCED SUBSTANCE   This quality (described in Ch. 8) is a sign of Lung qi deficiency, the degree measured by the amount of Reduced Substance [1-5].

FEEBLE-ABSENT   Moderate to severe Lung qi deficiency associated with deficient Kidney qi, with overworking the Lungs by excessive talking or singing, or with poor breathing techniques over a long period of time. Another common cause of this deficiency is the gradual depletion of Lung qi used in an attempt to overcome stagnant qi in the Lungs.

ROUGH VIBRATION   This is a sign of parenchymal damage and functional impairment of the Lungs. The Rougher and Deeper the Vibration, the greater the degree of damage, impairment, and concomitant Lung qi deficiency.

DEEP   This is a sign of severe deficient Lung qi and may be due to any of the reasons cited above for the Feeble-Absent quality.

CHANGE IN QUALITIES, EMPTY, CHANGE IN AMPLITUDE   Each of these qualities is a sign of the separation of Lung yin and yang, the first two of extreme Lung qi deficiency and chaotic impairment of Lung function. With any of these findings, further investigation is immediately required due to the danger of subsequent tumor formation. Of the three qualities, even a high degree of Change in Amplitude [5] is still much less serious than either of the other two.

A Yielding Empty quality (especially when also found at the left distal position) can be a sign of unresolved grief.

THIN   Clinically this is a sign of mild to moderate Lung blood deficiency. There is no literary reference to Lung blood deficiency; however, the Lung exposes specialized blood vessels to the air and has an important function with regard to blood by supplying it with oxygen (cosmic qi).

MUFFLED   A sign of qi stagnation associated with repressed emotion (possibly grief), especially if found simultaneously at the left distal position. If found at the right distal and Special Lung positions it could indicate a neoplastic process of the lungs.

ROBUST POUNDING   A sign of accumulating excess heat in the Lungs, it is often associated with allergies and is most often a sign of the body's unsuccessful attempt to overcome stagnation.

Special Lung position

According to Dr. Shen, this position reveals the past medical history of the Lungs, with the left Special Lung position telling us about the right Lung and vice versa. Dr. Hammer has also found it to be revealing of current conditions.

Theoretically its absence is a sign of health, however clinical correlation has found that its absence can also be a sign of serious pathology. Due to its ability to reveal predominantly the history of the Lungs, this position must always be considered in relationship with the qualities found at the right distal position. The presence of many of the following qualities at the Special Lung position (SLP) indicates great susceptibility to Lung disease.

Qualities at the SLP indicating extreme stagnation, especially a high degree of Muffled, can also inform us about tumors in the breast.

Location

This position is actually found at the superficial palmar branch of the radial artery, which extends from the radial artery in a medial and upward direction toward the trapezium bone, and can be found somewhere approximately between acupuncture points LU-9 (*tài yuǎn*) and PC-7 (*dà líng*). As this small anomalous branch can vary in location from person to person (and even from side to side in the same person), it is best to use the flat pad of the index finger to lightly search for its position.

The position usually has two depths. By varying finger pressure and rolling medially or laterally, one can often discern different qualities in the different parts and varying depths of the Special Lung position.

Keep in mind that smoke or toxic inhalants from any source (tobacco, industrial, moxibustion) will ultimately call forth all of the following qualities.

FLOATING   Rarely found here, this is a sign of an acute external pathogenic factor. Tense Floating and Slow is found with wind-cold, and Yielding Floating and Rapid with wind-heat. The same qualities are more often found at the right distal position.

SLIPPERY   While the Slippery quality at the right distal position refers to a current ongoing process, when found at the Special Lung position it represents an older process of stagnation of dampness in the Lungs. Usually preceded by qi stagnation and excess heat, it may be the result of anything that interferes with the dispersing and downward-directing action of the Lungs, the water metabolism function of the Triple Burner, Spleen qi deficiency, or diminished blood circulation from the Heart.

TIGHT OR WIRY   Tight or Wiry qualities in this position are a sign of Lung yin deficiency, spasm of the bronchi, or even pain (especially when Wiry). The Wiry quality indicates that whatever the pathology, it is more advanced than if the quality were Tight.

ROUGH VIBRATION   This quality reveals that the Lungs have been a site of repeated disease, that Lung alveolar function is impaired, and that the Lungs are highly vulnerable to more serious illness.

EMPTY   This is easily confused with the Floating quality. Remember, however, that whereas the Floating quality is very superficial and on pressure often reveals other qualities, the Empty quality is slightly less superficial and on pressure reveals no qualities. The sudden appearance of a Yielding Empty quality here usually suggests a recent and profound personal loss and unresolved grief.

YIELDING INFLATED   A sign of 'trapped qi' in the Lungs, it is often associated with Lung qi deficiency due to overuse (singing, talking) or misuse (incorrect breathing or meditation). When also found at both distal positions, birth trauma such as a breech birth must be considered.

TENSE-TIGHT INFLATED   If also found at the right distal position, this combination may reflect 'trapped heat'. (See the description of the Tense Inflated quality at the right distal position above). It is associated with emphysema.

NARROW   The Special Lung position is thin. Narrow is a term used only at this position as a substitute for 'thin' to avoid confusion; elsewhere on the pulse thin is a sign of blood deficiency, whereas here it is a sign of qi stagnation, as explained below under Restricted.

RESTRICTED   Restricted (short) is a sign of a more serious form of stagnation than Narrow (thin); both are signs of chronic Lung disease with reduced alveolar capacity. This can result from cigarette smoking or other inhalant toxins, or a neoplastic process. More rarely this quality can indicate premature birth or idiopathic pulmonary fibrosis.

MUFFLED   This quality commonly indicates a neoplastic process, and its degree determines the stage of the disease.

CHOPPY   This quality, once rare, is occurring more and more frequently in this position as a sign of inhalant Lung toxicity.

LEATHER-HARD   This quality, once very, very rare, is increasingly present and is associated with non-ionizing radiation, probably from cell phones, wi-fi, microwave ovens, and the many other electrical devices that are part of modern living.

Pleura position

Location

This position is located superficially at the distal end of the right Diaphragm position, between the right distal and middle positions. The presence of a pleural pathology is discernible when the distal aspect of the right Diaphragm position is either more Inflated and/or Rougher than the proximal aspect. Less often, a deeper Tight quality has been found at this position with a history of pleurisy in the distant past.

According to Dr. Shen, this is a sign of qi stagnation between the Lungs and the chest musculature that can be equated with the biomedical condition of pleurisy. If there is also activity at the right distal position, such as Tight Tense, Pounding, Slippery, and Rapid, and chest pain on breathing, the pleurisy could be active; otherwise it is most likely a sign of previous pleurisy.

LEFT MIDDLE POSITION

This pulse position represents the Liver, which, more than any other yin organ, is our first line of defense against stress (physical, emotional, or chemical). It is the organ most responsible for detoxification. Liver qi and blood provide the body's 'second wind' and allow us to recover our spent energy.

When the Liver cannot contain stagnant qi or heat, they will move to the most vulnerable organ or area. Likewise, if there is a separation of yin and yang, the yang will leave the Liver in the same manner. Once there, the qi, heat, and yang serve no useful purpose and create functional chaos in that organ or area. If the energy that the Liver cannot contain moves to the Lung, there may be asthma; to the Heart, palpitations at rest; to the Bladder, interstitial urethritis; to the Stomach, qi and food stagnation and ulcer; to the Esophagus, Barrett's esophagus; and to the Large Intestine, explosive diarrhea.

Liver qi is also the constraining qi of the body, restraining our impulses and maintaining a balance between our feelings and their expression; this makes it possible for us to function as part of a civilized society.

In our time, Liver qi deficiency is the most commonly occurring Liver condition. It creates problems in many other body systems that depend upon the Liver's moving function, such as peristalsis or the descending of Stomach qi.[1]

In addition to the principal left middle position, there are also distal and ulnar aspects (these are some of the complementary positions, discussed below). They become clinically relevant when they reveal a different quality than that of the principal position.

COMMON QUALITIES

TAUT, TENSE, TIGHT, WIRY, THIN All of these qualities are usually related to repressed emotion (often anger and frustration), which the Liver contains in order to maintain social order, and which causes constrained Liver qi. These qualities represent the worsening results of this repression, from qi stagnation (Taut) to excess heat (Tense), and finally to stages of yin deficiency (Tight, Wiry) and blood deficiency (Thin).

Found here, the Wiry quality could be a sign of abdominal pain, early hypertension, or diabetes (especially if the proximal positions are also Wiry). A Wiry quality present at both the left middle and left distal positions is associated with the use of cocaine. A Tight-Wiry quality at the left middle could be a sign of late-stage alcoholism.

ROBUST POUNDING This is a common sign of excess heat in the Liver usually associated with an attempt by the body to use metabolic heat to release repressed emotions. Sometimes, Robust Pounding occurs simultaneously with the Flooding Excess quality in this position with acute and chronic infection (hepatitis).

BLOOD UNCLEAR, BLOOD HEAT, BLOOD THICK, TENSE HOLLOW FULL-OVER-FLOWING   These reveal increasing amounts of excess toxic heat in the blood and in the Liver, which stores the blood (see Ch. 13 for further discussion).

REDUCED SUBSTANCE   This quality is a sign of mild to moderate Liver qi deficiency.

DIFFUSE   This is a sign of mild to moderate Liver qi deficiency, often found in combination with the Reduced Substance quality.

CHANGE IN AMPLITUDE   This is a sign of mild to moderate 'separation of Liver yin and yang.' It is a precursor to the more serious physiological chaos indicated by the following group of qualities.

EMPTY, CHANGE IN QUALITIES   These are more serious signs that the yin and yang of the Liver have separated, revealing chaos in Liver physiology with progressive Liver qi and yang deficiency, and an increasing vulnerability to tumors, lymphomas, and chaotic endocrine activity. These qualities may be the result of chronic use of cooling drugs like marijuana, chronic subclinical hepatitis and mononucleosis, the chronic presence of parasites, or overwork for a great period of time.

MUFFLED   A sign of neoplastic activity, the degree of which is measured by the degree of the Muffled quality [1-5].

SLIPPERY AT THE BLOOD DEPTH   Here, the Slippery quality is usually associated with turbulence in the blood caused by toxic conditions in the Liver and blood. At all three depths in the left middle position, especially at the organ depth, it is a strong sign of infection, including parasites, subclinical hepatitis, or chronic mononucleosis.

ROUGH VIBRATION   A sign of parenchymal damage and consequently possible Liver qi deficiency.

CHOPPY   A Choppy quality in the left middle position is usually a sign of residual toxicity that the Liver has been unable to excrete. Less often this quality can indicate Liver necrosis. When also found with a positive Liver Engorged position, this quality may indicate blood stagnation in the Liver.

LESS COMMON QUALITIES

TENSE INFLATED IN THE LEFT MIDDLE POSITION   This quality is associated with a recent episode of great but repressed anger. In the extreme, this quality can dominate most of the pulse.

YIELDING PARTIALLY HOLLOW   Usually the sensation of Hollowness is partial, being felt as Yielding at the qi depth and separation on pressure at the blood depth, rather than total absence of sensation in the middle. It is a sign of Liver blood deficiency.

FLOODING EXCESS AND ROBUST POUNDING   These are signs of internal excess heat, usually accompanied by a Rapid rate, due to fulminating liver infection (possible hepatitis or mononucleosis). If the rate is Slower, the infection may be more chronic.

FLOATING TIGHT   This quality has been found with internal Liver wind. This may be accompanied by wind in the channels and is a precursor sign to serious vascular accidents such as stroke.

SPREADING   This is a sign of Liver qi deficiency and early Liver blood deficiency (see Ch. 8).

LEATHER-HARD   A sign of depletion of Liver yin, blood, and especially essence, the etiology of this quality appearing in this position by itself is not yet understood. However, it often appears here and in other positions, or on the First Impression of the pulse, as a sign of radiation toxicity (perhaps as a result of cancer therapy or electromagnetic fields).

Uncommon qualities

LEATHER-HOLLOW   This Hollowness is absolute rather than separating at the blood depth. If the rate is Rapid it is a sign of impending hemorrhage from the liver. If the rate is Slow, it represents a recent hemorrhage. In either case, emergency room evaluation is required immediately.

DEAD   Indicates advanced or terminal cancer of the liver or bile ducts.

Liver Engorgement positions

When Liver blood is moderately stagnant beyond just heat in the blood, these positions will be present. The morphological liver itself is not necessarily physically engorged but the process is underway.

Distal Engorgement

The Distal Engorgement position is located at the proximal aspect of the Diaphragm position. The presence of Distal Engorgement of the Liver is discernible when the proximal aspect of the left Diaphragm position is either more Inflated or Rougher than the distal aspect.

Ulnar Engorgement

This position is found by first locating the left middle position with the middle finger, and then rolling the finger in an ulnar direction so that the extreme tip of the finger can feel the gap between the flexor carpi ulnaris tendon and the radial artery. There should be no pulse at this position, but if a distinct Inflated quality is present, one can say that there is Ulnar Engorgement of the Liver.

Radial Engorgement

As previously noted, this position is no longer considered reliable and will be suspended from our system of pulse diagnosis until more information is available.

GALLBLADDER POSITION

Location

Found by laying the right middle finger medially and proximally along and on top of the radial artery, between the left middle and proximal positions; it is felt with the ulnar side of the area of the first (distal) interphalangeal joint of the middle finger. The position may vary from medial to lateral, but it is usually very medial and can be close to the tendon.

Qualities

TENSE, SLIPPERY, LONG WITH ROBUST POUNDING   These are signs of damp-heat in the Gallbladder, usually without any or only very early symptoms of Gallbladder dysfunction.

TIGHT AND SLIPPERY WITH ROBUST POUNDING   These are signs of greater inflammation than Tense Slippery, and are also an early indication of stone formation. They are probably accompanied by digestive discomfort after meals, gas, and bloating.

INFLATED   This quality occurs with 'trapped heat and gas' in the Gallbladder. Inflated is a sign of significant progression of an infectious (excess heat) process. The gas is the by-product of bacteria. Referral for ultrasound of the gallbladder is urgent.

MUFFLED, WIRY, CHANGE IN AMPLITUDE, CHOPPY   At this stage the Gall-bladder has severe infection, or is necrotic (or nearly so), and there are possibly stones. Muffled is most often associated with tumor formation, although there is some question as to whether it is another sign of the deterioration process. The Wiry quality accompanies severe pain as well as necrosis. The Choppy quality is a sign of microbleeding, always present with the deterioration of an organ's wall.

RIGHT MIDDLE POSITION

In our pulse system, the Stomach is the only yang organ to co-occupy a principal position, sharing its position with the Spleen. All of the others occupy complementary positions.

The harder and more robust qualities that suggest stagnation and heat, such as Tense and Robust Pounding, are more closely related to Stomach function. The more pliable qualities, such as Feeble-Absent and Empty, are signs of Spleen qi deficiency. If we have only one or the other pathology, then the entire right middle position will be dominated by its relevant qualities.

More often, both Spleen qi deficiency and Stomach heat exist simultaneously. A Change in Qualities occurs in which the right middle position changes back and forth between the qualities that reveal the state of the Spleen and those related to the state of the Stomach. The Stomach Pylorus Extension position reveals information about the condition of the lower part of the stomach and the pylorus.

Qualities

TENSE-TIGHT   This is a sign of qi stagnation plus the resulting excess heat and growing yin deficiency (Tight). The yin deficiency occurs as a result of the attempt to balance the excess heat with cooling fluid. With excess heat, there may also be some Pounding. Stagnation is associated with the difficulty of digesting and moving poor quality and/or excessive food. The Tight quality is usually the result of eating too quickly due to constant emotional tension and pressure.

SLIPPERY-HOLLOW   Over time the Slippery and Hollow qualities may also appear either at the right middle or Stomach Pylorus Extension position, indicating ulcer formation.

ROBUST POUNDING   This is a sign of excess heat, usually the result of the stagnation of qi and food. Robust Pounding is commonly found in this position as a result of excessive intake of often poor-quality food that seems to make up the American diet.

INFLATED   Resuming physical labor immediately after eating, lifting after eating, sitting in a bent position for long periods of time, or trauma may create the qi and food stagnation reflected in this quality.

FLAT   This quality is a sign of stagnation that can be associated with early tumor formation and must be considered serious. The Dead quality is a much more advanced sign of the same condition.

REDUCED SUBSTANCE   This quality is a sign of mild to moderate Spleen qi deficiency depending upon its degree of severity [1-5]. This quality is discussed in Ch. 8. The Diffuse quality often accompanies Reduced Substance and is a sign that the deficiency is more severe.

DEEP FEEBLE-ABSENT   Anorexia or bulimia, thinking excessively while eating, eating irregularly and excessively, and eating junk food are some of the conditions that will deplete Stomach-Spleen qi and result in one or both of these qualities. Over time, or with a worsening of these etiologies, the pulse will become Feeble-Absent due to the depletion of Stomach-Spleen qi in its efforts to digest the indigestible.

EMPTY   The Empty quality is a sign of the 'separation of yin and yang' and of the extreme deficiency of either yin or yang, or both. Gastrointestinal function is chaotic and greatly compromised.

   The signs of Spleen qi-yang deficiency—Reduced Substance, Diffuse, Deep, Feeble-Absent and Empty (especially Empty)—are found in this position in patients suffering from anorexia and bulimia, which are increasingly common and very serious, even life-threatening, conditions. When these qualities are accessed, one must seriously consider these etiologies.

LEATHER-HOLLOW   The Hollowness is absolute rather than separating at the blood depth. If the rate is Rapid it is a sign of impending hemorrhage from the Stomach, often due to an ulcer, sometimes from a tumor. If the rate is Slow, it represents a recent hemorrhage. Emergency room evaluation is immediately required.

LEATHER-HARD   The interpretation of this quality by itself in this position is not yet understood. However, it often appears here as well as in other positions or on the First Impression of the pulse, and is a sign of radiation toxicity.

COMPLEMENTARY POSITIONS OF THE RIGHT MIDDLE POSITION

Esophagus position

The presence of esophageal qi stagnation is discernible when the proximal aspect of the right Diaphragm position is either more Inflated, Rougher, or Tighter than the distal aspect. If the body is deficient, the Inflated quality will be more Yielding, which is a sign of a loss of tone in the walls of the esophagus. A Slippery quality in this position is a sign of esophageal food stagnation.

   Stagnation in this position is often due to habitual obsessive thinking or repeated emotional stress while eating, although one major episode of emotional shock while eating could give rise to the same condition. Heavy lifting while eating, or bulimia, are other possible etiologies. Qi stagnation in the esophagus sometimes occurs with regurgitation, a serious medical issue with an increase in occurrence of Barrett's esophagus and adenocarcinoma of the esophagus. Finding this pulse sign can lead to early diagnosis and treatment.

Spleen position

This position is accessed by placing the left middle finger on the right middle position and rolling it medially toward the ulna. If present it is found between the vessel and the flexor carpi radialis, and is felt by the area of the finger that is just beneath the nail as an Inflated quality.

An Inflated quality here suggests a form of Spleen qi deficiency rooted in a constitutional Kidney yang deficiency, indicating a profound vulnerability. It requires a more strict nutritional lifestyle in order to avoid gastrointestinal disharmony. The presence of a pulse at the Spleen position may also be an indicator of vulnerability rather than frank deficiency.

Stomach-Pylorus Extension position

This position is proximal to the most proximal part of the right middle position and is found by rolling the left middle finger medially and laying the ulnar edge of the distal interphalangeal joint along and on top of the radial artery.

If the quality here is different from that of the principal position, there may be pathology. A Yielding Inflated quality indicates a probable stomach prolapse. Though such a prolapse may not be discernible by x-ray or ultrasound, symptoms include abdominal discomfort several hours after eating and insomnia after the evening meal. The cause is usually Spleen qi deficiency, specifically loss of its lifting function.

Tense, Robust Pounding qualities indicate excess heat in the Stomach, and Tight to Wiry qualities are signs of inflammation. Changes in Amplitude, Rough Vibration, Feeble and Reduced Substance qualities are found with impaired function, and the Choppy quality is seen with microbleeding due to excessive irritation and inflammation.

Occasionally, inflammation or ulcer of the lower stomach, pylorus, or duodenum will result in a Tight-Wiry Biting Hollow Slippery set of qualities. A Leather-Hollow quality found in the Stomach-Pylorus Extension position is a danger sign of hemorrhage, usually from a bleeding ulcer. The interpretation of the Leather-Hard quality in this position is not yet known.

Peritoneal Cavity (Pancreas) position

The simultaneous presence of both the Spleen and Liver Ulnar Engorgement positions should alert one to the presence of pathology in the pancreas, such as pancreatitis or a pancreatic tumor, and/or in the peritoneum, such as peritonitis, tumor, or ascites. A less auspicious pulse sign associated with these conditions is the presence of very similar qualities at the left and right middle positions.

Duodenum

If there are qualities indicating pathology in the Stomach-Pylorus Extension position and the same qualities appear at the Small Intestine position, there is probably a similar pathology in the duodenum.

PROXIMAL POSITIONS

....

PHYSIOLOGY

In order to understand some of the meanings of the pulse qualities that follow, it is important to keep in mind that Kidney energy is complex, with a seemingly infinite variety of Kidney functions. Summing it up as Kidney yin, yang, essence, and qi, is a massive oversimplification. How can a person born with such obvious Kidney essence deficiency symptoms as spina bifida have a powerful will, good teeth and bones, an intact endocrine system, good fertility and sexual function, and be a genius?[2]

Our answer is that even Kidney essence—normally associated with Kidney yin—has multiple aspects such as yin-essence, yang-essence, and even a combination of the two, Kidney qi-essence. To add to this complexity, each of the proximal positions is able to reflect multiple Kidney pathologies including the state of Kidney yin and Kidney yang, as well as fulminating conditions in the Bladder, Intestines, and pelvis/lower body, including the prostate.

DEPTH AND ROOT

Root refers to the Kidney position. Because the Kidneys are associated with the fundamental basal energy of the body, if their pulse has some strength, the body has root. This implies a greater resistance to disease, or, if a disease has occurred, that the prognosis will be better.[3] Dr. Hammer refers to these positions as the foundation on which our entire physiology and psychology rests.

LEFT AND RIGHT PROXIMAL POSITIONS

In some of the classical literature, the left proximal position is associated with Kidney yin and the right proximal position with Kidney yang and qi. However, clinical experience indicates that deficiencies of both Kidney yin and yang can be found at either or both proximal positions, with the former accompanied by a Tight and the latter by a Deep and/or Feeble-Absent quality.

Left proximal position

It should be noted that acute inflammatory conditions found on the Large Intestine or left Pelvis/Lower Body positions can temporarily overwhelm the usual qualities on the left proximal position. For example, as a result of fulminating colitis the pulse here is often Flooding Excess and Robust Pounding. The accompanying symptoms will usually help to differentiate the cause.

TENSE   This quality in this position is usually a sign of mild qi stagnation and excess heat in the Kidneys. It can also be an early sign of internal heat associated with subacute infection of the pelvic area or intestinal tract. Far less often, a Tense quality here, unless found uniformly over the entire pulse, is a sign of invading external heat in people who frequently walk barefoot or sit on hot sand or rocks for long periods in scant clothing such as bathing suits.

TAUT   Sometimes called 'Buddha's pulse', this quality is found at this position as a result of long-term sexual abstinence. The appearance of this quality was formerly a test in Buddhist monasteries to determine the degree of adherence to the vow of abstinence.

TIGHT-WIRY

Yin-essence deficiency

This quality is often a sign of yin-essence deficiency resulting from overwork of the mind, which drains the Kidney yin and creates Kidney yin deficiency. Other organs such as the Heart, Stomach, Lungs, and Liver will call upon the Kidney to supply yin when they become depleted of it. Likewise, Kidney yin deficiency will tend to exacerbate yin deficiency in these organs. Persistent sex beyond a person's 'energy' can cause a Tight-Wiry quality that in later stages will turn to qualities indicative of more qi-yang deficiency. This quality may also be a result of cocaine use.

With the Wiry quality incipient diabetes and/or essential hypertension should be considered, especially when these qualities are also present at the left middle position.

Pain

A Tight-Wiry quality here, together with a Choppy quality in the Pelvis/Lower Body position, can indicate pain associated with blood stagnation in the lower burner (such as menstrual pain), or invading cold.

Cold stagnation in the lower burner

Although now less common in developed countries, invasion of the lower burner by cold from excess, perhaps from exposure to cold water, ice, or snow, can manifest as a Tight quality in both proximal positions.

REDUCED SUBSTANCE AND DIFFUSE   These are mild to moderate signs of Kidney qi deficiency and are discussed in Ch. 8.

DEEP AND FEEBLE-ABSENT   Common in the elderly, these qualities are otherwise associated with severe constitutional Kidney qi-yang-essence deficiency. With excessive sex or heavy physical labor, these signs of Kidney qi-yang and essence deficiency can appear—especially if the Kidneys are already vulnerable—for constitutional or for other reasons. These qualities may also be signs of a propensity to long-term depression.

Since a Feeble-Absent left proximal position is most likely constitutional in all but the elderly, the patient should understand that he does not have the innate strength to do certain things that others can do easily. Unexpectedly, this has proved to be welcome and freeing information by the many who have pushed themselves, and been pushed by others, to work beyond their innate ability.

CHANGE IN QUALITIES OR AMPLITUDE, EMPTY Though once uncommon in this position, these qualities are appearing more and more often in younger and younger people, probably due to the increasing frequency of in utero 'insults', possibly from escalating environmental toxicity and substance abuse.

They are signs of the 'separation of Kidney yin and yang' and of chaotic Kidney function with a serious inability to sustain other organs. This is probably equivalent to a severely compromised immune system. Such qualities are part of a 'nervous system weak' condition (see Ch. 15 and the Glossary).[4]

The Change in Qualities and Empty signs reveal a much more advanced and serious state than the Change in Amplitude quality

FLOODING EXCESS, ROBUST POUNDING, SLIPPERY With acute (or an exacerbation of chronic) colitis, pelvic inflammatory disease, or prostatitis, the qualities in the proximal positions will be Flooding Excess, Robust Pounding, Slippery, and Tight-Wiry, with a Rapid rate. These qualities reflect disease processes of the intestines, prostate, or pelvic cavity rather than the innate condition of the Kidneys. Once the acute condition passes, the qualities that reflect the true condition of the Kidneys will return.

Right proximal position

Bladder position

The right proximal position is associated in the literature with Kidney qi-yang, although, as mentioned above, defects of Kidney yin or yang can appear in either the left or right proximal position. Bladder, urethra, and ureter function, including Kidney stones, only become an issue at this position when the quality there is very Tight-Wiry.

When there are signs of a more acute process (Flooding Excess, Robust Pounding, Slippery, Tight-Wiry and a Rapid rate), one should consider disharmony not only in the Bladder, but also in the Small Intestine (and, less frequently, the Large Intestine), prostate, and genital organs.

Common qualities

TENSE When not also found over the entire pulse, this can be a sign of developing subacute excess heat that if unattended may become an acute inflammatory condition in the Bladder, Small Intestine, or organs of the pelvis. The

Tense quality may also be associated with external heat due to walking on hot surfaces.

FLOODING EXCESS, ROBUST POUNDING, SLIPPERY   Each of these qualities indicates an acute fulminating inflammatory process involving damp-heat in either the Bladder, Small Intestine, or pelvic organs. The pulse may also be Rapid.

TIGHT-WIRY

Yin-essence deficiency

Although yin-deficient heat is revealed first as Tightness in the left proximal position, as it develops in severity it has been found to appear simultaneously in the right proximal position. Diabetes and essential hypertension must be considered, especially when the Tight quality is present at both the left and right proximal positions.

Pain

This quality can also be a sign of pain in the lower burner, either musculoskeletal or urogenital. The more Wiry the quality, the greater the pain.

Cold stagnation in the lower burner

Refer to the comments above under the left proximal position.

REDUCED SUBSTANCE AND DIFFUSE   These are mild to moderate signs of Kidney qi deficiency and are discussed in Ch. 8.

DEEP AND FEEBLE-ABSENT   These qualities are a sign of severe qi-yang deficiency.

CHANGE IN QUALITIES OR AMPLITUDE, EMPTY   The reader is referred to the discussion of these qualities under the left proximal position.

LARGE AND SMALL INTESTINE COMPLEMENTARY POSITIONS

Location

By rolling the ring finger distally and medially from the proximal position, the Intestine positions are accessed with the radial edge of the finger tip. In this manner, the Small Intestine is found distal to the right proximal position, and the Large Intestine distal to the left proximal position.

Common qualities

These positions are always considered in connection with findings at the Stomach, Spleen, and middle burner complementary positions (Stomach-Pylorus Extension position).

With a mild and short-term disharmony, the qualities listed below are limited to the Intestine positions. When the process is more acute and fulminating, or is a flare-up of something more chronic, then one or both of the proximal positions may also be affected.

TENSE   Although this quality is usually a sign of some qi stagnation and mild excess heat, there are often no associated symptoms when it is found at this position.

TIGHT   This quality is found with symptoms of irritation, irritability, and inflammation of the bowel. The bowel movements are usually frequent and loose.

BITING   The Tight quality is accompanied by a nipping sensation at the tip of the fnger when there is abdominal cramping, discomfort, or pain.

SLIPPERY   A Slippery quality indicates a damp condition, possibly with symptoms such as very loose, mucus-containing stools. Its presence usually occurs as the body attempts to balance inflammatory heat .

ROUGH VIBRATION   This is a sign of parenchymal dysfunction of the Intestines. If present to an excessive degree [4-5], biomedical investigation is warranted for silent pathologies such as polyps or cancer, and for more overt conditions such as diverticulitis, colitis, and symptomatic tumors.

CHOPPY   Normally related to blood stagnation, Choppiness in the Intestine positions seems to indicate microbleeding associated with more advanced bowel irritation and inflammation.

CHANGE IN AMPLITUDE   This is a sign of functional impairment which, if found to an excessive degree [4-5], warrants biomedical investigation.

ROBUST POUNDING   This is a sign of excess heat in the Intestines usually found with significant inflammation, and can indicate conditions such as early fulminating enteritis or colitis if the degree of Pounding is excessive [4-5].

INFLATED   A sign of trapped qi or heat in the Intestines, which usually manifests as trapped gas with abdominal discomfort and bloating.

MUFFLED   Although this quality has been found with the presence of some degree of fecal impaction and loss of peristaltic activity, it is most often found with stagnation of qi and blood and possible neoplastic activity.

PELVIS/LOWER BODY POSITIONS

Location

The left Pelvis/Lower Body position is found by laying the right ring finger along the radial artery, medial and proximal to the left proximal position. The area of the finger that is actually used is closer to the distal interphalangeal joint. The right Pelvis/Lower Body position is felt in the same manner on the right wrist using the left ring finger.

Qualities

This position primarily informs us about stagnation of qi, blood, and dampness in the lower part of the body and legs, providing very general information about acute and chronic conditions in these areas. Recent evidence suggests that qualities on one side may indicate conditions on the opposite side.

The Slippery quality is a sign of damp stagnation and often infection (PID, HPV, herpes, candida), and, together with the Choppy quality, of prostatic hypertrophy in men. The Tense quality reveals qi stagnation and excess heat. The Tight-Wiry quality is a sign of an inflammatory process, possibly with pain. The Robust Pounding quality reflects excess heat, the Choppy quality blood stagnation, and the Change in Amplitude quality represents significant functional impairment, depending upon degree. The Muffled quality in this position is the one most often associated with neoplastic activity of the ovaries, uterus, testicles, and prostate.

TRIPLE BURNER POSITION

According to Dr. Shen, the function of the Triple Burner is found in all three burners and has no single pulse position. If the qualities are generally uniform between the principal and other positions within a burner, the Triple Burner is considered to be functioning well. If, on the other hand, the qualities vary considerably from position to position within a burner, and especially between positions in more than one burner, the functioning of the Triple Burner is greatly stressed. This chaos is often associated with autoimmune diseases.

DIAPHRAGM POSITION

Location

Activity in the Diaphragm position is considered to be present when an Inflated quality is accessed in both directions, by rolling the finger proximally from the distal position and also distally from the middle position. If it is felt to be coming primarily from only one of these principal positions, it has an additional meaning (as explained in the sections on the Heart Enlarged, Pleura, Distal Liver Engorgement, and Esophagus positions).

Physiology and pathology

Dr. Shen conceived of this position as relating to the area "between the muscle and the skin." He felt that over time and without resolution, the pathology that resides there goes deeper, ultimately to the Liver qi or esophageal qi. We have found no clinical evidence to support this. A mild Inflated quality is considered normal.

Interpretation

When the left Diaphragm position in particular is Inflated, or the Inflated quality is present in both Diaphragm positions, it is usually due to repressed tender feelings replaced by anger during and following an acrimonious separation. From any single such incident, the Inflated quality will diminish over time, and is usually gone after seven to ten years.

If activity in the Diaphragm position is found to be present only on the right, the cause is probably repeated episodes of very heavy lifting beyond one's energy. There is also a link between significant qi stagnation in the diaphragm and hiatal hernia.

Musculoskeletal positions

We tend to ignore these positions, since patients readily report pain; however, by rolling the fingers to the radial side of the area between the burners one can access the musculoskeletal positions. The pulse here is usually very Tight-Wiry when there is pain and discomfort in the associated area.

Distal and radial to the distal positions we can access the neck. Radial to the area between the distal and middle positions we can access the shoulder-arm area. Radial to the area between the middle and proximal positions we can access the hip, and radial to the area between the proximal and Pelvis/Lower Body positions, we can access the knees.

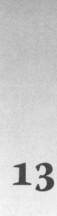

13

The Depths and Common Qualities
Found Uniformly over the Entire Pulse

Oliver Nash, L.Ac., M.B.Ac.C.

INTRODUCTORY REMARKS

Traditionally, Chinese medicine identified three principal depths: qi, blood, and organ (Fig.13-1). The pulse system developed by Dr. John Shen, drawn from his Ding family lineage, further refined this to nine depths (Fig. 13-2). In this system, the organ depth is divided into three distinct parts: organ-qi, organ-blood, and organ-substance. The other four depths are named for the specific pulse quality with which each is associated: Floating, Cotton, Firm, and Hidden. This nine-depth system was adopted by Contemporary Chinese Pulse Diagnosis (CCPD) and is used in this book.

Most of the remarks in this chapter refer to just five of the nine depths: qi, blood, organ-qi (O-Q), organ-blood (O-B), and organ-substance (O-S). When the pulse is assessed at an individual principal position, these five main depths tell us about a particular organ's contribution to the body's total qi, blood, and yang and about the yin substance of the organ associated with that position. When the pulse is taken simultaneously at all six of the principal positions, using six fingers, the entire pulse is being assessed, and each of these five depths reveals information about the qi, blood, yin, and yang of the body as a whole.

Locating the exact position of these depths requires subtle variations in finger pressure, the distance between them being approximately one tenth of a millimeter (though slightly more in larger or heavier people). The distance

Fig. 13-1 The three depths

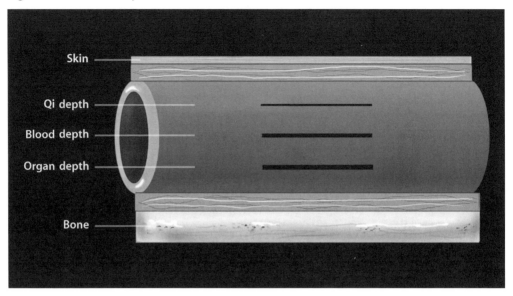

from the surface of the skin to the qi depth is about one third greater than the distance between the qi and blood depths, and between the blood and organ depths. Independently of at which depth the impulse is first encountered on the patient, each depth can be found at a fixed location accessed by a precise movement of the wrist of the pulse-taker. With advanced skill, it is possible to reproduce the exact pressure required to locate correctly each of the depths. In doing so, a uniformity is created that makes comparisons between patients and between practitioners relatively precise.

It must be emphasized that unless this technique is mastered, the information felt through the fingers during pulse diagnosis is unreliable within the model of Chinese medicine to which this book subscribes.[1] The sensations and interpretations of each of the qualities that comprise the substance of this book are applicable only if these depths are correctly accessed. Furthermore, if we initiate our examination of a pulse where we first encounter the principal impulse, and if that pulse is relatively deep, we will miss all the information about the more superficial qi and blood depths, not realizing that those depths are diminished or absent.

In this chapter we will discuss the meaning of particular qualities when they are found over the entire pulse, at all depths and also at certain depths only. In order to present this material, artificial divisions have been made when classifying pulse qualities. For example, pulse qualities revealing the progression of qi deficiency often involve depths other than the qi depth alone. Also, in order to avoid too much repetition, qualities that involve more than one depth are discussed under the heading of the depth at which they are first felt. For example, although the Inflated quality encompasses all five of the main depths, it is listed under the heading of the qi depth as it is first encountered there.

Finally, the presentation of pulse qualities in this chapter is extremely abbreviated. Further information can be found in the sections of this book that deal specifically with the individual pulse qualities.

INTERPRETATION OF THE THREE PRINCIPAL DEPTHS

To some extent, each of the depths reflects qi, blood, and yin. However, one of these aspects will predominate at any one depth. Qi is the lightest of the three aspects, tending to rise on the pulse and predominate over the superficial or qi depth; blood is somewhat heavier and is felt at the middle or blood depth; yin, or the substance of the organ, is the heaviest and is palpated at the deepest of the five depths, the organ depths (organ-qi, organ-blood, or organ-substance).

The natures of qi, blood and yin also explain why the pulse typically feels thinnest and lightest at the qi depth, becoming heavier, wider, and increasingly resistant as the fingers press down through the blood depth to the organ depths. As we shall see, when assessing all of the depths, any other progression of sensation, in either direction, is abnormal.

When interpreting the state of qi, blood, yin, yang, and essence it is important to remember that the pulse presents a pathological picture that is somewhat ahead of symptomatology. It is this time lag that makes the pulse such a valuable tool for preventive medicine, and is also the reason why even an Absent quality does not indicate a total absence of qi, blood, and yin.

THE NINE-DEPTH MODEL

As previously noted, in this system there are actually nine depths (see Fig. 13-2). This is because sometimes the pulse can be felt at a depth that is above the qi

Fig. 13-2 The nine depths

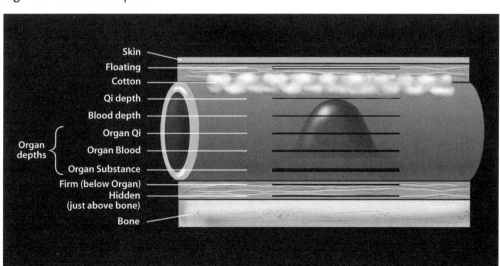

depth, or at a level deeper than the organ depth. The two depths above the qi depth are the Floating and Cotton qualities, and the two deeper than the organ depth are the Firm and Hidden qualities.

Within these nine there are two depths that students of this system study when they reach more advanced stages of the learning process. These are termed the organ-blood depth and the organ-substance depth. They form part of the tripartite subdivision of the organ depth: the qi of the yin organ, the blood of the yin organ, and the yin (parenchyma) of the yin organ. At these two depths, evidence of retained pathogens and toxicity are found.

THE HARDER AND MORE PLIABLE QUALITIES

In this chapter, under the headings of the various depths, the qualities most commonly encountered are listed. These qualities fall into two broad categories of sensation, hard and pliable.

The pliable or yielding qualities that separate and give way to pressure and can occur at any depth represent deficiency, usually of qi. These include Diminished, Spreading, Reduced Substance, Diffuse, Deep, and Feeble-Absent qualities. Empty and Changing qualities are signs of the separation of yin and yang.

The pulse qualities that are more resistant to pressure and relatively harder to the touch feel that way because of excess heat, a lack of fluids or a lack of yin in the body, or a combination of both. These include the Floating Tense, Flooding Excess Wave, Tense Full-Overflowing, Taut, Tense, Tight, Wiry, Leather, Choppy Rough Vibration, and Ropy qualities. (The only pulse that might indicate fluid excess is the Slippery quality, which slides under the finger in one direction.)

As with the individual positions, one should bear in mind that harder qualities found at one depth (over an entire position or the entire pulse) can override some of the more pliable (softer) qualities. These will be inaccessible until the condition represented by the hard quality is resolved. In such cases it is important to remember that the pathologies represented by both harder and softer qualities exist simultaneously.

Etiology of Disharmonies

The entire pulse helps us to assess the overall state of substances within the body. In simple terms, there are two broad causes of disharmony: stagnation of substances and deficiency of substances. Each can have multiple etiologies and can manifest as a variety of different pulse qualities.

Stagnation of substances can arise from: internal emotional repression and suppression (or resignation), an inability to eliminate external pathogenic factors, trauma (physical or emotional), chronic stagnating postures, or chronic deficiency.

Deficiency of substances can result from a variety of factors: constitutional or congenital defects, drained energy as a result of previous or current illness, excessive hemorrhage, vomiting, sweating, diarrhea, physiologically harmful drugs/medications, overwork or over-exercise of the body or mind, irregular living habits (lack of sleep, poor nutrition, sudden lifestyle changes and sudden cessation of exercise), inadequate digestion, absorption and transportation of food, or chronic stagnation due to deficiency or excess.

STABILITY AND ACTIVITY

Although discussed more fully in Ch. 7, it is worth reiterating the importance of rate and rhythm when assessing the pulse. In our system, alterations in the normal rate and rhythm are considered to be primarily signs of Heart disharmony. And since the Heart is the 'emperor', the diagnosis and treatment of this organ is prioritized. We often find that unless some degree of order and balance is brought to the rate and rhythm, all efforts to deal with other signs and symptoms tend to be less effective.

Classically, changes in rate are linked to acute external pathogenic factors or chronic qi and yang deficiency. However, an alteration from the normal rate is often a sign of more far-reaching processes, and unless it can be confirmed otherwise, is more likely a result of a shock to the Heart or an alteration in the circulation of blood and qi that ultimately affected the Heart.

CIRCULATION

The general circulation of qi and blood obviously has an impact on the entire pulse and organism. Dr. Shen associated problems of the 'circulatory system' with such symptoms as being easily tired, having cold hands and feet, migrating joint pain that worsens when inactive and improves with movement, passing or persistent pain and swelling in the joints, a chronically uncomfortable body and a tendency to anger, especially when the pulse is Inflated. Conditions such as fibromyalgia are frequently due to problems of the 'circulatory system'.

Circulatory problems manifest for one of two reasons: either Heart qi depletion is affecting the circulation, or insults to the circulation such as trauma and shock have affected Heart qi. The symptoms of both etiologies are similar, but when the cause is qi depletion the symptoms develop slowly and tend to come and go according to the changing strength of the person's qi. The effects of shock and trauma are sudden, and persist according to the ability of the organism's qi to restore circulation.

QI DEPLETION AFFECTING THE CIRCULATION

In adults, the principal cause of circulatory dysfunction is a deficiency of Heart qi that begins in utero. This may be the result of illness (rheumatic fever), or develop over a long period of time during adult life: usually the result of overwork, over-exercise, protracted emotional stress, or long-term serious illness. The pulse is Slow and ranges from Diminished at the qi depth (mild) to Deep or Absent (serious). The tongue body is pale.

If an etiology has its beginnings in childhood, the syndrome is more serious; this may happen when children are subjected to the same conditions as those listed under the adult etiology. The immature organism of a child is highly vulnerable to work beyond its energy levels, which are primarily meant for growth. The resulting qualities over the entire pulse reflect a 'qi wild' condition of varying severity, roughly determined by the age at which the problem began.

Circulatory Problems Affecting the Qi and Blood

A severe accident, extraordinary exertion, sudden emotional shock, sudden cessation of heavy exertion or exercise, or a profound climatic event can create stagnation in the circulation of qi and/or blood. In the case of qi stagnation, pain migrates and is milder and less persistent than in instances of blood stagnation. However, when blood stagnation is present, the pain is more likely to be fixed, severe and persistent, and the pulse tends to be harder and more Tight-Wiry than the Tense quality of qi stagnation.

If circulatory problems are caused by the sudden cessation of excessive work or exercise, one finds the more serious qualities of Yielding Hollow Full-Overflowing and Rapid.

The 'Circulatory System'

Dr. Shen differentiated three conditions involving problems with the 'circulatory system'. These are the circulation of qi, the circulation of blood, and the circulation of qi and blood together.

Liver qi circulation

An inconsistent, occasional Change in Amplitude over the entire pulse is a sign of a problem with the circulation of qi. It is usually the result of stress affecting the Liver and its involvement in qi circulation. Levels of qi rise and fall for many reasons, one of which is the varying degree of emotional stress that the Liver has to deal with. Thus when qi is reduced or stress is elevated, the condition worsens and the Change in Amplitude becomes more obvious on the pulse.

Blood circulation

A consistently present Change in Amplitude over the entire pulse reflects problems with the circulation of blood, and is either a sign that the Heart is affecting the circulation or that the circulation is affecting the Heart.

Heart affects blood circulation

Along with the Change in Amplitude, sometimes the entire pulse tends toward Feeble with the left distal position presenting as more Feeble-Absent than the rest of the pulse. The pulse rate tends to be between 60-70 bpm. Here the Heart qi is deficient and the effect on the circulation of blood is secondary.

Blood circulation affects the Heart

A shock to the circulation can result from many factors: trauma, sudden and powerful emotion, an abrupt episode of over-exercise or of work beyond one's energy, sudden cessation of long-term heavy labor or exercise, heavy labor especially before puberty, or overexposure to extreme climates. Eventually this deficit to the circulation affects the Heart, which controls the circulation.

Apart from a Change in Amplitude, the entire pulse also tends to be uniform except perhaps in that part of the pulse representing the area of the trauma. If the person was strong at the time of the insult, the left distal position can be a little Inflated and Tense. In a person who was less robust at the time of the insult, the left distal position will be Flat.

RATE

RAPID RATE Together with heat signs on the tongue and the color of the face (red) and eyes (injected), this can represent a febrile illness. However, the Rapid and Very Rapid Rates can be a sign of Heart qi deficiency in which the Heart has to work harder to maintain circulation.

VERY RAPID RATE This quality may accompany an acute anxiety or panic attack, usually involving the Heart. The tongue and eyes are usually normal.

ROBUST POUNDING AND BOUNDING WITH RAPID RATE Stimulants such as coffee and many medications such as ephedrine create this combination of pulse qualities. Until the stimulant is completely metabolized and excreted, the pulse signs are without diagnostic value.

STABILITY

The entire pulse also reveals the degree of stability within the organism as a whole. When one of the following four qualities appears at all five of the main depths over the entire pulse, the level of instability has become serious. This is a 'qi wild' condition in which the yin has lost control of the yang, which is then ungovernable and nonfunctional.

CHANGE IN QUALITY Qualities that are changing in many positions indicate a severe 'qi wild' condition, signifying a serious imbalance in which the patient is at great risk. This quality has also been observed in seriously mentally ill patients on heavy medication.

CHANGE IN AMPLITUDE The Amplitude of the pulse wave is a sign of the yang force (i.e., basal metabolic functional heat). High Amplitude reflects a strong yang force, while low amplitude is a mark of diminished yang force. In any one position, a Change in Amplitude is a sign of physiological instability, a 'separation of yin and yang' within the organ represented by that position. A Constant Change in Amplitude over the entire pulse is a sign of Heart qi-yang deficiency.

EMPTY INTERRUPTED OR YIELDING HOLLOW INTERRUPTED   These pulses represent a most severe form of 'qi wild' disorder as the instability is already in the yin organs and is complicated by severe Heart qi deficiency. If severe disease is not already present, the potential for its occurrence is great.

YIELDING HOLLOW FULL-OVERFLOWING AND RAPID   This form of 'qi wild' involves a dilation of blood vessels and contraction of blood volume. The symptoms are depersonalization, anxiety, widespread increasing organ dysfunction, and fatigue. The prognosis for severe illness within six months is moderately great if the condition remains unresolved.

QUALITIES AT EACH OF THE DEPTHS

The exact position of the nine depths is very subtle, and poorly conveyed in words. While the depths are best learned through demonstration, Fig. 13-1 will be our best visual guide. As the distance between the depths is only about a tenth of a millimeter, they are accessed by very precise, small increases or decreases in pressure by the practitioner's wrist, and therefore fingers, on the patient's pulse.

We find the Floating and Cotton qualities in the space between the surface of the skin and the qi depth. The distance from the surface of the skin to the qi depth is about one-third greater than the distance between the qi and blood depth, and the blood and organ depth. The qi depth is just below the surface at a precise point, and the organ depth is well above the bone at another precise point; the blood depth is halfway between the two. (We ignore for the moment the three divisions within the organ depth.) The Firm quality is found about halfway between the organ depth and the bone, and the Hidden quality is found just above the bone.

As noted above, the location of these depths depends on the proper positioning of the practitioner's wrist and the application of a precise pressure. They are not located by first finding the most superficial sensation of the radial artery and assuming it is the qi depth, nor by finding the deepest sensation and assuming it is the organ depth. By learning to calibrate and standardize our wrist movements, it is possible to locate the position of a depth even when the pulse there is Absent. The entire system described in this book depends on mastering this technique.

All Depths

Many pulse qualities can be found at any of the depths at one time or another.

These include Taut, Tense, Tight, Wiry, Robust Pounding, Slippery, Smooth Vibration, Rough Vibration, Reduced Pounding, Reduced Substance, Diffuse, Feeble, Absent, Thin, Tight, Wiry, Choppy and Leather-Hard. Some of these are discussed below, and others in the appropriate chapter (see the table of contents and index). Whenever the Muffled quality is found, it is usually accessed at all depths, either at one or more positions or uniformly over the entire pulse.

Other qualities are found at all of the depths simultaneously and are subsumed under Uniform qualities. These include Ropy, Inflated, Intermittent, Interrupted, Change in Rate at Rest, Change in Rate on Exertion, and Change in Amplitude. Anomalous variations of rate and rhythm from one position or burner to another have been observed in patients on medication.

ABOVE THE QI DEPTH

COTTON   This quality represents superficial qi stagnation and is palpated as an amorphous presence above the qi depth in the space between the surface of the skin and where the pulse is first encountered. It is found in the connective tissue there and feels as if the fingers are passing through a substance lacking in form. Over time, with increasing qi deficiency and a Deeper pulse, the Cotton quality can occupy the qi and blood depths. However, the degree of the Cotton quality is measured by the degree of resistance it offers and not by how deep it permeates. Obese individuals have a thickening of the connective tissue that is distinguished from the Cotton quality by its sensation of hardness.

This quality can be caused by emotional suppression, severe trauma affecting qi and blood circulation, or a combination of both. Dr. Shen called it the 'sad pulse' as it usually involves the conscious suppression of emotions in individuals who feel helpless to change a life situation that they know is not good for them. Dr. Hammer refers to it as the 'resignation pulse'.

The long-term physical consequences of an unresolved Cotton quality can be any chronic disease associated with prolonged qi stagnation, including arthritis or cancer, endocrine disorders such as adrenal insufficiency or hypothyroidism, and disorders of the reproductive system.

FLOATING   By its nature the Floating quality is felt above the qi depth at the skin and separate from the main impulse. It represents a process in which the protective and nutritive qi of the body rise to meet an outside challenge, usually from external wind, cold, or heat (or from internal wind if also Tight). If it lasts just a short time, this quality is normal; however, if the process lasts long enough it reflects the invasion of an external pathogenic factor that ultimately creates internal stagnation.

FLOATING TENSE AND SLIGHTLY SLOW   This indicates that the qi has risen to the surface as the organism attempts to defend itself against an external pathogenic factor, usually wind-cold.

FLOATING YIELDING AND SLIGHTLY RAPID   Like the previous quality, this one also indicates that the qi has risen to the surface as the organism attempts to defend itself against an external pathogenic factor, but here it is usually wind-heat.

FLOATING TIGHT   This quality is a sign of internal wind, usually associated with Liver excess or (yin) deficient heat and Liver blood deficiency. With this quality there should be concern for wind in the channels, and stroke.

FLOATING SLIPPERY   This combination can be encountered with a wind-damp condition such as hives.

FLOATING AND SMOOTH VIBRATION   This combination is associated with Heart qi agitation.

Floating vs. other superficial qualities

The sensations of the following pulse qualities are often confused with those of the Floating quality. They are listed here with the qualities that differentiate them.

FLOATING VS. INFLATED   The Floating quality is always found above and separated from the qi depth. Though expansive, the Inflated quality does not rise above the qi depth.

FLOATING VS. FLOODING EXCESS OR TENSE FULL-OVERFLOWING   The Flooding Excess and Tense Full-Overflowing qualities represent expansion due to heat, and although they can be felt above the qi depth, they both have a distinctive wave pattern (described in Ch. 9) that is missing from the Floating quality. Unlike the Floating pulse, they are connected to the main impulse.

FLOATING VS. EMPTY, LEATHER-EMPTY, EMPTY AND THREAD-LIKE, OR SCATTERED   The Floating pulse is found 'floating' above the qi depth just under the skin and separated from the main impulse that is always present beneath it. These other Empty-type qualities are felt only at the qi depth, above which they do not rise, and below which they are completely or partially vacant (see Ch. 9).

FLOATING VS. YIELDING HOLLOW FULL-OVERFLOWING   This quality has a normal sine wave that appears to be coming up from the blood depth and rising above the qi depth. Unlike the Floating quality, its sensation above the qi depth is connected to the main impulse. It is Yielding, as it separates easily under pressure. This is a 'qi wild' sign and reveals that yin and yang have separated in the 'circulatory system'.

FLOATING VS. TENSE HOLLOW FULL-OVERFLOWING   This quality has a normal sine wave that rises above the qi depth. It is different from the sensation of the Floating quality in that the sensation above the qi depth feels connected to the rest of the main impulse, which feels strong, forceful, swollen, and blown-up; rising powerfully from the blood depth, it feels both wide and expansive.

The expansiveness felt at the blood depth moves vigorously upward to above the qi depth, where the finger feels as if it is being pushed away from the wrist. On pressure from above it is slightly Hollow between the qi and blood depths before it resumes its forceful sensation at the organ depth. It is a sign of extreme heat in the blood associated with the hypertensive process.

FLOATING VS. FLOODING EXCESS   The Flooding Excess quality feels like the Hollow Full-Overflowing quality described above, however the sine wave lacks its second half, dropping off sharply when it reaches its peak. It too rises above the qi depth, but has a stronger base at the organ depth than does the Hollow Full-Overflowing and is never Yielding nor Hollow. Both Floating and Flooding Excess can be felt in the space above the qi depth. However, with the Flooding Excess quality the sensation above the qi depth is felt as an extension of the main impulse below; the Floating quality feels separate and unconnected to the qualities below it.

QI DEPTH

At this depth over the entire pulse, both the overall status of the moving or functional qi of the body (i.e., protective and nutritive qi) and the status of the 'nervous system' are being assessed. The qualities found here reveal information about qi stagnation, fluid stagnation, agitated qi, qi deficiency, carbohydrate metabolism and the 'nervous system'. As long as the pulse is present at the qi depth, the condition of the true qi is probably relatively good, because it is as the true qi becomes depleted that the qi and blood depths tend to disappear.

Qi stagnation qualities at the qi depth (see Ch. 11)

TAUT   The Taut pulse is slightly more resistant to pressure than normal, and represents the first stage of resistance to the free flow of qi through the channels. Usually the cause is repression of emotion, however any excessive or prolonged stress on the Liver (physical, chemical, or emotional) will interfere with the free flow of qi.

TENSE   As the body attempts to overcome stagnation, it generates excessive internal heat. The result is the Tense pulse, which represents equal degrees of stagnation and excessive heat. This is clinically different from the Taut quality, which represents only stagnation, and from the Tense-Long quality, which represents more heat.

TENSE ROBUST POUNDING   The addition of Robust Pounding to the Tense quality is a sign that the body is attempting to rid itself of excessive heat (see Tense quality above) by pushing it outward from the yin organs to the blood and qi depths. There are several possible etiologies, partly distinguished from one another by the pulse rate, the most common of which are: emotional repression, Stomach-Spleen working beyond their abilities, heat-producing foods (spices), and drugs (notably cocaine).

THIN AND TIGHT WITH A NORMAL OR SLIGHTLY SLOW RATE   This is a 'nervous system tense' condition that is constitutional or congenital in origin. This indicates that the 'nervous system' has been overworking since birth in the service of vigilance. Note that the rate does not change at rest or greatly upon exertion—unlike those qualities created by Heart shock—and that the eyes and tongue are normal.

THIN AND TIGHT AND SLIGHTLY RAPID RATE   This is a 'nervous system tense' condition that is attributable to life experience. The tongue and eyes will be slightly red.

TENSE ROBUST POUNDING SUPPRESSED   This presentation may be the result of synthesized chemicals, usually prescription, though possibly recreational. Robust Pounding only at the organ depth is another pulse picture with the same etiology. Often the pulse readings only become reliable when the substances have been metabolized and excreted.

INFLATED   The Inflated quality over the entire pulse is a sign of trapped qi throughout the organism, often due to trauma-related shock to the circulation, but also infrequently found with extreme repressed rage.

LEATHER-HARD   This hard quality is a sign of blood, yin, and essence deficiency that can be found at any or all depths, now often related to electromagnetic field radiation.[2]

SUPPRESSED WAVE   This quality can appear with the suppression of feelings, often if the patient does not wish to reveal himself.

Fluid stagnation quality

SLIPPERY   This pulse moves quickly under the fingers in one direction. Found at the qi depth with a Slow rate and a Yielding quality, it is a sign of qi deficiency. If, however, the pulse is also Tense or Tight with a Normal or slightly Rapid rate, it is a sign of excess sugar in the blood.

When found at all three depths over the entire pulse, Slipperiness can be a sign of pregnancy, elevated blood lipids and glucose, septicemia, steroid use, Heart qi deficiency, hypertension, or blood dyscrasias. The Slippery quality and other qualities that are frequently confused with it are discussed more fully in Ch. 11.

Agitation quality

SMOOTH VIBRATION   This is usually a sign of transient worry, anxiety, and lack of sleep. As the severity of the condition increases, the Smooth Vibration quality spreads to all depths and all positions on the pulse.

Qi deficiency qualities

There is a progression of pulse qualities in the evolution of qi, blood, and finally organ deficiency. The earliest sign appears at the qi depth as a Yielding and Pliable quality, becoming Diminished Feeble and Absent as the qi weakens. As it progresses further, qi deficiency goes on to affect the blood depth, in the form of the Spreading quality, and later deteriorates into the Flooding Deficient Wave, the Diffuse and Reduced Substance, Deep, Feeble, and Absent qualities.

YIELDING (PLIABLE)   Gradual increase in the pliability of the qi depth marks the initial stage of qi deficiency. This quality results from mild work or exercise beyond a person's qi, or appears during the recovery phase of a moderately severe illness.

DIMINISHED FEEBLE OR ABSENT AT THE QI DEPTH   These qualities mean that the protective, and some of the nutritive, qi has been compromised. In a biomedical sense the person has a slightly weakened immune system. In Chinese medicine terms, the person is more susceptible to attack from external pathogenic factors or any form of external stress (chemical or physical). Found at the qi depth, these qualities are usually the result of overwork or work beyond a person's capacity.

FLOODING DEFICIENT WAVE   This pulse rises just up to, but not beyond, the qi depth, and then suddenly recedes, lacking the force of the Flooding Excess pulse. It appears in individuals who push themselves beyond their energy levels.

Yin deficiency qualities

TIGHT AND THIN   At the qi depth these qualities are a sign of an overworking 'nervous system', a 'vigilance pulse' wherein the patient uses his mind excessively to be on guard. If found only at the qi depth, they also reflect yin deficiency as the body begins to expend yin to balance the heat used to overcome qi stagnation.

BLOOD DEPTH

The blood depth over the entire pulse reveals the general state of the blood for the entire organism, and specifically, information regarding the condition of blood in the vessels.

Beginning at the qi depth and increasing one's finger pressure down through the pulse, the blood depth should feel wider and offer more resistance than the qi depth, but less resistance than the organ depth. Beginning at the organ depth and releasing finger pressure, the pulse should become increasingly narrow. Different conditions can be delineated depending on whether one's finger is coming from the surface or from the organ depth.

Impaired blood circulation in the blood vessels

The following qualities—Blood Unclear, Blood Heat, Blood Thick, and Tense Hollow Full-Overflowing (Fig. 13-3)—are all accessed by slowly releasing pressure from the organ depth to the qi depth and above. Instead of the orderly diminishment of substance as one moves from deep to superficial, the opposite trend is encountered, and the substance increases. The degree and the depth to which the substance increases, as finger pressure is released, determines the quality. (The Tense Hollow Full-Overflowing requires that one apply pressure in the opposite direction, from superficial to deep, to identify the Hollow quality.)

Fig. 13-3 Progression of heat and toxicity in the blood

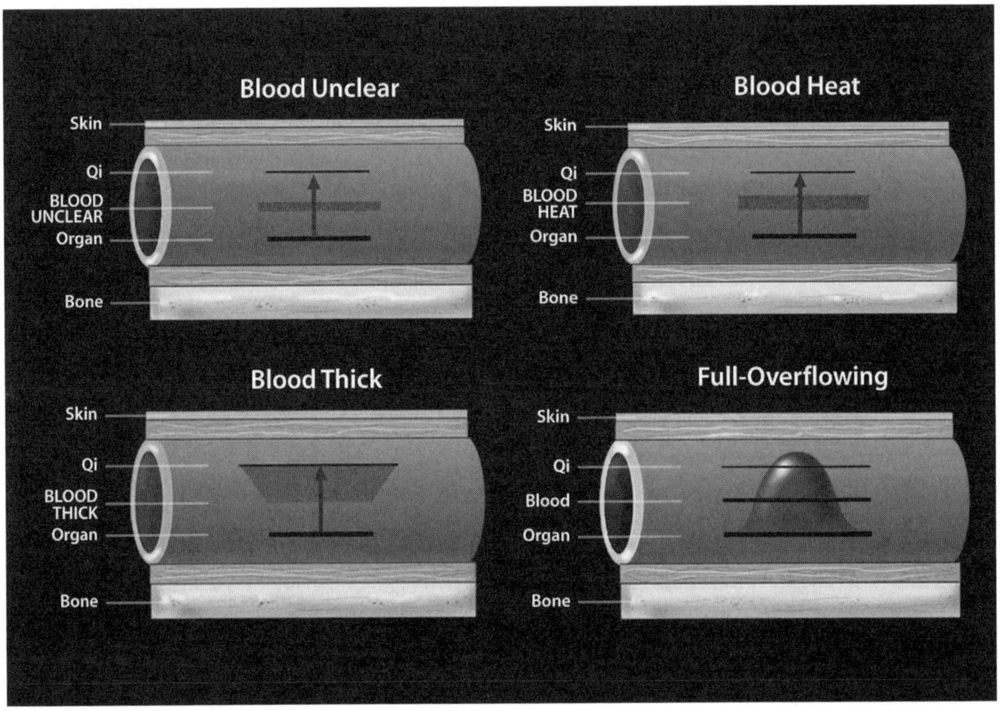

BLOOD UNCLEAR (TURBID BLOOD)   There is a barely perceptible increase, rather than decrease, in the size of the blood depth compared to the organ depth as one's fingers are raised from the organ depth toward the qi depth (see Fig. 13-4). As one releases one's fingers from the blood to the qi depth, the size diminishes again.

Dr. Shen likens the meaning of this quality to a glass of water in which dirt is suspended; it is a sign of toxicity in the blood. Symptoms often include fatigue and skin-related problems such as eczema and psoriasis.

The most common cause of this quality is exposure to environmental toxins, especially inhalant solvents. Another possibility is Liver stagnation or deficiency that prevents this organ from detoxifying adequately, thus contaminating the

Fig. 13-4 Blood unclear quality

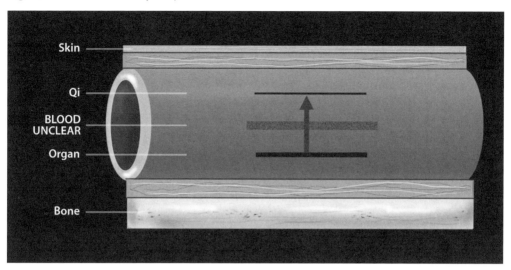

blood. Skin symptoms are an attempt by the body to discharge the toxicity.

BLOOD HEAT   As one raises one's fingers from the organ to the blood depth, the pulse expands even more in the blood depth than it does with the Blood Unclear quality. Again, as one continues to release pressure to the qi depth, the pulse diminishes. This is a sign of excess blood heat (Fig. 13-5), which, according to Dr. Shen, is usually the result of an over-working 'nervous system'; however, with excess blood heat, the heat has been found coming from both 'nervous system' and digestive sources. When the blood depth is also Slippery, the blood heat is due to inadequate digestion and metabolism of lipids. The Choppy quality at the blood depth signals further obstruction and deterioration of the blood vessel walls.

Fig. 13-5 Blood Heat quality

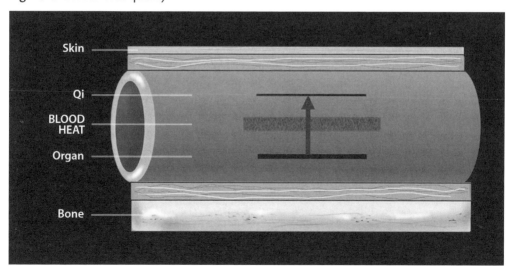

With regard to the digestive system, there is excess heat associated with heat-generating foods such as spices, wine, shellfish, coffee, chocolate, etc., usually affecting the Liver, Stomach, Heart, and Lungs. Excess heat is generated when the Spleen-Stomach is engaged in working beyond its energy, as with excess or difficult-to-digest foods.

BLOOD THICK (EXUBERANT BLOOD)   Raising one's fingers from the organ to the blood depth the pulse becomes extremely Wide, with Robust Pounding and sometimes Slippery and/or Choppy qualities. However, unlike the Blood Unclear and Blood Heat qualities, as one continues to raise one's fingers from the blood depth to the qi depth, the pulse does not diminish, but continues to widen (see Fig. 13-6).

Fig. 13-6 Blood Thick quality

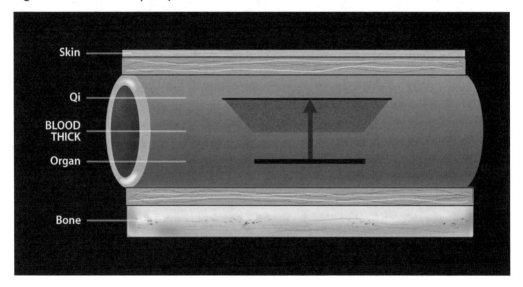

According to Dr. Shen, an early sign of this condition can be persistent acne after adolescence. The later signs are usually of a cardiovascular nature, such as hypertension and coronary occulsion. In either case, the sclera and vessels of the lower eyelids are very red and the tongue is scarlet.

Blood Thick may develop from heat in the blood (described in the entry immediately above) in which the etiologies are greater in degree and last longer. This also includes Liver-Spleen-Stomach dysfunction and an excessive dietary intake of fat and sugar, and is a process that gradually interferes with Heart function by increasing resistance in the circulation. Heat gradually depletes the compensating yin, drying out the intima and media of the vessels, and leading to a Ropy pulse.

TENSE HOLLOW FULL-OVERFLOWING   This quality (Fig. 13-7) feels swollen, rising wide and expansive above the qi depth in a sine wave curve, with a Robust

Fig. 13-7 Tense Hollow Full-Overflowing quality

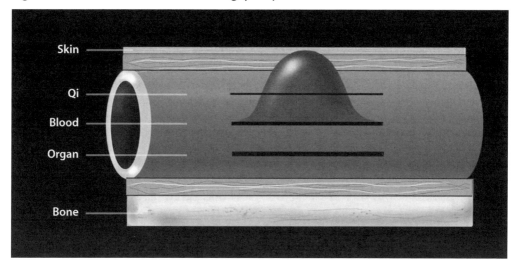

Pounding and often slightly Rapid rate. Its expansiveness is felt strongly in the blood depth, moving upward vigorously to and above the qi depth where the finger feels as if it is being pushed away.

When one presses from the surface toward the organ depth, the Hollow aspect causes this quality to give way with pressure at approximately the blood depth, and then resume its expansiveness as one presses from the blood depth to the organ depth.

The Tense Hollow Full-Overflowing quality is a sign of severe excess heat that the body is attempting to eliminate from the blood. Since the heat can no longer be contained in the blood, it invades the qi. When found over the entire pulse, this is a sign of potentially serious hypertension, and when very Tense or very Tight Hollow Full-Overflowing, it is a sign of imminent stroke and even death (see Ch. 9).

SLIPPERY   Slipperiness at the blood depth is a sign of turbulence and is found whenever there is some alteration in the normal strength or direction of the flow of blood or fluids. It may be due to increased resistance or decreased propulsion. Occasionally the Slippery quality has been found together in patients with the Blood Unclear, Blood Heat, or Blood Thick qualities with blood dyscrasias, such as sickle cell anemia.

ROUGH VIBRATION   When confined to the blood depth, Rough Vibration is a sign that heat in the blood is drying out and damaging the blood vessel walls. This is an early stage of arteriosclerosis.

ROPY   The Ropy quality is specifically a sign of the drying of the intima and media of the blood vessel walls due to either heat or lack of nourishment (see Ch. 11). There are two types of Ropy pulse: one that is also Tense and the other that is Ropy Yielding.

TENSE ROPY   The Tense Ropy quality is associated with excess heat, where the heat has damaged the blood vessel walls, causing a loss of elasticity in the smooth muscle fibers. Such deterioration encourages the development of arteriosclerotic plaques on the vessel walls.

YIELDING ROPY   The Yielding Ropy quality is the result of exercising beyond one's energy for a very long period of time. As blood is consumed in maintaining the exercise, the vessel walls and the flowing blood lose some contact and a separation of yin and yang occurs within the vessel, depriving the walls of yin nourishment and resulting in a process of drying-out and consequent fragility. This also leads to the arteriosclerotic process, but without the heat phase of the Tense Ropy quality (see Ch. 11) and only rarely leads to hypertension.

Blood deficiency

THIN   Thinness alone at the blood depth is associated with blood stagnation and is a rare form of blood deficiency due to decreased delivery of blood rather than deficiency of blood.

SPREADING (ON SLIGHT PRESSURE)   The qi depth is Absent, the blood depth separates with mild to moderate pressure, yet the organ depth remains substantial. This quality represents increasing depletion of nutritive qi, particularly from working beyond one's energy without sufficient rest. This quality has been found in relatively young, healthy people who overwork and have little chance to recover, and also in young women who have had multiple pregnancies, abortions, and miscarriages, in whom this quality represents both qi and blood deficiency.

DEEP (ABSENCE OF THE BLOOD AND QI DEPTHS)   Absence of the blood and qi depths over the entire pulse is a sign of both serious blood and especially qi-yang deficiency.

YIELDING PARTIALLY HOLLOW   The qi and organ depths are present, and the blood depth separates on pressure but is not entirely Absent. This indicates slight blood deficiency that may be due to gradual bleeding. The degree of blood deficiency is less than the Deep quality and much less than the Thin quality.

LEATHER-HOLLOW   The qi and organ depths are present and there is no sensation at the blood depth. More often this quality appears in one position when one organ can no longer control its blood, for example, the Stomach with a bleeding ulcer. When the pulse is also Rapid, the bleeding is imminent or in progress, and when Slow, the bleeding has already passed.

Found over the entire pulse, this quality is usually a sign of notable and even massive hemorrhage. The lack of control of blood and the shock that frequently accompanies it is usually of sudden onset and calls for emergency measures.

VERY TENSE OR TIGHT HOLLOW FULL-OVERFLOWING   When found over the entire pulse the appearance of either of these qualities can indicate true hypertension, and insulin-dependent diabetes when found only at the left middle and proximal positions. Over the entire pulse, these qualities represent another form of 'blood out of control', and the potential for cerebral bleeding or stroke is great.

Organ Depth

This, the deepest aspect of the pulse within our system, is located well above the bone and reflects the integrity of the yin organs, the basic functional units which, working together, create fluid, blood, and qi and govern all the functions of life in our bodies. This is why any alteration at the organ depth of the pulse is clinically very significant.

Organ qi, blood, and substance and retained pathogens

The qualities that appear uniformly over the entire pulse at the organ depths inform us about the presence and the nature of retained pathogens. Of the three organ depths (organ-qi, organ-blood, and organ-substance), it is the deeper two that are particularly informative with regard to retained pathogens. These pathogens are substances that the body considers a threat to the integrity of vital organs, and so diverts them through the divergent and *luo* channels to places that are less immediately threatening to the essential functioning of things such as the solid organs. The joints, skin, and sinuses are common areas of the body in which retained pathogens may be kept. Over time, these pathogens can do great damage, and the energy required to retain them deprives the body of energy that would otherwise be available for growth, development, and function. Qualities commonly found at the organ-blood and organ-substance depths are Tense, Robust Pounding, Choppy and Slippery.

The following are abbreviated descriptions of other conditions and associated pulse qualities found at the organ depth. More detailed information is presented in other chapters.

Stagnation at the organ depth

The following qualities may be the result of stagnation of qi (from either excess or deficiency), blood, fluid (dampness), or other substances such as phlegm or food.

Qi stagnation from excess

TAUT-TENSE   While frequently strongest at the organ depth, this quality is usually found simultaneously at all three depths. The Tense pulse is an early indication of qi stagnation together with excess heat.

Qi stagnation from deficiency

FLAT (TRAPPED QI)   This is a Deep pulse with a notably diminished wave. It occurs when a physical or emotional shock restricts the circulation of qi, preventing it from reaching an area of the body. This quality also suggests that the qi in the area was deficient prior to the shock. Clinically, except in the distal positions, it may be associated with a neoplastic process that develops over a very long period of time.

Blood stagnation

These qualities fall under two broad categories, stagnation in body tissues and cavities, and stagnation in the blood vessels, discussed above. The term blood stagnation refers to slowed or impaired circulation of blood. When this occurs in body tissues or cavities, it is expressed primarily by the Choppy quality and, rarely, a Very Tense Inflated quality that can indicate blood stagnation as a result of gradual bleeding into a body area.

CHOPPY   Sometimes confused with the tingling, buzzing, moving sensations of the Rough Vibration quality, the Choppy quality is coarser and uneven, like rolling one's finger across a washboard ('scraping bamboo'). When found at the organ depth, it is a sign of either blood stagnation or toxicity. (See discussion above and in Ch. 11.)

Since the body has given us a limited number of qualities, the Choppy quality has different meanings at different positions (see Ch. 11). Over the past twenty years, the Choppy quality has gone from being a rare to a common quality. This has been associated with the increasing levels of toxicity to which we are all exposed. Perhaps the best answer to the question of whether the Choppy quality indicates blood stagnation or toxicity is that most toxins create, and ultimately kill, through blood stagnation.

VERY TENSE INFLATED   This is a rare occurrence that is caused by gradual bleeding into an area or organ, such as with a subdural hematoma in the brain.

Stagnation of fluids (dampness)

SLIPPERY AND RAPID   When found only at the organ depth with a Rapid rate, Slipperiness is a sign of damp-heat in the yin organs or the biomedical equivalent of chronic bacterial, viral, or parasitic infection. Slipperiness at all three depths with a very Rapid rate indicates a more fulminating kind of infection, whereas when the rate is only slightly Rapid, pregnancy may be the associated condition.

SLIPPERY AND SLOW   When found only at the organ depth with a Slow rate, Slipperiness is a sign of damp-cold and represents chronic systemic infection of a yeast or fungal nature. A Slippery and Slow pulse at all depths has been observed in chronic blood dyscrasias such as leukemia, with iatrogenic damp-ness related to Heart and Kidney disease, and with the use of water-retaining medications. When present with Heart qi deficiency, the Slipperiness may be the result of turbulence in the circulation, in which case it is more common for the Slipperiness to be encountered at the blood depth. Recently it has been reported from China that this quality is found in patients with terminal cancer of the lung or large intestine.

Deficiency at the organ depth

Blood deficiency

Blood deficiency, other than from hemorrhage or chronic illness, has its roots in Spleen qi deficiency, digestion, and Kidney essence deficiency (marrow). How-ever, conditions where the Lung does not properly oxygenate the blood, the Liver does not store it, or the Heart does not circulate it can also play a part in the blood deficient syndromes.

THIN YIELDING   This quality reflects blood and qi deficiency, often due to Spleen qi deficiency as a result of inadequate digestion, absorption, storage, and metabolism of nutrients, or any of the above in combination with Kidney essence deficiency. In women of child-bearing age, hemorrhage associated with menstruation, abortion, miscarriage, or multiple childbirths is a possible etiol-ogy. Kidney essence deficiency must be considered due its influence on the bone marrow and thus the production of red blood cells.

THIN TIGHT   This quality is usually associated with overwork of the 'nervous system' due to overthinking for a long period of time, and is a sign of blood and yin deficiency, especially of the Kidney.

Yin and essence depletion

TIGHT   Tension turns to Tightness as excess heat evolves into a yin-deficient condition. This happens because the yin of the body exhausts itself trying to balance the heat.

Most often a Tight pulse reflects yin deficiency as a result of a person's overthinking (overworking the 'nervous system') for a period of years. However, intense pain throughout the body can also result in a uniformly Tight pulse that occasionally has the addition of a sharp, Biting quality (common in the Intes-tine positions). A Tight quality in certain positions, such as at the Intestines, Gallbladder, Special Lung, and Stomach Pylorus Extension, can be a sign of an inflammatory process in their associated organs.

WIRY   The Wiry pulse represents one step beyond the Tight pulse in the de-pletion of body fluid. It is the principal sign of the depletion of essence, the en-ergetic substance associated with bone marrow, as well as with the development and maintenance of the 'nervous system.' This quality reflects overworking of the 'nervous system' and exhaustion of Kidney yin-essence. It can also be associated with pain. When found in the left middle and left proximal positions, early diabetes and/or hypertension may be indicated. The Wiry quality, especially in the left distal and middle positions, is also found in patients with long-term cocaine use.

Qi and yang deficiency

The following six qualities occur when yin and yang are still in contact and can be differentiated from those qualities that indicate 'qi wild' conditions, where the yin and yang are separated.

SHORT YIELDING   This pulse can be felt at any depth as being discontinuous from the distal to the proximal position. It reveals an obstruction to the circulation between the organs or burners that is due to qi stagnation from excess or deficiency. When it is Short Weak[3] it is a sign of even more severe deficiency and reduced qi and blood circulation between the organs (see Ch. 10). This is sometimes the cause of a Heart-Kidney disharmony.

REDUCED POUNDING   An organism that is approaching exhaustion manifests a Reduced Pounding pulse which, on pressure, lacks force. This is a sign of a desperate attempt by a weakened and stressed body to maintain homeostatic function despite severe qi and yang deficiency.

DEEP   This pulse is accessed only at the organ depth and reflects a chronic internal disharmony of advanced qi deficiency that may be difficult to heal and portends relatively severe illness within a few years. It should be noted that the pulse of an obese person is normally slightly deeper than that of a thinner individual. Dr. Shen confirmed in a personal communication that his Hidden quality (described in his 1980 book) and the Deep quality described by Dr. Hammer are the same. There is some debate as to whether the Deep pulse in a seemingly healthy individual may simply be a constitutional quality.

DEEP REDUCED SUBSTANCE   Here the Deep pulse maintains its form but seems to lose its resilience, matter, and buoyancy. It is a further sign of qi and blood deficiency of the yin organs.

FEEBLE-ABSENT   The pulse becomes increasingly Yielding to finger pressure, and the deficiency increases in severity until one can find little (Feeble) or no (Absent) evidence of the pulse at any depth. When the entire pulse is Feeble-Absent there is deficiency of the true (*zhen*) qi; in other words, the qi, yin, and blood of all of the yin organs is deficient. There is weakened resistance and increased vulnerability to disease.

This pulse is found in those with impaired immune systems and chronic fatigue syndrome, and in women who have gone beyond their energetic ability in giving birth and child-rearing. This quality can also be a sign of what Dr. Shen terms 'nervous system weak' when found at the proximal positions.[4]

Empty qualities

Separation of yin and yang (yin and yang out of contact)

While the following qualities are not felt sensationally at the organ depth, they all involve the organ depth. When found over the entire pulse, the following types of Empty qualities are signs of a 'qi wild' disorder, signifying that the qi of the whole organism is in chaos. There are several stages of the Empty quality, each being more serious than the last, discussed and illustrated in Ch. 9.

SEPARATING AT ORGAN DEPTH The qi and blood depths are present, but the organ depth has a sensation that gives way to finger pressure by moving to the sides of the fingertips. It represents a severe depletion of qi and blood in the organ and a 'separation of yin and yang'. It becomes more serious when the Empty quality is combined with various Interrupted-Intermittent qualities.

SEPARATION OR ABSENCE AT THE BLOOD AND ORGAN DEPTH With these qualities, a sensation is palpable at the qi depth, separating or no sensation at all is felt at the blood and organ depths. This is a more serious stage in the process of organ deficiency than the previous quality. It indicates that there is increasing loss of functional interaction between yin and yang. The yin cannot nourish the yang or yang cannot move the yin, or both. As a result, the yang floats to the surface of the body and scatters aimlessly or moves to the most vulnerable organ or area.

A combination of an impoverished environment (including inadequate nutrition, shelter, and clothing), overwork, excessive sex (especially between the ages of fifteen to twenty) and/or constitutional deficiency are possible etiologies. Another increasingly common cause is excessive exercise at a young age, which leads to profound qi depletion and in many cases severe anxiety and difficulty with attention. Other increasingly common causes are drug abuse, especially marijuana and heroin, and mononucleosis and liver infections such as hepatitis.

LEATHER-EMPTY This is similar in form to the Empty quality, except that the surface is much harder and wider. The Leather-Empty quality represents a more severe deficiency of essence, yin, or blood than the Empty quality (the 'qi wild' condition is more advanced).

EMPTY THREAD-LIKE (SOGGY) This quality feels "like a thread floating on water."[5] The pulse is felt only at the qi depth but disappears on pressure. It is a sign of extreme deficiency of blood, essence, and yang.

SCATTERED   A more extreme form of the Empty quality, it is felt only discontinuously at the qi depth, like an Empty quality that appears and disappears as one rolls one's finger proximally-distally. This quality signifies a further disintegration in the continuity of qi within both yin and yang, and of the blood circulation. It is found in terminal AIDS patients where it has been referred to as 'ceiling dripping'. The prognosis is poor. It has been found that with the advent of new drug therapies, this quality is now more rare.

MINUTE   The sensation of this quality is found only at the blood depth (there is no accompanying sensation at the qi and organ depths). It is discontinuous, resembling the Scattered quality, Thin, and Yielding with little resistance to pressure. It is a sign of extensive qi and yang deficiency in a seriously ill person. In terms of a 'qi wild' disorder, it is a stage beyond the Scattered pulse (described above) and indicates that there is not enough yang left to rise to the surface.

YIELDING HOLLOW FULL-OVERFLOWING   The Empty and the Hollow qualities are frequently confused. The Hollow pulse is felt at the qi and organ depths, but much less in the blood depth, whereas the Empty pulse is felt consistently at the qi depth and as separating or absent at the others.

When the Yielding Hollow Full-Overflowing quality appears with a Slow pulse it reflects physiological damage beginning sometime between the ages of ten and fifteen. This form of 'qi wild' is considered less serious than the two types involving the Interrupted quality.

The Yielding Hollow Full-Overflowing pulse which is also Rapid can occur later in life following excessive exercise during which the blood vessels dilate and the Heart pumps with greater vigor. When such exercise is suddenly discontinued, the blood vessels remain dilated while the blood volume dramatically decreases. This leaves a separation of yin (blood) and yang (vessel walls) that is experienced on the pulse as a Hollow quality. More rarely, an episode in which a person is called to suddenly lift a weight far beyond his or her capacity can also cause a Yielding Hollow quality. For a more complete discussion, see Ch. 9.

EMPTY INTERRUPTED-INTERMITTENT, YIELDING HOLLOW INTERRUPTED-INTERMITTENT   These qualities represent the most severe forms of 'qi wild' in that the instability is already in the yin organs, combined with chaotic qi in the Heart. The presence or imminence of serious, even terminal, disease is great.

BENEATH THE ORGAN DEPTH

FIRM   This quality is found just below the organ depth (no pulse is perceptible at the qi, blood, or organ depths) and represents serious stagnation of qi, blood, and fluids due to extreme invasion of cold. This is seen with serious hypothermia.

HIDDEN EXCESS   This quality is only felt far beneath the organ and Firm depths and is accessed only by the deepest pressure "to the level of the bone."[6] Li Shi-Zhen describes it as stagnant internal yin cold. This quality has only been found with life-threatening hypothermia.

CONCLUSION

It is worth repeating that one major premise of this system of pulse diagnosis is that the large segment of the pulse takes clinical precedence over the small segment. That is, the larger picture of the pulse should be looked at before exploring the more specific. Before attempting to cope with the individual deficiencies and excesses in particular organ systems, we must first resolve the disharmonies in rate, rhythm, and stability; in the general depletion of the true qi in its various forms, as described in this chapter; in the disorders that involve the entire blood and circulation; or in the general separation of yin from yang. Otherwise, little of lasting value will be accomplished since the issues that affect the entire pulse (or large segments of it) are the ones of greatest significance to physiology and survival. Furthermore, the unresolved qualities involving large aspects of the pulse render the qualities on the lesser aspects unreliable indicators of disease patterns.

14

Uniform Qualities on Other Large Segments of the Pulse

Karen Bilton, L.Ac.

UNIFORM QUALITIES ON LEFT OR RIGHT SIDE

In this section are listed the most common disorders associated with each of the individual pulse qualities when they are found uniformly over one or the other side of the wrist.

LITERATURE: HUSBAND-WIFE BALANCE

There are several interpretations in the literature concerning the relationship of the right and left sides of the pulse. One view is that a husband-wife (i.e., right and left pulse) imbalance is a sign of eternal difficulties with interpersonal relationships, especially with intimate partners, a phenomenon that Dr. Hammer corroborated clinically through work with many patients. Another view is that a husband-wife imbalance is a reflection of being unbalanced physically, mentally, or both. Dr. Hammer once encountered a forty-five-year-old woman with neck and back pain since childhood. She also complained of feeling unbalanced and "discombobulated down my left side all my life." The moment the left and right side pulses were balanced after treatment, she broke down and began to cry and to talk about her relationship with her husband. Following this, she had no further symptoms.

According to Van Buren,[1] the laws of nature operate to continuously maintain balance. Yang conforms to the right side of the body and yin to the left side.

However, in the service of balance, polarized cosmic energy enters a woman's body with the yang distributed to the right side and the yin to the left; in a man, yang is distributed to the left side and yin to the right. Although not explicitly stated, the inference is that in a woman the right pulse—and in a man, the left pulse—should be more Robust. Van Buren believes that in order to maintain balance, in a woman, yin points are needled on the right side and yang points on the left, and in a man, yin points on the left and yang points on the right.

Dr. Hammer's information concerning Worsley's practice with regard to husband-wife balance and imbalance has been obtained from his students over a period of twenty-eight years. From 1971 through approximately 1981, Worsley taught that normally, in a woman, the right pulse should feel more Robust than the left, and in a man, the left should feel more Robust than the right. Any deviation indicated disharmony. Then in the 1980s, the message changed. The view now seems to be that the left pulse should always be more Robust than the right, the reason being that the yin organs on the right side are more concerned with nurture, and those on the left more with function. Since function is more active than nurture, the functional pulse should normally have a more Robust quality. In fact, any deviation is considered extremely serious, and Dr. Hammer has been informed that in Worsley's view, without correction, an individual with a husband-wife imbalance in which the right pulse is more Robust than the left could be expected to live only six months. Some students of Worsley who also consider this imbalance to be serious take a less cataclysmic view: they speak of grave consequences within three to fifteen years. More importantly, they view (as does Dr. Hammer) the husband-wife imbalance as a sign of constant difficulties with interpersonal relationships, especially with the opposite gender.

Li Shi-Zhen's[2] view of the imbalance in left and right pulses is set forth in the following passage:

> Both men and women have a slight yin-yang imbalance which is reflected as a slight difference between the right and left pulses. The left is yang and the right is yin. Men have more yang qi. So, provided their qi is will regulated, their left hand pulse is stronger. Women have more yin blood. In women, provided their qi is well regulated, their right hand pulse is stronger.

It should be mentioned that Worsley's[3] original thesis regarding the relationship between the right and left pulses in men and women seems to reflect Li Shi-Zhen's view.

Amber[4] also lists certain conditions in which there are disparities between the left and right pulses:

> Aneurysm of the arch of the aorta; cervical rib; embolism of the brachial artery; atheroma of the brachial or subclavian artery; aneurism of the subclavian, axillary, brachial, and innominate arteries; mediastinal tumor; fracture of the arm; cicatrices of the arm; tumor or enlarged gland of axilla; pneumothorax; pleural effusion.

Hammer

Dr. Hammer examined a number of people in which either the left side or right side were much more deficient than the other. One patient, a woman Five Element practitioner, whose right side seemed so extraordinarily less than her left, had been tortured for over twenty years by the Worsley label of a severe husband-wife disharmony, inferring that she could not gainfully participate in an intimate relationship.

Dr. Hammer's finding was that on her right side she had an anomaly commonly known in Chinese medicine as a *fǎn quán* pulse, one in which, in her case, the anomaly on the right side was much greater than on the left.

One of the defects of the Worsley system is the absence of the perspective of the vast knowledge that exists outside of that system and cannot inform it.

Shen-Hammer

Dr. Shen's views about the right- and left-side pulses are an integral part of his 'systems' theory in which the right side represents the 'digestive system' and the left side the 'organ system.'[5] When the right pulse is more Robust than the left, the inference is that the 'digestive system' is overworking to compensate for a deficient yin 'organ system'. When the left pulse is stronger than the right, the inference is that the 'digestive system' is more deficient than the 'organ system', either from poor nutrition or eating habits in a young person, or through working too soon after eating in an older person. Dr. Shen appears to view the integrity of the 'digestive system' as a predictor of whether a person can or cannot recover from an illness. In other words, while the preference would be for equality between the sides, if the 'organ system' is impaired and the left pulse is reduced, the preference is for the right-side 'digestive system' to be more Robust than the left side. This is in direct contrast to Worsley's view of the husband-wife imbalance, in which the left side should normally be more Robust for both men and women.

'Systems' model synopsis

Please refer to Ch. 14 of the source text, *Chinese Pulse Diagnosis: A Contemporary Approach*, as well as *Dragon Rises, Red Bird Flies*.[6]

Change in Amplitude and Qualities from side to side

Patients in whom a Change in Amplitude or other pulse qualities change from side to side, first only on one side and then only on the other, have great current difficulty with interpersonal relationships, which are dominating their lives at the time. Other causes are a sudden excessive expenditure of energy beyond one's available true qi. An example is firefighters battling forest fires for days or weeks on end with little rest (less exertion in a physically weaker person would yield the same result). Dr. Shen has used the expressions 'qi wild', 'circulation of qi and blood not balanced', and 'relation to organ not good' to describe this phenomenon. He has indicated that when the qualities are changing first on one side and then the other, it is a weak 'nervous system' disorder similar to a 'qi wild' state, and is much more serious. This is one of the pulses that is reminiscent of the husband-wife imbalance, the significance of which requires further investigation.

UNIFORM QUALITIES BILATERALLY AT THE SAME POSITION

In contrast to the presence of a quality in just one position, the presence of a quality bilaterally at the same position is regarded as being more a sign of pathology in an *area* of the body, rather than in a specific yin or yang organ (Table 14-1). However, both types of pathology can of course occur at the same time. For example, trauma or heavy lifting can affect the entire chest while sparing or damaging either the Lungs and/or the Heart.

Qualities appearing bilaterally at a particular burner are usually more serious signs than when they appear on only one side.

Each bilateral position, hereafter referred to alternatively as a burner, is discussed in terms of the following commonly-found qualities. Many of the etiologies of these multiple qualities are similar. The variables that determine the differences in pulse qualities are the strength of the person when the etiology began, and the amount of time that has passed since the event, or the duration of the detrimental activity.

This body of information is summarized in the following table. For elaboration please see Ch. 14 in the source text.

Table 14.1 A: Similar Qualities Found on the Sides **245**

Table 14.1
A. Similar Qualities Found on the Sides

QUALITY	CONDITION

■ LEFT SIDE 'ORGAN SYSTEM'

Robust:

QUALITY	CONDITION
Cotton	1. Sign of short-term resignation ('sad pulse') > 5 years; Cotton spreads to the right side
	2. Trauma to that side
Left side Uniformly Tight to Wiry with a Rapid rate	Pain: location corresponds to the position which is Tightest
Left side Tight Hollow Full-Overflowing with Slippery blood depth	Later stage diabetes
Left side Rapid and very Tight Hollow Full-Overflowing	Hypertension – precursor to a paralytic cerebrovascular accident (stroke) on the left side of the body
Left side Slippery at the blood depth	Liver blood toxicity, turbulence in blood
Left side Slippery and Tense at the organ depth	Infection (parasites or low grade hepatitis), especially in the Liver
Left side Yielding Slippery at the qi depth with a Slow rate	Organ system qi deficiency.
Left side Yielding Slippery at the qi depth, Tense with a Normal or Rapid rate	Elevated sugar levels in the blood
Left side Tight Floating	Moderate Liver wind condition

Reduced:

QUALITY	CONDITION
Left side Deep and Feeble-Absent, Empty or Slow Yielding-Hollow Full-Overflowing	1. Constitutional 'nervous system weak'
	2. Prolonged recovery from a serious illness that has weakened the yin organs
	3. Ongoing, chronic draining illness such as paraplegia; or a degenerative disease such as multiple sclerosis

A. Similar Qualities Found on the Sides, *cont.*

QUALITY	CONDITION

■ RIGHT SIDE 'DIGESTIVE SYSTEM'

Robust:

QUALITY	CONDITION
Right side Tense and slightly Rapid	Eating too quickly from a constitutionally 'nervous system tense'
Right side Tight, especially in the right middle Stomach position (also a Tense quality on the left side - 'nervous system tense')	'Nervous system' is affecting the nervous innervation of the digestive system – stagnant Liver qi is unable to assist the Stomach to move qi down
Right side Rapid and very Tight Hollow Full-Overflowing	Hypertension – precursor to a paralytic cerebrovascular accident (stroke) on the right side of the body
Right side Slippery and Tense	'Digestive system' damp-heat and/or infection
Right side Slippery at the qi depth	Elevated sugar levels in the blood
Right side Slippery at the blood depth	Elevated sugar and lipids in the blood, causing turbulence in the blood

Reduced:

QUALITY	CONDITION
Right side is very Reduced: Deep and Feeble-Absent	Irregular eating: eating when the 'digestive system' is not ready, and not eating when it is
Right side Slippery and Feeble	Severe damp-cold disorder in the 'digestive system' indicative of decreased metabolism and regulation of fluids in the Spleen, Lungs, and especially Kidneys
Right side Empty or Yielding Hollow Full-Overflowing and Slow	Sign of extreme deficiency from chronic resumption of physical labor immediately after eating; indicates that the qi in the 'digestive system' is 'wild'

Table 14.1 A: Similar Qualities Found on the Sides **247**

A. Similar Qualities Found on the Sides, *cont.*

QUALITY	CONDITION
■ **RIGHT AND LEFT SIDES**	
Changing:	
Change in Amplitude from side to side, first on one side and then the other	Sign of 'qi wild,' 'circulation of qi and blood not balanced.' Indicates 1. Great current difficulty with interpersonal relationships (especially the opposite gender), which are dominating their lives at the time 2. Sudden excessive expenditure of energy beyond one's available true qi
■ **LEFT > RIGHT SIDE**	
Robust:	
Rapid, Robust Pounding and uniformly Tense, which remain the same after treatment; more pronounced on left side due to the Liver mediating the 'nervous system'	Constitutional 'nervous system' tense, hyper-vigilance over many generations
■ **LEFT > RIGHT SIDE**	
Robust:	
Tense and more Rapid than the constitutional type; the depth of tension depends on the time and intensity of the stress, which becomes less Tense after treatment. More pronounced on left side due to the Liver mediating the 'nervous system'.	Nervous system tense from situational stress, constant worry, being on guard, over thinking, drug abuse and over work

B. Uniform Qualities Bilaterally at Same Position

QUALITY	DISTAL POSITION	MIDDLE POSITION	PROXIMAL POSITION
Floating			
Floating Yielding and Rapid	Current wind-heat	Rare	Rare
Floating Yielding and Slow	Unresolved external pathogenic factor in deficient person		
Floating Tense and Slow	Current wind-cold	Rare	Rare
Floating Tense with Normal or Rapid rate	Unresolved cold from excess causes internal stagnation and heat in strong person		
Cotton (very rare finding, isolated in one burner)	Recent emotional trauma	Emotional stress while eating; ruminating while eating (Cotton and Tight)	Mild Kidney qi deficiency
	Minor accident to chest	Sitting in one position continuously; resuming work too soon after eating; minor trauma to abdomen	Minor trauma to lower body
Muffled The Muffled quality is a sign of the stagnation of all substances, qi, yin, blood. More specifically, it is associated with the neoplastic process from its inception [1-2] to its culmination in a tumor [4-5].	1. Tumor in the breast 2. Tumor in the mediastinum 3. Hiatal Hernia 4. Trauma to the chest	1. Pancreatic tumor 2. Esophageal tumor 3. Stomach tumor 4. Ascites	1. Uterine tumor 2. Uterine prolapse

Table 14.1 B: Uniform Qualities Bilaterally at Same Position   **249**

B. Uniform Qualities Bilaterally at Same Position, *cont.*

QUALITY	DISTAL POSITION	MIDDLE POSITION	PROXIMAL POSITION
Hollow Full-Overflowing	Headaches w/ hypertension	Hypertension and/or diabetes	Hypertension or diabetes
Flooding Excess Heat from excess in organ	Acute fulminating myopericarditis Acute bacterial pneumonia	Acute infection, peritonitis, hepatitis, cholecystitis, pancreatitis	Fulminating PID, prostatitis, nephritis, urinary tract infection, colitis
Inflated Trapped qi or heat in organ or area in a person who is strong at the time the qi is trapped. Qi cannot get out of organ or area. Trapped blood	1. Yielding • talking, breathing or singing incorrectly • unresolved grief 2. Mildly Tense • breech birth 3. Moderately Tense • Liver qi moving upward • breast pathology • trapped heat (invading cold turns to heat) • emphysema 4. Tense • sudden extreme anger and active • one major episode of lifting beyond one's energy • trauma or surgery to upper burner 5. Very Tense • extravasated blood in chest	1. Yielding Trapped qi • Spleen qi deficiency with distention • ruminating during meals 2. Tense Trapped heat • frequent lifting of heavy objects after eating • Liver-GB –escaped qi and heat interfere w/ Spleen-Stomach function • trauma-surgery 3. Very Tight • pancreatitis or peritonitis • Stomach fire 4. Very Tense • extravasated blood in peritoneum	1. Rare: excessive gas in intestines from obstruction: • Inflated but Slow • Bean (Spinning) with total obstruction 2. Rarer: acute episode in chronic PID, prostatitis or colitis: • mild Tight-Wiry and Rapid • usually severe Flooding Excess 3. Very Tense • extravasated blood in peritoneum

B. Uniform Qualities Bilaterally at Same Position, *cont.*

QUALITY	DISTAL POSITION	MIDDLE POSITION	PROXIMAL POSITION
Flat Qi cannot get into an organ or area in a person deficient at the time of the causative event	1. Severe disappointment when very young; event outside of awareness –loss of parent before age 8 2. Cord around neck at birth 3. Physical trauma to the chest when energy not strong 4. Improper breathing, misuse of voice 5. Mediastinal or breast tumor 6. One episode of excessive lifting by a weak person	1. Sitting position leaning forward for a long time (e.g., typists) 2. Abdominal trauma or surgery 3. Lifting frequently too soon after eating	Rare: standing in one place or walking for a long time on hard surfaces
Very Tense Qi stagnation and heat from excess, usually in strong person	1. Moderate or less recent chest trauma 2. Unresolved cold with internal heat from excess: asthma 3. Excessive use of voice by strong person for a relatively short time 4. Lifting: single extraordinary episode beyond one's energy (Very Tense)	1. Emotional stress with errant Liver qi interfering w/Spleen–Stomach function 2. Trauma and surgery w/ pain 3. Qi and food stagnation or excess cold with slight pain 4. Repeated prolonged bending 5. Physical work during or right after eating	Pain from: 1. Trauma or surgery to lower burner or pelvis 2. Overexposure to heat in lower burner, especially feet 3. 'Buddha's pulse' (sexual abstinence over a long period of time: Taut-Inflated) 4. Early stage of inflammatory condition in lower burner (more Rapid)

Table 14.1 B: Uniform Qualities Bilaterally at Same Position   **251**

B. Uniform Qualities Bilaterally at Same Position, *cont.*

QUALITY	DISTAL POSITION	MIDDLE POSITION	PROXIMAL POSITION
Tight-Wiry Diminishing yin-essence due to overwork, especially of 'nervous system' Pain Hyperactivity and infection	1. Cardiac asthma and chronic lung asthma (Rapid rate, Wiry with medication) 2. Hypertension and/or headache 3. Trauma with pain 4. Special Lung position: long-term yin deficiency 5. Cocaine abuse (Wiry) 6. Excessive emotional stress & yin depletion in upper burner, esp. shock & mania 7. Febrile disease in upper burner consumes Kidney yin, which fails to nourish Heart & Lung yin 8. Severe pain in upper burner: local tumor	Severe yin-essence deficiency: 1. Nervous tension w/ Liver qi stagnation, errant Liver qi interferes w/Stomach function 2. Hypertension or diabetes 3. Infection in area or organ, pancreatitis (Slippery) 4. Pain due to: • excessive eating (long time) • lifting too soon after eating • sitting in bent position • eating rapidly • tension while eating 5. Trauma 6. Tumor 7. Inflammation, ulcer 8. 'Running piglet disease' (rare)	1. Kidney yin deficiency & heat from deficiency 2. Infection in area or organs (e.g., colitis), especially with Rapid rate 3. Pain due to: • blood stagnation: Choppy at Pelvis/Lower Body position • qi stagnation in Intestines • kidney stones • trauma • inguinal hernia • over-exposure to cold (feet) 4. Very early diabetes or hypertension
Slippery	1. Asthma w/ damp-heat in Lungs and chest: Slippery & Rapid 2. Phlegm or phlegm-fire in Heart obstructing Heart orifices: Slippery Tense and slightly Rapid 3. Phlegm-cold disturbing orifices of Heart: Slippery Tense and Slow 4. Special Lung Position: phlegm in Lungs	1. Spleen qi deficiency: Slow rate 2. Spleen & Liver-GB damp-heat: Rapid (w/ infection of local organs: liver parasites, gallbladder, pancreas, appendix, peritoneum) 3. Ulcer: Tight Hollow and Rapid, esp. Stomach-Pylorus Ext. position 4. Stagnant food: Slippery at SPEP and especially at Esophagus position	1. Kidney stone w/ severe pain: Wiry & Rapid 2. Infection w/ colitis, enteritis, PID, prostatitis (Flooding Excess)

B. Uniform Qualities Bilaterally at Same Position, *cont.*

QUALITY	DISTAL POSITION	MIDDLE POSITION	PROXIMAL POSITION
Thin Blood deficiency	1. Blood deficiency in Heart and Lungs 2. Qi and blood deficiency (Deep Thin Feeble) 3. Heart yang deficient (Thin, Slow, Arrhythmic); yang deficient cardiac asthma 4. Heart & Lung yin and blood-deficient type asthma (Thin Tight and slightly Rapid) 5. More severe Lung yin deficiency asthma w/ obstruction of blood circulation in Lungs and Heart (Thin Wiry) 6. Heart blood deficiency & Heart, Lung phlegm 'misting the orifices' (Thin Slippery)	Prolonged Spleen qi deficiency w/ consequent Heart & Liver blood deficiency	Kidney essence-blood deficiency (bone marrow) usually due to constitution (Thin Deep Tight-Wiry and slightly Rapid)
Feeble-Absent Long-term qi deficiency in a very deficient person due to Kidney essence deficiency and very prolonged drain on qi for following reasons	1. Found later in life in those with large emotional shock in early childhood out of awareness (e.g., loss of parent) with stagnant qi due to suppressed breath from unconscious sadness. Depletion comes from attempt to overcome stagnation. 2. Physical trauma in distant past—overcoming stagnation 3. Long-term overwork of Lungs such as excessive singing or talking 4. Tuberculosis: Floating Slippery at Special Lung position (Dr. Shen)	1. Spleen qi deficiency from Kidney Essence def.; poor nutrition or irregular eating habits in childhood affecting Liver 2. Sitting in bent position for long time, possibly from sadness, especially during mealtime 3. Resuming work too soon after eating (long-term) 4. Mild anorexia, bulimia or extreme diet 5. Rumination while eating 6. Parasites 7. Liver attacks Spleen long-term	1. Constitutionally deficient Kidney qi, essence, yang affecting many systems 2. Long-term excessive sexual activity 3. Menorrhagia or chronic active or quiescent colitis

Table 14.1 B: Uniform Qualities Bilaterally at Same Position   **253**

B. Uniform Qualities Bilaterally at Same Position, *cont.*

QUALITY	DISTAL POSITION	MIDDLE POSITION	PROXIMAL POSITION
Empty Separation of yin & yang; advanced qi deficiency found with long-term conditions (in a very deficient person) or profound yin deficiency, or both	1. Extreme overwork of Lungs & Heart 2. Physical trauma to chest in very distant past 3. Emotional trauma as child, found in later years as exhaustion due to overcoming stagnation, Flat quality 4. Grief for recent loss of loved one, especially Special Lung position, lasting only for weeks or months, unless grief turns into melancholy	1. Impoverishment in childhood 2. Kidney essence deficiency fails to support Spleen 3. Sitting in bent position (e.g., secretary, sadness) very long time 4. Rumination while eating—very long time 5. Working too soon after meal—very long time 6. Trauma to abdomen a long time ago 7. Severe anorexia-bulimia (or very destructive dieting) 8. Chronic parasites 9. Pancreatic enzyme function fails 10. Drug abuse	1. Serious yin & yang deficiency in greater & lesser yin stages of six stages 2. Constitutionally deficient Kidney essence affecting many systems 3. Long-term excessive sexual activity in weak person 4. Menorrhagia for long time 5. Multiple pregnancies and deliveries 6. Chronic sub-clinical colitis for long time

Hollow
 	
1. Leather-like Hollow
  a. Rapid: imminent bleeding
  b. Slow: bleeding in recent past
 	
2. Yielding Hollow Full-Overflowing: separation of yin & yang
 	
3. Tight Hollow Full-Overflowing: heat in blood
	1. Trauma to chest with possible bleeding: Leather-like Hollow
	
	2. Lifting very far beyond one's energy (once): Yielding Hollow Full-Overflowing
		1. Bleeding in abdominal area: Leather-like Hollow
		
		2. Heavy physical labor after eating:Yielding Hollow Full-Overflowing
		
		3. Hyperacidity in Stomach: Tight Hollow; with ulcer: Slippery Tight
		
		4. Hypertension, diabetes: very Tight Hollow Full-Overflowing if also in proximal position, usually left
			1. Leather-like Hollow: acute sudden bleeding in pelvis
			
			2. Yielding Hollow Full-Overflowing:
			  a. Slow: menorrhagia
			  b. very diminished intestinal function from heavy work after eating
			
			3. Hypertension, diabetes: very Tight Hollow Full-Overflowing, especially if also found in middle position, usually left

B. Uniform Qualities Bilaterally at Same Position, *cont.*

QUALITY	DISTAL POSITION	MIDDLE POSITION	PROXIMAL POSITION

Vibration
 	
1. Smooth superficial: worry
 	
2. Rougher & deeper: serious pathology, usually organ parenchymal damage
	1. Smooth & Superficial:
	  a. Distal position: worry & anxiety; Heart qi agitation & anxiety
	  b. Neuro-psychological Position: Heart qi agitation & anxiety
	
	2. Rougher or Deeper Vibration:
	  a. Distal position:
	   • 'Heart disease'
	   • mediastinal disease (tumor)
	   • very severe trauma (rare)
	  b. Neuro-psychological position
	   • central nervous system (essence) damage
		1. Serious physical illness in abdominal area
		
		2. Severe trauma to the abdomen
			1. Serious physical illness in Kidney or pelvic area, including tumor
			
			2. Severe trauma to pelvis/ lower body area

Table 14.1 C: Similar Qualities Bilaterally at Same Position   **255**

C. Similar Qualities Bilaterally at Same Position

■ STAGNATION BETWEEN BURNERS, BILATERALLY

INFLATED BETWEEN UPPER AND MIDDLE BURNERS (DIAPHRAGM POSITION)	MUSCULOSKELETAL
1. Separation and suppression of tender feelings with anger a. Tense Inflated is more recent b. Yielding and less Inflated is less recent 2. Repeated episodes of lifting beyond one's energy using upper part of body 3. Hypertension when Liver and Heart are strong (rare) 4. Strong, sudden, unexpressed anger when Heart and Liver are both strong	Tight at radial side of area between burners Above distal position: neck Between distal and middle positions: shoulder girdle Between middle and proximal positions: hip Between proximal and Pelvis/Lower Body positions: knees

■ CHANGE IN QUALITIES, BILATERALLY

DISTAL POSITIONS	MIDDLE POSITIONS	PROXIMAL POSITIONS
1. Separation of yin and yang of Heart and Lungs: severe asthma or allergies 2. Breast tumor 3. Extreme abuse of voice or improper meditation breathing techniques 4. Mediastinal and lung tumors usually associated with excessive tobacco abuse	Neoplasms of stomach or pancreas	Neoplasms of uterus, ovaries, intestines, bladder, kidneys

■ CHANGE IN AMPLITUDE, SHIFTING FROM SIDE TO SIDE

FIRST ONE SIDE HAS IT AND THEN THE OTHER, NEVER AT THE SAME TIME

MOST COMMON	LESS COMMON
Current severe interpersonal dislocation	Recent work beyond one's energy

15

Qualities as Signs of
Psychological Disharmony

by Brandt Stickley, A.P.

THE BENEFITS OF USING Contemporary Chinese Pulse Diagnosis in the identification and management of psychological disharmony assume a number of forms. As much as the pulse itself is a medium of communication from the body to the practitioner, it may equally be employed as a means of returning the grace of that message to the patient.

As an objective mode of diagnosis, reference to the findings of the pulse avoids provoking the reactions typically classed as resistance in many psychotherapeutic paradigms. As such, it offers the practitioner a sensitive and immediate avenue into the patient's experience of the world. Additionally, the pulse quite simply offers a means of diagnosing psychological disharmonies. Of course, due to the ineffable mystery of human emotion and its myriad manifestations, these pulse qualities can be taken as signs providing direction for further exploration, but cannot be taken as the terrain itself. A quality neither guarantees certain consequences, nor does a given state guarantee the appearance of a specific pathognomonic quality. We must make allowances for the general condition of the patient as well as the influence of etiological factors in the expression of conditions and pulse qualities alike.

THE HEART AND NERVOUS SYSTEM

A word is in order regarding the relationship between Dr. Shen's concept of the 'nervous system' and the more conventional role of the Heart in consciousness. In Dr. Shen's usage, the 'nervous system' is the fastest moving and most readily affected qi of the organism, prone to influence from both internal and external pathogens. If the 'nervous system' is strong, it will divert these pernicious influences to a vulnerable organ, and cause only physical disorders that carry less social stigma than psychological ones. If the 'nervous system' is weak, a Kidney essence deficiency, the disturbance will have a more global impact on the entire organism and psychological problems may result.

The Heart is home to the spirit (*shén*), which is received from above and controls the 'mind', while the 'nervous system' is derived from the more material basis of Kidney essence. Balance between these two poles is necessary and mediated by the Triple Burner's regulating function. The Heart and the 'nervous system' may be robust or deficient; their status will affect the body's response to stressors. If the Heart is strong, stress will produce agitation as an adaptive response by alerting the mind to action. However, in its extreme form, agitation becomes anxiety, panic, and neurosis. A mildly deficient Heart and mind will be expressed in mild and transient depressions. If the condition is more tenuous and the deficiency more severe, mild psychotic states may appear, especially with the accumulation of phlegm in the Heart. With more severe psychotic states, the deficiency of Kidney essence as well as Heart qi and blood, and phlegm misting the orifices, is implicated.

If either the 'nervous system' or Heart are deficient, stress can easily induce psychological problems. The capacity to resist stress and to keep psychological function intact has obviously important benefits, especially considering the negative repercussions of mental illness in our current cultural milieu. One should not be misled by specific emotional states such as anger, depression, or mania into treating these states without first or simultaneously addressing the larger issue of the 'nervous system' and the Heart.

THE CENTRAL ROLE OF THE HEART IN HUMAN PSYCHOLOGY

The significance of the Heart in all disruptions of awareness is paramount. The tendency to associate emotions solely according to the conventional correspondences fails to recognize that the integrity of the Heart and 'nervous system' mediates any such expression. This is true primarily because of the Heart's preeminence in all aspects of awareness. Almost all psychological disorders can and must be understood in terms of awareness and communication. When there are issues with communication, the associated Fire energies of the Heart, Pericardium, Triple Burner, and Small Intestine are likewise involved.

It should be noted that all of the following psychological disturbances are maladaptive maneuvers. They are functions of Pericardium yin, the protector of the Heart, as described in *Dragon Rises, Red Bird Flies*.[1] The withdrawal of Liver yin excess, and less often the aggression of Liver yang excess and the fanaticism of Kidney qi excess, are associated with this Pericardium function.

THE PULSE: SUMMARY

The following summary focuses on the pulse signs of disturbed Heart function. Experience has shown that most psychological conditions associated with Heart function include some 'phlegm misting the Heart orifices' even when no Slippery quality is found at the left distal or Pericardium positions. It must also be kept in mind that the psychological rather than physical manifestations of stresses to the 'terrain' are a function of a vulnerable 'nervous system' ('nervous system weak', Kidney essence deficiency) condition, another aspect of Kidney-Heart disharmony.

STRESS AND SHOCK—THE LIVER AND HEART

As a general rule, emotion associated with ongoing stress is contained by the Liver (thus qi stagnation). In our time, when the Liver is so compromised by drugs and environmental toxicity, this containment is less effective and increasing amounts of calming, mind-altering substances are required with again a further diminishment of Liver function, a vicious cycle.[2]

Shock, on the other hand, affects the Heart.

The primary initial effect seems to be Heart yin deficiency, thus the traditional herbal formula Generate the Pulse Powder *(shēng mài sǎn)* that restores Heart-Lung yin. This may be a consequence of the Heart's immediate response to shock by sending blood from the periphery to vital organs, perhaps thereby depriving itself of blood-yin. Perhaps it transforms its yin into blood to meet the emergency. Most Heart conditions, qi agitation, qi and blood deficiency and stagnation, and phlegm misting the orifices, seem to begin with Heart shock. Shock in utero and at birth have the most profound lasting effects, even including all physical trauma.

MILD TO MODERATE PSYCHOLOGICAL DISORDERS

Less serious states of psychological disharmony, including anxiety, mild transient depressions, situational and habitual worry, and irritability, are associated with varying degrees of 'Heart qi agitation' characterized by Smooth Vibration over the entire pulse; occasional Changes in Rate at Rest; a Rapid rate; Tight at the Pericardium position; Tight and occasionally Slippery at the left distal position; and Smooth Vibration at the Neuro-psychological positions. The Muffled quality at the left distal position is a sign of depression and a 'closed' Heart with emotional withdrawal, associated with a loss of joy in life and with heart-felt hurt and pain. This is often accompanied by an inflated left diaphragm position, discussed later in this chapter, where the softer tender emotions are replaced by harsher angry ones in response to hostile interpersonal separations.

Impaired memory, poor concentration and attention, and one type of insomnia are associated with Heart blood deficiency. This is attended with a Thin quality at the left distal position and/or an increase in rate on exertion of greater than 20 beats per minute.

Heart yin deficiency is characterized by a more severe form of restlessness and agitation and is accompanied by very Tight qualities at the left distal position. A Hesitant Wave is also a sign of a moderate Heart yin deficiency associated with obsessive thinking and compulsive behavior.

While the ongoing stress associated with the 'nervous system tense' condition primarily affects the Liver, the consequent excess of stagnant qi or heat in the Liver often affects the Heart, attended by palpitations at rest, Tightness at the Pericardium position, and extreme Tenseness at the left distal position.

Severe psychological disorders

More serious and less transient mental and emotional problems are associated with Rough Vibration over the entire pulse (associated with Heart Shock, terror, and guilt); the Bean (Spinning) quality (associated with terror); and moderate to severe Slipperiness at the left distal position (phlegm misting the orifices). In mental-emotional disorders, it is often necessary to address phlegm misting the Heart orifices even in the absence of the Slippery quality. Slipperiness at the Mitral Valve position is a sign of panic and phobia disorders associated with a Mitral Valve prolapse.

Very severe psychological disorders

'Qi wild': disrupted circulation, separation of yin and yang in the entire organism

The Yielding Hollow Full-Overflowing quality, along with constant Changes in Quality over the entire pulse, suggest a 'qi wild' state with pervasive 'separation of yin and yang' and chaotic circulation. The Yielding Hollow Full-Overflowing quality with a Rapid rate is associated with depersonalization and dissociated states of consciousness, and severe anxiety and panic associated with impaired Heart qi-yang and blood. Signs of severe Heart dysfunction, such as the arrhythmic Intermittent and Interrupted qualities, are also often identified with severe mental and emotional disturbance.

Separation of Heart yin and yang

Chaos and instability in Heart function can be associated with a variety of severe mental and emotional disturbances evidenced by pulse qualities such as Interrupted and Intermittent rhythms, Unstable, Change in Qualities, Empty (rare), or Bean (Spinning), often accompanied by the Slippery quality and all found at the left distal position.

Pathogenic influences

Pathogenic influences such as phlegm and fire, as well as chaos, are associated with the most severe and overwhelming disruptions of the Heart and mind including severe depression, mania, psychosis, and schizophrenia. All of these conditions usually present with an intense Slippery quality at the left distal position.

NEGATIVE EMOTIONAL STATES

Negative emotion primarily affects the most vulnerable organ, and only secondarily seems to influence the organ associated with the conventional five phase correspondences. It is noteworthy that the suppression or repression of emotions is largely what creates pathology. Other variables, such as positive life experiences and a relatively robust body condition (terrain), may often mitigate the pathological impact of negative emotion.

GRIEF, MELANCHOLIA, ANGUISH, AND SADNESS

A distinction is made between grief and melancholia, both in duration and intensity. Grief is self-limiting and naturally attends the experience of loss, while melancholia is grief that persists for a long time and beyond its natural function.

Recent grief and anguish

Dr. Hammer has observed Empty Special Lung positions to be found shortly after profound loss. The Split quality may also be noted if death is involved with the loss.

Long-term unexpressed grief and anguish

Sadness experienced early in life that is unexpressed most often affects the upper burner, presenting with a bilaterally Flat distal position, reflecting the inability of qi to enter into the Heart, and possibly Feeble much later in life, reflecting depletion due to the attempt of the qi to enter into the Heart.

Melancholia

Inflated and Muffled qualities found bilaterally in the distal positions, or one or the other, may suggest prolonged grief or melancholia. Kidney qi deficiency sapping the potential to move beyond grief would be expressed with a Deep and/or Feeble-Absent quality in the proximal positions.

Grief associated with a past loss later in life

Here the body condition at the time of the loss will affect the pulse picture. In a vulnerable individual or very young person, a Flat quality may be found at the distal positions. In a more robust person and an older person, the quality would be Inflated Yielding.

Depression

The 'nervous system' is developed and sustained by Kidney essence. Most of the depressions under discussion have their roots in failures of Kidney essence, which may be either genetic, intrauterine, or very early life insults in origin, such as birth trauma or prematurity. They have been described in lucid detail in *Dragon Rises, Red Bird Flies*. The contribution of Kidney essence may be differentiated in its yin, yang, and qi aspects. Kidney yin gives the 'life' (substance) to the life force; Kidney yang gives the 'force' (power) to the life force, and Kidney qi is the blend of the two into the 'balanced function' of the life force. If Kidney essence—just now described as the life, force, and function—is adequate, depression is a more remote scenario. If, however, Kidney essence is inadequate, the incidence of all types of depression increases, as described below.

When the life force drives one's development into progressive evolutionary stages where the encounter of significant obstacles will become the scene of a powerful struggle in which a person might feel "If I cannot be myself, I will be nothing," depression and suicide can be the outcomes of the accompanying great emotional pain. It is a monumental paradox that we find, in depression, "the stronger the 'life-force' the greater the pain and the risk of an individual taking their own life."[3]

Endogenous depression

Whether due to nature (genetics, intrauterine, or very early life events) or nurture (post partum), the principal deficit that governs the expression of the most enduring and profound depressions is that of Kidney essence. Depression with these etiologies is characterized by the apparent absence of precipitating events and the inability to sustain will and drive in the face of defeat or despair. Endogenous depression is the black hole of despair.

Pulse
The proximal position reflects the state of the Kidneys, and deficiency of yin and/or yang essence can manifest on either side or even on both at the same time.

Kidney qi and yang-essence deficiency in the proximal positions may be shown by Deep, Feeble-Absent, very Reduced Substance and/or very Reduced Pounding, Diffuse, Empty, and very large Change of Amplitude or Qualities. This is the most common cause of endogenous depression characterized by fatigue, psychomotor retardation, lassitude, and severe emotional pain. The substance (yin-essence) is present but the drive is absent.

In the less common case of endogenous depression due to yin-essence deficiency, agitation predominates, and the Wiry quality is present in the proximal positions.

OTHER FORMS OF DEPRESSION DESCRIBED IN
Dragon Rises, Red Bird Flies

Primary anaclytic[4] depression

Resulting from lack of maternal bonding, occurring by definition in infancy, this condition leads to extreme disruption of Heart function with qualities such as arrhythmic Interrupted, Intermittent, Yielding Hollow Interrupted, or Yielding Hollow Intermittent.

Cyclothymic depression

Associated with inconsistent maternal bonding, one finds that a large occasional Change in Rate at Rest with a Normal or Slow rate suggests this condition. These people are subject to extreme mood swings (now identified as borderline personality).

Agitated depression

With agitated forms of depression, often found with Liver qi stagnation (due to excess or deficiency), there will be evidence of suppressed emotion (impotent rage) such as a Tense and Robust Pounding left middle position and mild Liver fire that moves to the Heart. Mild Heart fire from this etiology is reflected in a Tight Pericardium and later a Tense and Robust Pounding quality at the left distal position, sometimes accompanied by palpations at rest. A Slippery quality will occur as phlegm is congealed from dampness in the attempt to cool the fire. Phlegm misting the orifices is a consequence attending some of the most severe mental illness, including schizophrenia and mania, and almost always neurosis.

Yin-deficient heat due to yin deficiency, evidenced by a Tight left distal position, presents with restlessness that is increased by deficiency of the Kidneys (demonstrated by a Tight-Wiry proximal position).

Hysterical or reactive depression

This person wears their 'heart on their sleeve' and is constantly in and out of love and relationships. The Pericardium position is Tight and possibly Slippery in this condition, with a small, occasional Change in Rate at Rest. The pulse picture changes depending on the patient's mental phase and overall condition. During the depressive phase, either the Flat or the Inflated quality appears at the left distal position, representing in both cases Heart qi stagnation. With the Flat quality, the patient is more vulnerable and disposed toward jealousy, envy, and spite. The more robust individual with the Inflated quality will be prone to anger. During the euphoric phase there may be Smooth Vibration as the patient worries about an inevitable rejection by others that may be a self-fulfilling prophecy.

Dysphoric depression (lack of joy) without fatigue

MUFFLED AT LEFT DISTAL OR OVER ENTIRE PULSE   Increasingly, the most common sign of a lack of joy is the Muffled quality at the left distal position. While the Muffled quality over the entire pulse alerts one to a possible neoplastic process, it can also indicate a great lack of joy that, at its extreme, is suffocating the entire organism.

FLAT   The mildly Flat quality bilaterally at the distal positions signifies chest qi stagnation, both Heart and Lung qi stagnation, and mild Heart blood stagnation.

The Flat quality may be due to an early loss or an often forgotten disappointment that occurred at a time when the individual was young, vulnerable, and deficient.

Sudden bad news or rejected love may be represented with a persistent Flat quality that suggests ongoing vengeance and spite, and unhappiness even when in 'love'.

Delivery with the umbilical cord wrapped around the neck will cause a Flat quality, often bilaterally, and generally has more severe consequences, including constant emotional difficulty, increased vengefulness and spite, fearfulness, and shooting chest pain. A blue-green color seen around the mouth is a corroborating sign. (The Flat quality at these positions could also be due to an early physical shock to the chest.)

INFLATED   Found at the left distal position, this quality signifies loss or chronic disappointment in love at a time when the organ qi was more mature. With the withdrawal of Heart feelings, and a tendency to quick anger, this individual will likewise be unhappy even when in a relationship. The Inflated quality at the left distal or bilaterally at both distal positions can also attend a single episode of great, unexpressed anger and the person becomes prone to quick anger. Sometimes the Inflation is also found at the Diaphragm positions, and even into the middle positions with extreme repressed rage.

Lack of joy with fatigue (including post-partum depression)

Thin or a Change in Rate on exertion in excess of about 20 beats per minute suggests Heart blood deficiency. Other symptoms include waking after four to five hours of sleep, and may derive from the classic scenario in which Spleen qi deficiency accompanies the Heart blood deficiency.

With Heart qi deficiency, the depressions are more profound, with a greater degree of psychomotor retardation. Signs of Heart qi deficiency at the left distal position include the Feeble-Absent, Change in Qualities or Amplitude (which is less serious), and Empty characteristics. There may be a Slippery or Vibration quality at the Mitral Valve position. The entire pulse may exhibit Change in Amplitude; in addition, the rate on exertion may rise slightly or remain the same.

(See phlegm misting the orifices, discussed above.)

Post-partum depression

Signs of qi and blood deficiency attend the profound loss of these substances through pregnancy and childbirth, especially in the absence of the nourishing safeguards (e.g., herbs) more common to traditional cultures.

Involutional depression

Intra-individual failure and loneliness in middle and old age are often associated with midlife crisis and represents a failure to individuate, including grieving for oneself, despair, and depression of the soul and spirit. A number of qualities indicate the extent of the effect on the individual including Muffled at the left distal position, commonly associated with lack of joy, and Empty at the left middle position.

A common scenario of suppressed emotion and resignation to a life of "quiet desperation" is demonstrated by the Cotton quality over the entire pulse, and can accompany a midlife depression.

At the later stages of an unresolved midlife crisis, Heart blood stagnation ('Heart small') can appear. A Flat quality, or Deep with Rough Vibration or Choppy, suggests this more advanced condition of blood stagnation associated with lifelong fear and coronary artery disease, which may be seen with men's heart attacks.

Post-chemical intoxication, post-hepatitis, or post-mononucleosis depression

The use of cold-natured drugs (like marijuana) or a history of hepatitis or mononucleosis can produce an inability to implement plans into action, leading to another type of midlife depression. An Empty quality ('separation of yin and yang') at the left middle position indicates functional chaos of the Liver and is often found in the later stages of this process. The Liver not only moves the qi, it also contains it. Impulse control is lost with this profound Liver yang deficiency and 'separation of yin and yang', with the obvious consequences.

Depression associated with a severe 'qi wild' condition

Depression is the late development stage of the anxiety, panic, and dissociation that attend having over-exercised beyond one's energy, either over a long period (Slow rate) or having then suddenly ceased such activity (Rapid rate). In either case, the Yielding Hollow Full-Overflowing or Yielding Ropy qualities demonstrate a 'separation of yin and yang'.[5]

CONDITIONS AND QUALITIES PATHOGNOMONIC OF ANXIETY

Heart qi agitation

Dr. Hammer, in collaboration with Dr. Shen, has documented the potential progression of Heart qi agitation from mild to more serious forms. There is usually a background of Heart shock and Kidney-Heart disharmony, and a progression of the symptoms. Facial color—blue at the chin if intrauterine, mouth if at birth, throughout the face or at the temples later in life—can be used to determine the onset and severity of this shock.

Smooth Vibration

Found at the qi depth, or limited to the left distal position, a Smooth Vibration quality suggests worry and is the mildest form of Heart qi agitation. As the condition worsens it can spread gradually to the entire pulse, at which time we have a person who will, even if there is nothing to worry about, find something. The rate at rest is generally stable.

With Heart qi deficiency, a Rapid, consistently elevated rate is a possible indicator of recent Heart shock and qi agitation, and, in our time, is a more common etiology than excess heat. Over time the rate will slow as Heart qi diminishes. Even then a small stress may be attended by a temporary but extreme elevation in rate. Anxiety, irritability, and worry are the emotional symptoms associated with this degree of Heart qi agitation.

OCCASIONAL CHANGE IN RATE AT REST   This quality is associated with a form of Heart qi agitation characterized by considerable instability in relationships, in thinking, concentration, focus, moods, and behavior that fit the once popular characterization of a 'grasshopper mind'. While the immediate etiology could be shock to the Heart or prolonged periods of worry, my experience indicates that the original insult was in utero or early in life and involves the Kidney essence deficiency 'nervous system weak' condition. Other symptoms of Heart qi agitation include a sleep pattern of frequent waking, anxiety, and palpitations with exertion. This is one form of Kidney-Heart disharmony.

Excess heat in the Heart

LEFT DISTAL POSITION TENSE WITH ROBUST POUNDING, OR PERICARDIUM TIGHT   Tightness in the Pericardium (in the middle of the left distal position) is felt as a sharp sensation, like a pencil point hitting one's finger. This is a sign of excess heat in the Heart, usually derived from Stomach or Liver heat ('nervous system tense') or overwork of the Heart in the face of chronic worry. With increases of excess heat uncontained by the Pericardium, the entire left distal position will be Tense with Robust Pounding. Symptoms include mild angina spasms, shortness of breath when anxious, palpitations with exertion, flushing and heat in the face, irritability, and being easily angered.

Heart yin deficiency

TIGHT LEFT DISTAL POSITION   This is a sign of Heart yin deficiency. The primary symptoms are nervousness and agitation with moderate to intense stress;

easily awakened from light sleep yet also able to quickly return to sleep, tossing and turning and therefore tending to be up and down all night; often a little tired in the morning; and some difficulty in focusing one's thoughts and actions. This condition can derive from a shock affecting the Heart, prolonged tension, or prolonged worry, all of which represent overwork of the Heart that drains its yin. More severe obsessive thinking and behavior is expressed on the pulse with a Hesitant Wave.

Heart blood deficiency ('Heart weak')

This is primarily a condition of Heart blood, with some element of Heart qi deficiency. Sleep is steady for a few hours, with early morning waking, no difficulty returning to sleep, and excessive dreaming. Symptoms include anxiety and some depression; impairment of memory, concentration, and attention; frequent tiredness in the morning (less so than with Heart qi deficiency); being easily startled; a roller coaster feeling and lack of focus (less than with Change of Rate at Rest); and unsettling palpitations upon mild to moderate exertion. There will be mild numbness and coldness in the extremities, and fatigue even without exertion, related to the disrupted sleep. Heart blood deficiency can derive from multiple causes, including excessive worry over a long period of time, Kidney essence deficiency, Spleen qi deficiency, chronic disease, excessive gradual blood loss over time, prolonged Heart qi agitation, and constitutional weakness.

THIN LEFT DISTAL POSITION; INCREASE IN RATE >20 BEATS/MINUTE The Thin quality at the left distal position represents greater Heart blood deficiency than the increase of rate on exertion greater than 20 beats/minute that likely will also be found. Greater increases of rate indicate a greater degree of blood deficiency.

THIN OVER ENTIRE PULSE When blood deficiency is more global, the entire pulse will be Thin, Thin and Feeble (with qi deficiency), or Thin and Tight (with yin deficiency), accompanied by symptoms of deficiency associated with other organs. (See discussion in Ch. 10 under Narrow Pulse Group – Thin.) Symptoms of diminished memory, focus, and concentration, characteristic of Heart blood deficiency, will manifest.

Heart qi deficiency

FEEBLE-ABSENT LEFT DISTAL POSITION This sign of significant qi deficiency suggests a susceptibility to anxiety and emotional fragility.

CONSTANT LARGE CHANGE IN AMPLITUDE OVER ENTIRE PULSE This is also an indicator of Heart qi deficiency. Symptoms include fatigue in the morning, emotional instability and easily becoming anxious, cold hands and feet, and migrating pains.

YIELDING HOLLOW FULL-OVERFLOWING   This quality may be accompanied by a Slow rate if due to prolonged work and/or exercise beyond one's ability and chronic fatigue, or by a Rapid rate if associated with the sudden cessation of long-term excessive exercise. Symptoms of sudden stopping include profound anxiety, depersonalization, dissociative experiences, and a tendency to explosive anger. Over time, severe physical deterioration is another sequellae too varied to characterize generally.

SLOW   Contrary to popular opinion, the Slow pulse rate associated with aerobic exercise is not a favorable condition and is a sign of Heart qi deficiency. Exercise temporarily ameliorates the lethargy and depression associated with diminished Heart function through increased circulation, but ultimately depletes it further, requiring increasing amounts to produce the same effect.

CHANGE IN QUALITIES AND CHANGES IN AMPLITUDE AT THE LEFT DISTAL POSITION   These are signs of the 'separation of Heart yin and yang' and more serious signs of Heart qi and/or yin deficiency, suggesting a greater instability. Change in Qualities is the much more serious sign of functional chaos.

SLIPPERY AND ROUGH VIBRATION AT MITRAL VALVE POSITION   Phobia, anxiety, and panic are associated with valvular prolapse and insufficiency. The Slippery quality indicates a more severe condition and the rough Vibration quality much less so. Both qualities suggest Heart qi and possibly blood deficiency. Findings here as well as elsewhere in this pulse system are often early signs of disharmony not yet detectable by biomedical methodology.

ARRYTHMIC QUALITIES   Although often overshadowed by a significant associated physical cardiac condition, the Intermittent and Interrupted qualities render one prone to anxiety, emotional fragility, and instability. Because the Heart controls the mind, chaotic Heart qi is not conducive to a quiet or even functioning mind.

Heart-Gallbladder deficiency

Symptoms include dizziness, blurred vision, timidity, palpitations, sighing, excessive dreams, being easily startled, and a quick temper. These symptoms may derive from the depletion of Heart qi due to excess in the Gallbladder according to the law of midday-midnight. The Gallbladder divergent channel passes through the Heart.

The left distal pulse position is Deep and Thin, the right middle position Feeble, the Stomach-Pylorus Extension position Slippery-Hollow, and the Gallbladder position is Tense and Slippery with Robust Pounding. (Spleen qi deficiency and Spleen damp-heat and Gallbladder damp-heat are almost always found together clinically.) The tongue has a yellow-white, moderately thick coating, especially in the vertical line if it exists.

WORRY

Consistent and excessive thinking while eating, including worry or academic ru-minations, drains the Spleen-Stomach. However, the principal impact is on the Heart, which controls the mind. With regard to thought, the Spleen-Stomach qi's function is to serve the Heart in terms of short-term memory, as with cram-ming for examinations whose information is quickly forgotten.

SMOOTH VIBRATION   Smooth Vibration is a reliable sign of worry that can be precisely interpreted based on its extent and location. At the left distal position, it as an early sign of worry, which over time can affect the whole left side of the pulse. At the qi depth it indicates transient worry, while at all depths it suggests a propensity to worry even in the absence of precipitating events. At the Neuro-psychological position the Smooth Vibration quality is associated with symp-toms of Heart qi agitation including anxiety and prolonged worry.

TIGHT AT PERICARDIUM POSITION, TENSE AT LEFT DISTAL POSITION   These are signs of profound worry over a longer period of time and reflect the effect that excess heat can work upon the Heart. This heat is a response to either over-working of the Heart or to the heat that accumulates when the attempt to over-come Heart qi and or blood stagnation fails.

OCCASIONAL CHANGE IN RATE AT REST   Change in Rate at Rest, at first oc-casional and later constant, demonstrates the progressive impact of worry and mild Heart shock.

FEAR AND TERROR

Dr. Hammer defines fear as the emotion that is signaled by the fundamental unknowns of our existence, such as all the great developmental transitions and transformations between birth and death. Fear and faith are two sides of a coin mediated by the water phase.[6]

Profound guilt and fear

CONSISTENT ROUGH VIBRATION OVER THE ENTIRE PULSE AT ALL DEPTHS
The Rough Vibration quality is indicative of severe Heart shock, guilt, and fear and can occur in those who have been party to rape, childhood sexual abuse, or other experiences of terror, either as perpetrator or victim.

BEAN (SPINNING)   The Bean (Spinning) quality at the left distal position is usually accompanied by severe Heart shock and terror. It is a more severe sign of this condition than Rough Vibration over the entire pulse.

'QI WILD' QUALITIES   The chaos of these pulses may be related to terror. These qualities include Empty, Yielding Hollow Full-Overflowing, Interrupted-Intermittent Yielding Hollow, and Change in Qualities. The Interrupted-Intermittent Yielding Hollow Full-Overflowing pulse represents the greatest instability.

Roller-coaster feeling

As mentioned above, signs of Heart qi agitation such as occasional Change in Rate at Rest suggest an unstable Heart and therefore an unstable mind. The mind races and thinking becomes capricious; there is confusion and a breakdown in the orderly conduct of life—this is the roller-coaster feeling and existence.

Post-traumatic stress disorder

Signs of acute stress and danger include a Rapid Bounding rate, a Change in Rate at Rest, a Tight Robust Pounding quality at the left distal position, Rough Vibration over the entire pulse, and even the Bean (Spinning) quality at the left distal position. In less acutely stressful and dangerous conditions, the Empty quality over the entire pulse is a marker of the instability and chaos of a temporary PTD that may disappear when the crisis is over.

Vengefulness and spite

Symptoms of Heart qi stagnation, associated with the Flat or even Inflated quality at the left distal position, reflect a tendency to vengefulness and spite.

Paranoid personality

Pulse signs associated with the paranoid personality may include signs of 'nervous system tense', such as a uniformly Tense quality over the entire pulse, and more importantly, Thin, Tight qualities at the qi depth. Paranoid personalities are highly organized to be defensive rather than directed toward enhancing relationships. This is because they expect, based on life experience, the worst rather than the best from human relations.

Psychosis, schizophrenia, and dissociated mental states involving boundaries

All of the signs mentioned above that are associated with instability, such as the 'qi wild' (Empty, Yielding Hollow-Full-Overflowing), 'circulation out of control' conditions (arrhythmias), and 'nervous system weak', are implicated. Severe disorganization, anxiety, terror, hallucinations, delusions, paranoia, depersonalization, and dissociation are some of the symptoms of the inner chaos associated with a defect in boundary delineations between the internal and external environments.

I have found that 'phlegm misting the orifices' is a key element in the cause and resolution of almost all severe mental-emotional conditions.

STAGNATION IN THE MIDDLE BURNER

Qi, food, and phlegm stagnation in the middle burner can result in different degrees of a consistency of symptoms that we describe as psychotic or as a loss of touch with reality.[7] As always with psychosis, a 'nervous system weak' condition may be implicated.

Qi stagnation

The pulse signs of qi stagnation in the middle burner are the Muffled, Tense, and Robust Pounding qualities in both middle positions, with changing degrees in both qualities depending on the amount of stress that the individual is experiencing. The symptoms of mental instability vary a great deal with the daily fluctuations in stress.

Food stagnation

The Esophageal position is Slippery or rough, and the middle positions, Stomach Pyloric Extension position, and Intestine positions are particularly Tense and Inflated with Robust Pounding.

Phlegm stagnation

Stagnant dampness (from Spleen qi deficiency or poor digestive habits, and Gallbladder damp-heat) accumulates and combines with excessive heat from Liver qi stagnation and/or Stomach heat to create phlegm. This phlegm goes to the Heart where it 'mists the orifices'. The psychotic symptoms associated with phlegm stagnation are more persistent.

The associated pulse qualities are Tense and Robust Pounding at both middle positions and the Stomach Pyloric Extension position (SPEP), as well as a great deal of Slipperiness at the Stomach Pyloric Extension and Intestine positions (and possibly some at the right middle position).

Phlegm-fire in the Heart

The left distal position is Tense-Tight and Slippery with Robust Pounding, the left middle position is Tense with Robust Pounding, the right middle position constantly changing from Tense and Robust Pounding to Feeble or Empty, and the right distal position is Feeble and/or Slippery.

Phlegm-cold in the Heart

The left distal position is Feeble and Slippery, the right middle is Feeble or Empty, the right distal may be Feeble. The lack of heat from the Liver is notable and the psychological symptoms are of a more quiescent nature, such as depression. This 'cold' is akin to yang deficiency and not external cold.

BIPOLAR DISEASE

During the manic phase, Liver fire is being transmitted to the Heart. The left middle position is Hollow Full-Overflowing with Robust Pounding and the left distal position is Tense to Tight with Robust Pounding and may also be Slippery.

The proximal positions will be Tight, especially the left proximal position, which will become Wiry due to the ongoing depletion of the water-essence of the Kidneys attempting to control the Liver-Heart fire.

In the depressive phase, after the 'wood' is burned, the qualities reflect deficiency. At the left distal position, Feeble-Absent, Change in Qualities or Amplitude, and Rough Vibration (indicating parenchymal damage) suggest Heart qi deficiency, while a Slippery quality is a sign of phlegm misting the orifices. The left middle position shows a Reduced Substance or possibly Empty quality, indicating qi deficiency. The left proximal position is usually Tight-Wiry.

This presentation reflects the interaction between the spheres of wood, fire, and water energies as mediated by the thermostat of the Triple Burner. The reader is directed to *Dragon Rises, Red Bird Flies*[8,9] for a fuller treatment of this pathogenesis. The disorder in the Triple Burner is manifested by less similarity in qualities at different positions, especially at the same burner.

'QI WILD'

The following pulse qualities meet the criteria of 'qi wild' provided they appear over the entire pulse at all or almost all positions. They include the Empty, Leather-Empty, Empty and Thread-like, Scattered, Minute, Yielding Hollow Full-Overflowing, Yielding Ropy, Change in Qualities, and the Yielding Hollow Full-Overflowing Interrupted and Yielding Hollow Full-Overflowing Intermittent qualities.

Patients will complain of emotional fragility, labile emotions, severe anxiety, quick temper, feelings of being 'spaced out', losing one's mind, and being out of control. Terrifying dissociated states may occur. In addition, they are easily fatigued and suffer extreme tiredness and migrating pains. The mental and emotional symptoms are particularly severe if the 'nervous system' is already weak. The result is physiological chaos and severely impaired function.

TENSION

Liver qi stagnation

TAUT OR TENSE AT LEFT MIDDLE POSITION   The Taut and Tense qualities are the most common signs of Liver qi stagnation. The Taut quality is the milder of the two. Robust Pounding is found as the condition worsens.

OCCASIONAL CHANGE IN AMPLITUDE OVER THE ENTIRE PULSE   The occasional Change in Amplitude can be due to stress affecting the Liver. The change will be more obvious when energy is reduced or if the stress level is raised.

'NERVOUS SYSTEM'

Throughout life, Kidney essence is a primary source of sustenance to the 'nervous system' (marrow).

'Nervous system tense' [10]

Dr. Hammer considers this pulse quality to be reflective of a state of vigilance, and regards it as a sign of a survival mechanism for certain people who are in a constant state of alertness against danger and therefore more likely to survive.

Symptoms of the constitutional variety include an ongoing tension unrelated to any particular current externally-generated life stress. It is commonly found in minorities that successfully survived persecution over a long period of time.

The organ most affected by this tension and generally by stress is the Liver, whose containment function is called upon to control emotions that might otherwise interfere with vigilance. Accompanying symptoms will depend on the vulnerability of other organ systems affected by excess heat in the Liver, a consequence of the qi stagnation associated with containment, especially the Heart (palpitations-agitation) and the Stomach (regurgitation-constipation). Ultimately, Liver qi deficiency is a consequence of enduring this condition over a long period of time.

Symptoms associated with 'nervous system tense' due to both types of conditions include enduring tension, mild flushing, intolerance of heat, hypertension, headache, dryness of eyes, thirst which is easily quenched, tendency to constipation, difficulty getting to sleep, ready perspiration, and eczema.

The principal pulse signs in both cases are the Tight and Thin qualities at the qi depth, and a uniformly very Tense quality over the entire pulse, often with Robust Pounding. With the constitutional type the pulse is Slower, and with the environmentally-related type, the pulse is more Rapid.

Intervention with the environmentally-related 'nervous system tense' condition can reduce the Tense and Robust Pounding qualities as well as the other tension symptoms, but intervention with the constitutional type can only reduce the symptoms and other physiological consequences of ongoing excess heat, but not change the pulse.

'Nervous system' affects 'organ system'

Over time, the 'nervous system' can affect the 'organ system.' Early symptoms include agitation, irritability, easily excitable, and the subsequent fatigue that may alternate with and then accompany the tense agitation. The pulse on the left side is only slightly Deep, but in the early stages there is a very Thin and Tight line at the qi depth on the left side.

'Nervous system weak'

'Nervous system weak' is primarily a Kidney essence deficiency condition though extraordinary events in early life, such as the anaclytic one in which an infant is essentially abandoned and/or nutritionally deprived, can create a similar condition.

The 'nervous system weak' person is vulnerable, easily disturbed, and unstable from childhood, at which time they were sickly, fragile, and physically unable to keep up with their peers. These symptoms can persist throughout life, along with continuously changing symptoms, needs, and persistent fatigue. In the past it was called neurasthenia in a person who had rapidly changing symptoms that were unsubstantiated by medical diagnostics.[11]

The pulse picture varies from early in childhood when it is described by Dr. Shen as superficial and Tight with a Rapid rate, to the mid-adult stage when Dr. Hammer finds extensive Smooth Vibration, the left side Deep, Feeble moving to Empty, especially at the proximal positions. In the late adult stage there are increasing signs of a 'qi wild' condition with Change in Qualities, especially on the left side and the proximal positions.

The left side of the pulse is Deeper, with Reduced Substance and Thinness, becoming Feeble-Absent, while retaining a Tight quality at the qi depth. There may also be Change of Qualities and Amplitude at the proximal positions, suggesting a separation of Kidney yin and yang.

Anger

Sudden anger: trapped qi in the Heart

The qualities associated with sudden, great, unexpressed anger tend to manifest mostly on the left distal, Diaphragm, and middle positions with a very Inflated quality. The more recent the sudden anger, the more pronounced the Inflated quality. On several occasions, Dr. Hammer observed the Inflation occupy most of the pulse.

Sudden, great, unexpressed anger that occurs when one is active causes the left distal position to be very Inflated. If it occurs when one is quiet, it will cause a very Inflated quality in the left middle position, and if it occurs while eating, it will produce a very Inflated quality in the right middle position.

Propensity to anger: trapped qi in the Heart

The Inflated Yielding pulse at the left distal position, sometimes in both distal positions and even at the Special Lung position, is a sign of trapped qi in the Heart, often beginning with a breech presentation at birth. The consequences are being quick to anger, lifelong fatigue, and bodily discomfort, with difficulty lying on one's left side.

Gradually developing anger, repression, and passive-aggressive behavior

The qualities associated with gradually developing repressed anger and frustration are Taut, Tense, and, much later, Tight, especially at the left middle position.

Poor impulse control

As noted above, the Liver is the master of qi, both in moving and containing it. With the increasing incidence of Liver qi-yang deficiency, largely due to the ubiquitous use of recreational substances, the cold herbs marijuana, LSD, and heroin, the Liver is failing to contain, acting on impulse, strangely offset somewhat by the simultaneous inability to move qi.

Here the left middle position exhibits one or another of the 'separation of yin and yang' qualities such as the Empty and Change in Qualities.

Explosiveness and impotent rage

The individual flies into a violent rage at the least provocation. Complicating the more traditional factors involved in explosive rage is the poor impulse control, attributable to Liver qi-yang deficiency. Those other factors are the degree of impotence that the person feels prior to the outburst, and the stability of his mind and nervous system. With regard to the stability of the mind, we are concerned with Heart qi agitation, trapped qi in the Heart, and especially with phlegm in the Heart (represented by the general Change in Rate at Rest and the Tense Inflated Robust Pounding Slippery quality at the left distal position). With regard to the 'nervous system', we are concerned with the basic integrity of Kidney essence (proximal positions may be both Tight-Wiry and Feeble) and with Liver qi stagnation transforming into Liver fire and wind (Tense Inflated Robust Pounding qualities at the left middle position, and possibly a Floating Tight quality above the left middle position, on the left side, or over the entire pulse). As with bipolar disease, Dr. Hammer finds the consistency of the thermostatic and homeostatic functions of the Triple Burner to be an essential factor in maintaining emotional balance.

A 'separation of the yin and yang' of the 'circulatory system' with the presence of the Yielding Hollow Full-Overflowing Rapid rate is attended by uncontrollable anger. People with trapped qi in the Heart are prone to anger and explosive rage throughout their lives, presumably expressed when some of the trapped qi suddenly escapes.

Separation and divorce

INFLATED AT DIAPHRAGM POSITIONS   The greatly Inflated quality at the left Diaphragm position is usually associated with a separation in which one's tender feelings are suppressed and replaced by anger, in the service of making the transformation emotionally possible. Inflation related to this reason can occur at both Diaphragm positions if it is severe, though Inflation at the right Diaphragm position is a sign of lifting beyond one's energy.

INDECISION

The Empty quality at the left middle position is associated with insults to the Liver, such as from excessive marijuana use, that renders the drive to execute plans inoperable.

Indecision can affect the Gallbladder and cause signs of pathology, including the Tight Robust Pounding, Choppy, Wiry, Muffled, Slippery, or Change in Amplitude qualities at the Gallbladder position.

Instability of the Heart causing a state of constant doubt of oneself will likewise make decisive action difficult. The occasional Change in Rate at Rest associated with what used to be called the 'grasshopper mind' is a related finding.

RESIGNATION

COTTON (RESIGNATION)   This 'sad pulse' (Dr. Shen's term) is a sign of hopelessness and helplessness in the face of adversity that Dr. Hammer calls the 'resignation pulse'. The person feels resigned to circumstances he believes to be beyond his control, and may have a tendency to blame others. It is a sign of superficial qi stagnation ('stuckness'), sometimes due to a lack of will associated with Kidney qi-essence deficiency (reflected by Deep, Feeble-Absent proximal positions). Henry David Thoreau expressed this best when he said "Most men lead lives of quiet desperation and go to the grave with the song still in them." (See also Chs. 9 and 13.)

OBSESSIVE THINKING (RUMINATION)

The Hesitant quality is associated with overwork of the mind tinged by worry (mild Heart yin deficiency), often derived from a sustained preoccupation and rumination on a single subject, often the patient's health. In its mildest form it suggests mild perfectionism, and in its highest, debilitating obsessive-compulsive behaviors. The left distal position may be Tight.

As noted earlier, obsessive thinking is a form of excess that depletes the Spleen qi if it occurs while eating. The associated clouding of consciousness is partly due to the accumulation of fluids owing to deficiency of the Spleen qi, which inhibits the rising of clear Spleen qi to the brain. Perhaps more important is the accumulation of these fluids in the Heart and 'misting of the orifices' that especially interferes with clear consciousness.

OBSESSED WITH DEATH

Beginning with the observation by Efrem Korngold in the mid-1990s of a Split pulse on the right side in a patient with brain cancer and six months to live, we have been observing this quality, especially in the left middle position, in people preoccupied with death. This has included concern about their own deaths or that of people about whom they care. It has also occurred with increasing frequency in people contemplating suicide. Recently we had two patients with undiagnosed cancer whose entire left side was Split.[12]

OBFUSCATION

People can manipulate their pulse to confuse the examiner in a variety of ways for short periods of time. In one of Dr. Hammer's cases,[13] the sensations under his fingers were constantly changing until it occurred to him that this was happening to mislead him. When this possibility was conveyed to the patient she said that she did not want him to know about her suicidal thoughts.

WITHDRAWAL AND THE DEEP QUALITY

It is possible for patients to present with a Deep quality over the entire pulse that may or may not persist, and is not a sign of severe qi deficiency. This indicates a pattern of emotional withdrawal when faced with stress; it is reversible, in Dr. Hammer's experience, with acupuncture used to raise the qi.

DENIAL AND THE EMPTY QUALITY

The Empty quality has been observed in those who mobilize all of their energy to the surface in the interest of presenting an acceptable face to the world, even in the midst of considerable inner pain and conflict.

PHYSICAL PAIN

The pulse is uniformly Tight to Wiry, and possibly a little Rapid, in painful conditions. For the exact location one would search for the position that is most Tight-Wiry, including the musculoskeletal positions.

Physical pain is an important emotional issue on many levels, including the irritability that accompanies it from day to day and the depression that ultimately sets in if it is not resolved. The Cotton quality can develop in people with chronic pain who are resigned to their condition. A Muffled quality at the left distal position, or even over the entire pulse, is a sign of depression characterized by dysphoria or lack of joy. Chronic pain is often repressed emotional pain that has been diverted via the divergent channels to physical pain, especially in the back and joints.

ADDICTIONS

There is no simple pulse picture related to the propensity to addiction. A few remarks can be made about the effect of different addictive recreational drugs on the organism.

In alcoholism the left middle position is Tight to Wiry due to the drying out of the liver parenchyma from alcohol abuse. In marijuana abuse the left middle position is Empty. With hallucinogens the left middle position is Empty and the Neuro-psychological position is Muffled.

In cocaine use the left distal and middle positions are Tense with Robust Pounding and Slippery with Rough Vibration until the burned-out stage, when this position exhibits all the qualities of deficiency, from yin-deficient Tight-Wiry to the much later qi-deficient Feeble-Absent. The pulse rate is Rapid in the Tense and Wiry stages and Slow when the pulse is Feeble-Absent.

CENTRAL NERVOUS SYSTEM DISORDERS

The Doughy quality at the Neuro-psychological positions is frequently a sign of pathology in the central nervous system that typically has emotional-mental sequelae. The Muffled quality at this position may be associated with the excessive use of hallucinogens. A Change in Amplitude has been tentatively associated with dizziness, and the Choppy, very Tight and Robust Pounding qualities at the Neuro-psychological positions have likewise been tentatively associated with trauma.

Likewise, the Arnold-Chiarri has been discovered by accessing the Neuro-psychological position with an extraordinarily Tight-Wiry quality that also appeared here simultaneously with an Inflated large vessel position, suggesting a brain aneurysm.

LEFT-RIGHT IMBALANCE

Imbalance between the expected and relative strengths of the pulse from left to right is termed a husband-wife imbalance. Generally, the left side is stronger in a man and the right in a woman. Reversal of these strengths is associated with difficulties in interpersonal relationships, especially in those with the opposite sex, as well as a feeling of being imbalanced physically, mentally, or both. A pseudo-imbalance, mistaken for this husband-wife imbalance, occurs with an anomaly of the radial artery such as the Three Yin pulse *(sān yīn mài)*. Dr. Shen interpreted this in a different manner, with the right side representing the 'digestive system' and the left side the 'organ system'.

CHANGES IN AMPLITUDE SHIFTING BACK AND FORTH BETWEEN SIDES   This pulse picture is a sign of current, ongoing interpersonal conflict. The amplitude changes first on one side while the other has no change, and then it shifts to exactly the opposite. It can, however, indicate work well beyond a person's energetic capacity.

KIDNEY-HEART DISHARMONY

The left distal and proximal positions on the pulse reflect Heart-Kidney disharmony.

FEEBLE-ABSENT AT LEFT DISTAL AND PROXIMAL POSITIONS, NORMAL AT LEFT MIDDLE POSITION WITH A SLOW OR RAPID RATE   In contrast to the common textbook presentation of yin deficiency as characterizing a Kidney-Heart disharmony, according to Dr. Shen, the principal combination associated with Kidney-Heart disharmony in our time is qi-yang deficiency. It is usually accompanied by anxiety and insomnia, but marked by fatigue and depression and is usually ascribed to an insult in utero or early in life.

FEEBLE-ABSENT AT LEFT DISTAL AND PROXIMAL POSITIONS, TENSE INFLATED AT LEFT MIDDLE POSITION   Stagnation in the middle burner inhibits the communication between the upper and lower burners and leads to a false Kidney-Heart disharmony syndrome that is easily resolved by moving the qi of the middle burner.

TIGHT AT LEFT DISTAL AND PROXIMAL POSITIONS, AND SLIGHTLY RAPID   If both positions are Tight it indicates that there is a disturbance of the spirit with Heart and Kidney yin deficiency, which is more likely due to emotional shock, lifelong excessive thinking often in the form of prolonged worry, and anxiety than to constitutional predisposition. With yin-deficient qualities there is greater agitation than with the qi-deficient qualities.

FEEBLE-ABSENT AT LEFT DISTAL AND TIGHT AT LEFT PROXIMAL POSITIONS Most likely, both positions were originally Feeble-Absent with a constitutional etiology. In a state of overwork of the mind and nervous system, yin is depleted and the dominant Kidney problem changes from qi to yin deficiency with a Tight quality at the proximal position.

TIGHT-WIRY AT LEFT DISTAL POSITION, FEEBLE-ABSENT AT LEFT PROXIMAL POSITION   Once rare, this combination is found more often now than before due to the increasing frequency of Kidney qi-yang deficiency in younger people. It can occur with shock to the Heart when there is Kidney qi deficiency and during the manic stage of bipolar disease.

Heart Patters Affecting Sleep

Heart excess heat ('Heart fire')

With the excess-type heat associated with Heart qi agitation, brought on by worry or Liver fire, it is hard to fall asleep. The mind is racing and worried, and the individual is restless. If one does get to sleep, one also tends to wake easily and be up and down all night. When one awakens, one is thinking obsessively about a real problem.

Heart yin deficiency and Heart qi agitation

With the Heart yin-deficient type of Heart qi agitation characterized by the Hesitant Wave and Tight left distal position, the Heart qi is excited and/or erratic. The individual is very sensitive to sound, restless, up and down all night, irritable, nervous, and of course tired. An individual with a Change in Rate at Rest type of Heart qi agitation may also have difficulty falling asleep if she is overworked, or has been under great stress the previous day.

Heart blood deficiency

Heart blood deficiency is characterized by a pattern of mild difficulty in falling asleep, and then waking after four or five hours, but usually able to return to sleep. Often there is nothing on the mind when one awakens, unless one also has some Heart excess heat or deficiency. There is a propensity to mild depression, especially around the time of waking. The person will feel less tired in the morning than those with Heart yin and qi deficiency, or either Heart qi or blood stagnation.

Heart qi and blood stagnation

People with stagnant Heart qi cannot sleep at all some nights, and are preoccupied with real or imagined hurts and thoughts of vengeance. Those with stagnant Heart blood wake up exhausted, even after sleeping through the night, but more often awaken after four or five hours of sleep and remain awake, experiencing considerable fear, especially in the early hours of the morning.

Trapped Heart qi/heat and Heart qi-yang deficiency

Those with trapped qi/heat in the Heart, Heart qi deficiency, and Heart yang deficiency find that their bodies are uncomfortable because they cannot lie flat, and they wake up to find a more comfortable position. They too awake tired in the morning, even when they have slept through the night. Those with Heart qi and yang deficiency are very depressed in the early morning after they awaken.

KIDNEY-HEART DISHARMONY AND SLEEP

If both the left distal and proximal positions are Tight, the individual will easily wake at the slightest sound or disturbance because, as Dr. Shen said, "the Heart is sensitive." This is the yin-deficient type of Kidney-Heart disharmony. If the left distal position is Tight and the left proximal position is Feeble-Absent, the essence is insufficient such that a person will only sleep about five hours, conforming to the Heart blood deficiency pattern. This may be due to the Kidney essence's control of the bone marrow that makes blood.

If both the left distal and proximal positions are Feeble-Absent, they will wake and go back to sleep frequently, but without the tossing and turning characteristic of the Heart yin sleep pattern. With qi deficiency, as well as with trapped qi, the individual is physically very uncomfortable in the reclining position, and accordingly finds it difficult to sleep for long periods of time.

TRIPLE BURNER

The Triple Burner is evaluated on the pulse for consistency and balance between sides. If the qualities at the burner are similar, the Triple Burner is said to be relatively intact. If the qualities over the entire pulse differ widely in all the burners, there is a severe Triple Burner deficiency and probably a 'qi wild' condition.

The lower burner reflects the foundation or root, a person's ground, which

Table 15-1: Pulse Qualities as Signs of Psychological Conditions **281**

may be either constitutionally weak or drained through life experience and life-style choices. The foundation tells us how well a person can recover and stand up again after being knocked down by life.

The middle burner reflects how centered the person is in life, his ability to handle stress, recover energy, focus and nourish himself. The upper burner reflects the capacity to reach out to the world with balance between communication and self-preservation.

Table 15-1 Pulse Qualities as Signs of Psychological Conditions

PULSE QUALITIES	PSYCHOLOGICAL CONDITIONS
■ I. Confirmed	
Rate Changing at Rest Occasionally	Racing "grasshopper" constantly shifting agitated mind, mood and behavior
Hesitant	Obsessive-compulsive
Yielding Hollow Full-Overflowing and Rapid	Rapidly developing anxiety, panic, labile emotions and easy to anger, depersonalization, delusions
Sides vary greatly in amplitude and/or substance (husband-wife imbalance)	Severe intra- and interpersonal conflict and anguish
Muffled left distal position	Depression, lack of joy
Yielding Hollow Full-Overflowing and Rapid	Rapidly developing anxiety, panic, labile emotions and easy to anger, depersonalization, delusions
Very high fever and very low rate and very low fever and very high rate	Delirium, coma
Amplitude shifting from side to side	Current significant interpersonal conflict
Inflated at left middle position (sometimes spreading to other positions)	Contained explosive anger
Flat: left distal	Vengeance, slow hidden rage, jealousy
Suppressed Wave at qi depth and Suppressed Pounding	Emotions muted

PULSE QUALITIES	PSYCHOLOGICAL CONDITIONS
Inflated:	
• Diaphragm	Inflated at the left Diaphragm often is found in a situation in which a person is attempting to, or is actually separating from a person who they find it necessary to feel very angry at in order to effect the separation.
• At left middle position (sometimes spreading to other positions)	Contained explosive anger, impotent rage
Pulse stronger at the qi depth than at other depths	Relates in a superficial and extroverted way as a coping mechanism, especially under stress
Slippery at left distal position	Range of psychological problems from neurosis to psychosis; phlegm misting orifices
Vibration:	
• Smooth	Worry and tendency to worry
• Rough at first impression	Guilt, fear, past shock

■ II. Reliable

Amplitude changing occasionally over entire pulse	Tension; occasional external stress responding with internal conflict
Amplitude changing over entire pulse constantly	Concentration impaired after moderate time; moderate mental lethargy
Bean (Spinning)	Profound unexpressed fear/terror
Taut-Tense (entire pulse)	Tense; vigilant; slight to moderate repressed internal conflict
Tight (entire pulse)	Agitated; pain

■ III. Reliability less established

Deep	Tendency to withdrawal, especially under stress
Rate: Rapid (Bounding)	Tendency towards anxiety
Rate: Slow	Tendency towards depression
Hollow Full-Overflowing	Suppressed hot labile emotions; hot temper expressed rarely and unpredictably
Flooding Excess w/ Robust Pounding	Sudden explosive but enduring outward rage
Interrupted-Intermittent (uncommon finding)	Fear; shifting moods

Table 15-1: Pulse Qualities as Signs of Psychological Conditions **283**

PULSE QUALITIES	PSYCHOLOGICAL CONDITIONS
Empty:	
• Middle Burner	Losing center; feeling unbalanced; cannot find place in life; feeling lost
• Either side for 3-4 weeks	Post-traumatic syndrome due to unexpected shock that passes
Yielding Hollow Full-Overflowing Slow (gradually developing)	Anxiety, panic, labile emotions and easy to anger, depersonalization, delusions
Empty, Quality Changing, Amplitude Changing *in one position* (all indicate separation of yin and yang):	
• Left distal (Heart)	Mental instability, confusion
• Right distal (Lungs)	Intractable grief; difficulty making transitions, taking in the new and letting go of past, due to deficient strength to change and evolve
• Left middle (Liver)	Tendency to live in mild delusional state with grandiose plans that are never executed; easy frustration; emotional liability (especially anger)
• Right middle (Spleen)	Tendency to ruminate aimlessly and unproductively
• Proximal positions (Kidneys)	Tendency to profound recurrent unexplained (endogenous) depression
Qi Depth Yielding, Feeble, Absent, Spreading (at blood depth), Flooding Deficient, Diffuse, Reduced Substance, Reduced Pounding, Deep, Feeble, Absent	Emotionally vulnerable; retreat as a way of life; avoiding stress

■ IV. Reliability least established

Rate on exertion:	
• Rate increases more than 20 beats per minute	Memory and attention span diminished; focus wanders mild to moderately
• Rate rises less than 8 beats/ minute, stays same or decreases	Concentration impaired after short time; severe mental lethargy
Empty Thread-like (moderate to severe)	Losing center; feelings unbalanced; cannot find place in life; feeling lost
Leather (moderate to severe)	Memory and attention span severely diminished; focus wanders in extreme; agitated; losing center; feelings unbalanced; cannot find place in life; feeling lost

PULSE QUALITIES	PSYCHOLOGICAL CONDITIONS
Leather-like Hollow	Emotions eating away at person inside (gastric and duodenal ulcer)
Minute and Scattered (very severe)	Losing center; feelings unbalanced; cannot find place in life; feeling lost
Empty Interrupted-Intermittent & Yielding Hollow and Interrupted-Intermittent	Possible immature stunted emotional development
Blood Depth partially Hollow	Mildly diminished memory and attention span, focus wanders
Blood Unclear	Thought and emotions imprecise and vague
Blood heat; blood thick	Repressed hot emotions
Tense Ropy	Emotional obdurate rigidity, especially under pressure
Yielding Ropy	Person is rigid but bendable under pressure
Thin: Thin Tight	Memory and attention span diminished; focus wanders moderately to severely; agitated
Thin: Thin Yielding	Memory and attention span diminished; focus wanders moderately to severely; tendency to depression; cannot protect self
Restricted (Special Lung position)	Difficulty making transitions, taking in the new and letting go of past due to rigidity
Long	Stable but slightly tense
Short (literature: brief)	Person whose personality is compartmentalized, not integrated, and each part out of touch with another; in the extreme, Dr. Jeckyl and Mr. Hyde or multiple personality
Choppy	Fixed, obstinate, unmoving
Tight-Wiry	High strung; agitated; becoming hardened against the world but supersensitive
	Extreme deficiency of Kidney yin-essence which in turn dries out the Pericardium. This makes it difficult to access or release Heart feelings.
	This manifests as an inability to accept or give love and tenderness.
	(As in diabetes, of which the Wiry quality in the lower and sometimes middle burner is an early sign, the body has lost control of sugar metabolism, the sweet taste, perhaps metaphorically of love.)

16

Prognosis and Prevention

Hamilton Rotte, A.P.

T HE CENTRAL THEME OF this chapter is how the pulse serves prevention while functioning as a prognosticator. It is true, of course, that the pulse provides information about acute and chronic conditions and about therapeutic progress. But just as importantly, it can reveal the not-so-obvious sources of a patient's symptoms.

PAST AND PRESENT

The future is a continuum with the present and the past. With regard to the past, qualities in the Special Lung positions tell us about past insults to the Lungs. A Rough Vibration over the entire pulse tells us of the likelihood of a previous shock to the Heart. For the present, a generalized Tight quality over the entire pulse usually tells us that a person has been overworking his mind for some time, unless he is very young, when it might indicate generalized pain. For the future, Muffled and Choppy qualities in the Pelvis/Lower Body position should alert us to the possibility of a neoplastic process in the uterus and ovaries in a woman and the prostate and testicles in a man.

THE LONG-RANGE VIEW

The pulse is a 'slice of life' and an in-depth catalogue of a person's physiology and pathology between birth and death at the moment it is examined, reflecting the results of the lifelong struggle between anabolism and catabolism and independent of the person's current complaints, however minor.

TIME LAG

A set of correlations has been recognized between what has been palpated and what concretely occurs as symptoms. These correlations are what we call the qualities. The signs accessed from the pulse are often several steps ahead of symptoms and thus are prognosticators, and potentially preventers, of pathology. At the same time a quality, such as Feeble, may convey qi deficiency, even though the appearance of disease may not occur for months or years, another opportunity for prevention. These time frames should give us a sense of the relative seriousness of the condition and the urgency of intervention. We must also realize that while Absent may be the quality observed at a position or even on a larger aspect of the pulse, if the person can show up in your office, he or she is still alive, and their organs are still functioning.

The predictive time periods that we offer have a wide tolerance, and are relative measurements. Constitution, vulnerability, life habits, treatment, fortune and fate are the principal variables involved—reflected in the saying that "man can cure disease but cannot cure fate."

SERIOUSNESS

All of the qualities discussed in this chapter are considered only as they appear consistently on the pulse from day to day and week to week. This consistency is in itself a sign of seriousness. The interpretation of the same qualities occurring inconsistently is different, and usually less consequential in terms of pathology. The degree of the quality measured, on a scale of one to five, is another determinant of the seriousness of the prognostication.

We consider children's pulses somewhat differently that those of adults. Chaos in the pulse may reflect a child's immaturity and state of constant growth rather than being a sign of serious disease.

Some of the qualities indicate a current pathology that the patient may deny. Informing people that their condition is indicated by an objective reading of their pulse, rather than as a personal impression, usually bypasses the resistance to interpretation that is encountered in psychotherapeutic practices, and hastens the rapid dissolution of the denial and flood of emotion and information. (See Ch. 15 and endnotes 4 and 5.)

QUALITIES

There are qualities that tell us about the very distant, semi-distant, and more immediate futures, and also about any time. The following discussions are meant to convey a flavor of the pulse as prognosticator and pillar of a preventive medicine.

ANY TIME

In some positions a quality can be a sign of danger at any time. A good example is the Inflated quality at the Large Vessel position, which is a reliable sign of an aneurism or disturbance in the circulation of cerebrospinal fluid, all of which are imminently dangerous to life.

DISTANT FUTURE

We roughly consider the distant future in terms of twenty to thirty years. Most disharmonies are progressive if not corrected either by the organism, a change in lifestyle, or therapeutic intervention.

COTTON This quality, associated with emotional resignation (discussed in Chs. 9, 13, 15), tells us that there is general stagnation of qi, which, if uncorrected over a very long time, will lead to those diseases, especially cancer, which are associated with the slowing of the circulation of qi. The cancer will occur in areas of the body that are vulnerable for other reasons (retained pathogens, severe deficiency and/or stagnation).

FLAT If the Flat quality (discussed in Ch. 8) is found bilaterally in the distal positions, the qi and blood circulation in the chest is impaired. Found bilaterally, unresolved grief or Heart shock may be the etiology. Mediastinal and breast tumors are of future concern and associated with this sign when it is present for a long time.

When found only at the left distal position, it is often associated with stagnant Heart qi (see 'Heart closed' in Chs. 12 and 15) in which the individual has withdrawn his Heart energy from the channels in response to some emotional trauma of the distant (and often long-forgotten) past, or to a birth with the umbilical cord tied around the neck, or to chest trauma at a young age. We can anticipate constant interpersonal problems, including a tendency to spitefulness and vengefulness, as often the longer term result.

Another form of a Heart closed condition is stagnant Heart blood identified at the left distal position with the Choppy quality. It is associated with Heart shock and with prolonged labor with the individual's head outside of the mother and the umbilical cord around the neck. Eventually, this quality is often found with symptoms of unexplained fear, tension, shortness of breath (especially on inhalation), and chest pain.

At only the right distal position, the Flat quality is a sign of Lung qi stagnation, possibly due to unresolved grief, that portends respiratory problems such as asthma, chronic bronchitis, or Lung cancer, and kidney problems, including nephritis, that ensues from the inability of the Lungs to cause the qi and fluids to descend.

INFLATED YIELDING IN LEFT DISTAL POSITION   Described in Ch. 8, the Inflated Yielding quality is a sign that qi is trapped in an organ or area of the body and cannot get out. Predictable symptoms are fatigue, depression, discomfort in the entire body, quick temper throughout one's life, and hypertension. Without correction, the heart could become enlarged.

YIELDING OR DIMINISHED QI DEPTH   This indicates early deficiency of true and protective qi. These qualities indicate that a person is vulnerable to mild ephemeral illnesses, and that the distant future holds the possibility, if the process is not halted, of chronic fatigue syndrome and other chronic diseases.

TAUT-TENSE   When found over the entire pulse, this quality (see Chs. 11 and 15) is a sign of an early 'nervous system tense' condition leading eventually to heat in the blood and hypertension. In an individual position it is an early sign of qi stagnation with some excess heat, for example, at the right middle position, foretelling a slowing of peristalsis with food stagnation, gas, and distention.

TIGHT   Common long-term effect of yin deficiency, associated with the Tight quality over the entire pulse, is arteriosclerosis with the drying and hardening of the blood vessels (see Ch. 11). If the Tight-Wiry quality is found simultaneously only in the left middle and proximal positions, one must consider glucose tolerance problems such as diabetes in the far future.

ARRHYTHMIA: CONSTANT CHANGE IN RATE AT REST   This is an early sign of potential Heart qi-yang deficiency that will manifest at first with anxiety and emotional vulnerability, and later with being easily fatigued, shortness of breath, dependent edema, spontaneous cold sweating with beading, coldness, and chest pain. (See Ch. 6.)

SLOW RATE   A rate under 55 beats per minute, depending on age, is a sign of deficient circulation and eventual vulnerability to disease, especially chronic fatigue syndrome, fibromyalgia, migrating arthritis, volatile anger, and circulatory disease. Although a slow pulse rate is associated with a healthy heart in biomedicine, it is our impression that exactly the opposite is true (see Ch. 7). The average life span of athletes is far less than that of the general population. A very Slow rate is also found with severe toxicity, usually of the inhalant type.

RAPID RATE   A persistently Rapid rate, for any reason (including Heart shock), will gradually cause an exhaustion of Heart qi. Symptoms include varying degrees of fatigue, even after long sleep. If uncorrected it can eventually lead to Heart yang deficiency and serious Heart disease and failure (see Ch. 7).

Semi-Distant Future

The semi-distant future is defined as roughly five to twenty years.

SPREADING OVER ENTIRE PULSE This quality (see Chs. 8 and 13) is a sign of a mild to moderate progression in the diminishment of qi, with some blood deficiency due to overwork, which is a step toward eventual chronic fatigue syndrome or some other chronic disease in the semi-distant future. Related outcomes are sudden heart attacks in vulnerable young adults, especially physicians, athletes, and driven young businessmen.

FLOODING DEFICIENT WAVE, DIFFUSE, AND REDUCED SUBSTANCE This pulse is a sign of moderate qi deficiency in an individual who is pushing himself far beyond his energy with overwork and sleep deprivation (see Ch. 8). In those with particular vulnerabilities, the possibility of sudden physical and emotional collapse, including heart attacks, fulminating blood dyscrasias, and neurological diseases in young men, is of special concern.

EMPTY AT LEFT MIDDLE POSITION In the young and early middle aged this is often a sign of the use of marijuana or hallucinogens, or of chronic hepatitis/mononucleosis, with gradually developing symptoms of lassitude, indecision, and inability to carry out one's plans and visions. There is eventually an increasingly frequent danger of primary liver cancer and lymphomas with an Empty quality at the left middle position.

THIN-TIGHT OVER ENTIRE PULSE Signs of blood and yin deficiency, circulatory and deficient-type heat symptoms will eventually be encountered with this pulse (see Chs. 10 and 11). This includes dryness, shortened menstruation, vision problems, throbbing headaches, palpitations, vertigo, parasthesias, afternoon fevers, very restless sleep, and later hypertension and adult onset diabetes. Found only at the qi depth, it is a sign of a current or developing 'nervous system tense' condition.

THIN YIELDING This combination (see Chs. 10 and 13) portends symptoms of blood deficiency, as listed just above, and symptoms of qi deficiency including being easily fatigued, shortness of breath, sleep with frequent waking/sleeping pattern, diarrhea or constipation, prolonged scanty menstruation, and urinary frequency.

BLOOD UNCLEAR This sign is identified with eventual skin diseases such as eczema and psoriasis, which can affect any part of the body, together with being easily fatigued and severe malaise, arthritis, and headaches. It is a sign of toxicity in the blood and stress on the Liver and Lungs; hepatic and pulmonary complications may be anticipated (see Chs. 10 and 13).

BLOOD HEAT   Symptoms of skin diseases with itching, sore throat, canker sores, tongue sores, bleeding gums, excitability, migraine headaches, hard and dry stools, and dark scanty urine are to be expected as early outcomes of this sign. It is also a sign of future hypertension and stroke. (See Chs. 10 and 13.)

BLOOD THICK   In adolescents, one will encounter persistent, severe acne. Severe hypertension and possible stroke later in adulthood are strong possibilities. (See Chs. 10 and 13.)

TENSE HOLLOW FULL-OVERFLOWING   When the pulse is Tense Full-Overflowing there is extreme excess heat in the blood that the body is having difficulty eliminating, sclerosing the arteries and thus putting a burden on the Heart, Liver, and Kidneys. There is a strong likelihood of eventual hypertension and stroke.

SLIPPERY AT ENTIRE QI DEPTH   If the pulse is slightly Rapid, this can be a sign of excessive sugar in the blood and an early sign of diabetes (see Ch. 11). If the pulse is Slow, it is a sign of general qi deficiency and mild immune system, protective qi deficiency with known vulnerability to external pathogenic factors.

SLIPPERY AT BLOOD DEPTH   This a sign of turbulence in the blood often found with the Blood Heat and Blood Thick qualities (see Ch. 11). The turbulence is an indication that the conditions for the laying down of plaque already exist and that arterio-atherosclerosis is well on its way. Damp-heat in the Spleen and Gallbladder is frequently involved.

ARRHYTHMIA: INTERRUPTED OR INTERMITTENT   When we find the Interrupted quality with more than five irregularly missed beats per minute, or the Intermittent quality that misses a beat regularly less often than every 15 to 30 beats per minute, we can predict that the onset of symptomatic Heart disease will occur within the next five to ten years (see Ch. 6).

ROUGH VIBRATION AT BLOOD DEPTH   This is a sign (see Ch. 11), usually found with the Slippery quality at the blood depth, indicating that the vessel walls are damaged, and which presages the development of arterio-atherosclerosis.

INFLATED   An Inflated quality (see Ch. 8) at the right distal position and/or the Special Lung position can be a sign of developing emphysema.

TENSE AND TIGHT-THIN AT THE QI DEPTH   When the Tense quality is found over the entire pulse in almost all positions and the qi depth is Tight-Thin, the condition is 'nervous system tense'. This leads to stagnation and ensuing excess heat that enters the blood to protect vital organs, creating blood heat and Hollow Full-Overflowing hypertensive disorders (see Ch. 11).

In an individual position, the Tense quality is a sign of increasing qi stagnation with some excess heat. At the left middle position, one will eventually find the symptoms of headache, irritability, quickness to anger, cold hands and feet, difficulty recovering one's energy, distention and pain on the sides, suffocating sensation in the chest, sighing, and agitated depression.

TENSE SLIPPERY AT THE GALLBLADDER POSITION   This combination at this position signifies developing cholecystitis and cholelithiasis (see Ch. 12).

WIRY   A Wiry quality over the entire pulse can be a sign of severe ongoing pain that will disappear when the pain is resolved. Found at the left proximal and middle positions it can be a sign of developing hypertension or diabetes (deficient yin-essence). A Wiry quality at the left distal and/or left middle position is a possible sign of cocaine abuse, potential or existing Grave's disease, or advanced manic-depressive illness (see Ch. 11).

YIELDING ROPY   The Yielding Ropy quality (see Ch. 11) is found in individuals who have exercised far beyond their energy over a long period of time. The vessel wall that expands to accommodate the increased blood flow associated with the exercise shrinks more slowly than does the quantity of blood when exercise is reduced, or deficiency results when the exercise exceeds the terrain. Thus, there is a separation of the yin (blood) from the yang (wall of the vessel) so that the less-nourished vessel wall becomes harder. This causes a hardening of the arteries for reasons other than heat or atherosclerosis, and it occurs with ensuing neurological sequelae such as Parkinson's disease.

CONSTANT CHANGE IN AMPLITUDE   Over the entire pulse, if the change is large, this sign indicates a significant deficiency of Heart qi that will ultimately result in heart disease and failure. If the change is smaller, the Heart qi deficiency primarily diminishes circulation or is the result of insults to circulation, such as physical trauma or emotional shock. The circulation responds to trauma with a spasm of the peripheral blood vessels that inhibits circulation, causing the Heart to overwork and drain the Heart qi and yin. With the latter, anticipated problems include migrating joint pain and cold hands and feet. Intermediate signs include disturbance in mental activities, insomnia, palpitations, emotional vulnerability, and fatigue (especially in the morning). (See Ch. 6 for further detail.)

When found at a principal position, it indicates an early to intermediate separation of yin and yang and deterioration in function of the yin organ associated with the position where it is found. At the left middle position, for example, it reveals potential problems with the recovery of energy and healing, detoxification, one form of chronic fatigue syndrome, menstrual difficulties, impaired planning and decision-making, and an inability to appropriately advance or retreat. Uncorrected, the ultimate consequence can be primary liver cancer and lymphomas. At complementary positions, Change in Amplitude is a sign of diminished function.

EXCESSIVE INCREASE IN RATE ON MILD EXERTION > 12-20 BEATS/MINUTE   This is a sign of Heart blood deficiency with eventual symptoms of palpitations, insomnia, weakness, fatigue, loss of memory and concentration. Over a moderate period of time, this will lead to Heart qi-yang deficiency. (See Chs. 6, 12, and 15 and the Glossary.)

RHYTHM DISORDERS   An Intermittent quality whose pulse misses more than one beat every thirty beats, or an Interrupted quality in which beats are missed more than once a minute, portends severe heart disease in the semi-distant future (see Ch. 6).

IMMEDIATE FUTURE

Less serious prognosticators

OCCASIONAL CHANGE IN RATE AT REST   This is a predictable sign (see Ch. 6) of impending emotional instability with a 'grasshopper' changing mind and roller coaster feeling, fear, borderline psychological states, palpitations, insomnia, and fatigue.

HESITANT WAVE   This quality (see Ch. 6) is a sign of a person who has a tendency to be obsessed with one theme such as money, health, or religion. Mild Heart yin deficiency symptoms of hyperactivity, irritability, insomnia, and palpitations should be expected. This quality has been associated with massive and often fatal heart attacks in vulnerable young professionals working mentally beyond their energy.

SMOOTH VIBRATION   A sign of worry, at all depths over the entire pulse, Smooth Vibration indicates that a person will find something to worry about even when there is nothing to worry about. They are always rehearsing for disaster (see Ch. 11).

More serious prognosticators

CHOPPY   The Choppy quality on first impression, right distal position, left middle position, right middle position, and Special Lung position indicates toxicity with anticipated chronic fatigue, malaise, skin, sinus, and joint disorders (retained pathogen). Usually associated with blood stagnation, its appearance with enormous toxicity was at first puzzling until it was discovered that many toxins kill through massive blood stagnation.

At the Gallbladder, Stomach-Pylorus Extension and Intestinal complementary positions it is a sign of microbleeding and irritation or inflammation in the mucosa of these organs, anticipating Crohn's disease (regional enteritis), colitis, and cholecystitis and cholelithiasis.

The Choppy quality at the Pelvis Lower Body positions, often together with the proximal positions, indicates lower burner blood stagnation. The following disorders can be anticipated soon after the appearance of this quality: fixed pain, especially menstrual, intermittent menstrual bleeding with purple clots, spider veins, purpura, ropy stools, flushing up with migraine headache (the qi and blood separate and the qi rises), and rectal bleeding with hemorrhoids (see Ch. 11).

FLOATING TIGHT   Especially at the left middle position or left side, it is associated with Liver wind (Liver yin deficiency and 'separation of yin and yang'), resulting in a rising yang condition attended by headache and flushing, 'wind in the channels', and by stroke in the very long term (see Ch. 9).

WIRY   The most serious consequences of a Wiry quality, a sign of serious essence deficiency, are diabetes and hypertension (see Ch. 11).

SLIPPERY AT THE MITRAL VALVE POSITION   Slipperiness at this position (see Ch. 12) is a sign of mitral valve prolapse, that blood is regurgitating into the left auricle. Panic disorder, anxiety, and palpitations can be predicted. Since this a moderate sign of Heart qi deficiency, one can predict heart disease if the condition is uncorrected.

SLIPPERY TIGHT AT THE GALLBLADDER POSITION   Together with the Tight quality (see Ch. 12), this is a sign of impending severe cholecystitis and cholelithiasis.

SLIPPERY AT THE LEFT DISTAL POSITION   This signifies that the Heart orifices are blocked by phlegm-heat or phlegm-cold, with severe emotional problems, psychosis, or, more remotely, epilepsy (see Chs. 11 and 12).

SLIPPERY AT ORGAN DEPTHS (QI, BLOOD, AND SUBSTANCE)   At these depths over the entire pulse, qualities often indicate retained pathogens. The Slippery quality is often found here with Robust Pounding and Choppiness, indicating a toxic damp-heat disorder associated with toxins, infection (e.g., chronic hepatitis), or parasites. The future concern is when the toxicity, infection, or parasites can no longer be retained and become acute diseases (see Ch. 12).

MUFFLED   Very pronounced Muffled quality (see Ch. 8) is associated with the process of tumor formation, malignancy, and severe autoimmune disease such as lupus. An active search for a tumor is recommended. This is easier when the extreme Muffled quality is concentrated in a particular area. In one instance when the Muffled quality (moving toward a Dead quality) was found at the Gallbladder position, a rare tumor of the gallbladder and liver bile ducts was found two-and-a-half years before biomedical confirmation.

MUFFLED AT THE LEFT DISTAL POSITION   Exceptionally, at the left distal position, it is a sign of the dampening of the spirit, of impending dysphoric depression, usually associated with a significant loss. This is often of a love relationship, though at least once it was associated with the sudden monumental loss of money and status.

ROUGH VIBRATION   Over the entire pulse this quality is associated with Heart shock, fear, and guilt. The consequence is significant emotional disturbance, depending upon the degree. In a principal position it is a sign of parenchymal damage and in a complementary position of functional impairment, the ultimate harm depending again upon degree and time lapsed.

FLOODING EXCESS   With the sudden appearance of this quality (see Ch. 8), there is excess heat in an organ or area with the possibility of an imminent deep infection such as a hidden appendicitis, colitis, peritonitis, and septicemia.

DEEP AND/OR FEEBLE-ABSENT   Over the entire pulse, it is another prognosticator of a near future, pervasive chronic fatigue syndrome or other chronic disease (see Ch. 8). When found at one position, it marks a qi deficiency in the associated organ and some loss of function within one year. If it is found at the left middle position, it will be accompanied by fatigue, especially later in the day, with difficulty recovering or getting one's second wind (see Ch. 12).

INFLATED AT THE LARGE VESSEL POSITION   With an Inflated quality at the Large Vessel position (see Ch. 12), one can expect defects in the circulation such as an aneurysm, especially in the ascending aorta. Less often, cerebral aneurysms and defects in the cerebral spinal fluid circulation have also been recorded.

INFLATED MORE AT THE DISTAL ASPECT THAN PROXIMAL END OF THE LEFT DIAPHRAGM POSITION   When this aspect is greatly Inflated compared to the middle position, it is at least a sign of an energetically enlarged heart, although a gross enlargement is also possible and should be biomedically investigated (see Ch. 12).

EMPTY   This quality found consistently over the entire pulse (see Ch. 9) portends a profound loss of contact between yin and yang ('qi wild'), with major illness predictable within three months to two years.

The sudden appearance of the Empty quality over the entire pulse can occur with post-traumatic stress syndrome, when a person brings all of his available energies to the surface in order to cope.

At individual positions, this quality reveals major dysfunction of the associated yin organ in which the yin and yang have lost contact. If found consistently at the left middle position, one could anticipate a vulnerability to major infection, autoimmune diseases, and neoplasms of the liver.

EMPTY THREAD-LIKE; LEATHER-EMPTY; MINUTE; SCATTERED; YIELDING HOLLOW FULL-OVERFLOWING AND SLOW   Increasing degrees of the 'qi wild' disorder, a profound separation between yin and yang, signifying either current major illness or its likely development within six months. These qualities appear in the fatal stages of illness.

LEATHER-HOLLOW   With a Rapid rate, this quality (see Ch. 13) portends imminent hemorrhage in the organ or area associated with the position in which it is found, and should be treated as a medical emergency. If it appears with a Slow rate, it suggests a recent past severe hemorrhage in the organ or area that could imminently recur.

LEATHER-EMPTY   This is a profoundly serious sign of the depletion of blood, yin, and essence associated with prolonged chronic disease and eventual damage to the bone marrow.

VERY TENSE, TIGHT OR WIRY HOLLOW FULL-OVERFLOWING AND RAPID   When this combination (see Ch. 8) is found at the left distal and left middle positions, or over the entire pulse, and the rate is very Rapid, a stroke may be imminent. If these qualities are accessed only on one side, there is imminent danger of a stroke on that side.

CHANGE IN QUALITIES   When found over the entire pulse, this indicates a serious 'qi wild' disorder with separation of yin and yang, in which case there will be serious illness within six months to two years. When found at an individual position, it indicates a separation of yin and yang with functional deterioration of the yin organ associated with that position, with illness possible within several months to a year (see Ch. 6).

YIELDING HOLLOW FULL-OVERFLOWING AND RAPID   Associated with the sudden cessation of extended and heavy exercise, with near-term rapidly developing severe anxiety, episodes of depersonalization and dissociation, severe fatigue, migrating joint pains, and other serious physical deterioration (see Chs. 6 and 8).

CHOPPY   The Choppy quality (see Ch. 11) in the left distal position is a sign of symptomatic or asymptomatic coronary artery blockage and a prognosticator of an early heart attack.

A blockage of the hepatic portal system to the heart with possible sudden fatal hemorrhage is associated with the Choppy quality at the left middle position. It is also increasingly found here due to the ubiquity of severe environmental toxicity.

The Pelvis/Lower Body positions are where the Choppy quality was once most commonly found, and is where it involves potential endometriosis, fibroid tumors, and ovarian cysts in women, and prostatic enlargement and prostatic tumors in men.

At the Gallbladder position, the Choppy quality is a sign of large gallstones and necrosis of the gallbladder with the threat of peritonitis.

BEAN (SPINNING)   While it is unlikely that the Bean (Spinning) quality will be felt without symptoms, it is mentioned in this context to alert the reader of its possible emergent seriousness, mostly indicating states of extreme terror or pain (see Ch. 11).

UNSTABLE   This quality (see Ch. 6) indicates imminent, extremely serious illness in the yin organ associated with the position in which it is found. At the left distal position, coronary occlusion or heart failure can be anticipated at any time.

INTERRUPTED OR INTERMITTENT   When the Interrupted quality is at a stage where the rate consistently cannot be accurately read, or the Intermittent quality occurs less than every five beats, this is a sign of serious heart disease and probably a shortened life (see Ch. 6).

YIELDING HOLLOW INTERMITTENT OR INTERRUPTED   Perhaps the most serious sign of heart disease, combining chaotic Heart function and a serious 'qi wild' condition, and portending a very shortened life (see Ch. 6).

DEAD   The sensation of this quality (see Ch. 8) is that of touching a dead body in which there is no movement. The diagnosis is usually a malignant carcinoma and the prognosis is early death.

POSITIONS

Left middle position

Slippery at the organ depth here and most generally at the organ-blood and organ-substance subdivisions indicates a retained pathogen such as a chronic infection, parasites, or hepatitis (see Ch. 12).

Right middle position and Stomach-Pylorus Extension position

A Tight Hollow and Slippery combination here suggests the onset of gastritis and an ulcer (see Ch. 12).

Esophagus position

An Inflated Rough or Slippery quality here may accompany short-term reflux and long-term Barrett's syndrome and esophageal cancer (see Ch. 12).

PARADOX

When the signs and symptoms correspond to each other in terms of their Robust or Reduced aspects, the illness is less serious. But when they vary, such that one is Reduced while the other is inappropriately Robust, the illness is more serious. In an acute illness, the pulse should be Robust and Pounding, and in a chronic disease, it should be Reduced.[1] (This is discussed more fully in Chs. 3 and 17.)

In a young person the Ropy quality, the Reduced qualities (Deep, Feeble-Absent, and all the Empty qualities), and the chaotic qualities (Interrupted-Intermittent, Change in Qualities, Unstable) are more serious than when found in an older person.

Likewise, finding one of the hard qualities (Tight, Rough Vibration, Choppy, Wiry, Leather-Hard) or the very Robust qualities (Hollow Full-Overflowing, Flooding Excess) in a young person would be inappropriate.

When, at any age, the rate stays the same, rises less than eight beats, or decreases on exertion, we can expect the occurrence of Heart disease (Heart qi-yang deficiency) relatively soon.

A Thin pulse in a man or a Wide pulse in a woman is usually a sign of current or at least certain-to-be serious illness.

Especially in the terminal stage of the six stages, the presence of a very high temperature and a very low pulse rate, or a very low temperature and a very high pulse rate, are signs of extreme physiological disorder ('qi wild') and imminent death.

LIMITATIONS

Determining the exact locations and type of neoplasms, infections (damp-heat), or endocrine disorders is difficult without the assistance of other signs and symptoms and biomedical assistance. We have not yet identified the exact location of excesses in the Bladder, Kidney, Small or Large Intestines reflected in the Flooding Excess and Robust Pounding qualities at the proximal positions. The same is true for the findings of the Slippery, Choppy, and Robust Pounding qualities at the organ-blood and organ-substance subdivisions of the organ depth.

SIGNS OF A POSITIVE PROGNOSIS

It is unfortunate that our discussion of prognosis is weighted so heavily in the direction of increasing pathology. It is true that the pulse record is a statement of a person's condition at a particular point along the continuum from birth to death, and that our principal concern as physicians is to diagnose and treat the disharmonies revealed by the record. Since we must all eventually die, the picture is usually not a pretty one, in as much as the record is telling us how we are dying and how far along we are in the process.

However, as discussed in Ch. 3, the pulse record also tells us about our *strengths*. Strong proximal positions (lower burner) tell us that we have root, ground on which to stand and heal. Strong middle positions (middle burner) tell us that we can focus on healing, restore and cleanse ourselves. Strong distal positions (upper burner) tell us that we can reach out to the world with awareness of our creative being, with the strength to communicate and protect our being, and to maintain mental and emotional stability despite the "slings and arrows of outrageous fortune" with which we are all constantly bombarded.

Even with signs of Heart disharmony, a Normal rhythm tells us that there is strength to recover. A Normal rate, consistent with the person's age, indicates the ability to maintain cardiovascular stability under stress.

Another important sign is the integrity of the right side of the pulse, especially the right middle position. This informs us that the digestive system and Spleen-Stomach qi (see Ch. 5) are capable of restoring qi and blood when the organism is under stress. And clearly, when overly Robust or Reduced pulses approach the signs that approximate those of the Normal pulse described in Ch. 5, we are on the road to healing.

The Tense quality and modest Robust Pounding over the entire pulse tells us that there is enough true (upright) qi, or sufficient metabolic heat, to sustain the organism under adverse circumstances. Normal complementary positions inform us that the pathology found in the associated principal positions is not as serious as it first seemed, and that the chances for restoration are favorable. The presence of a Normal sine wave within the qi depth is another positive sign when the person is ill.

A pulse that shows great instability in a person whose recent history indicates positive growth may be a sign of a general principle that physiological instability is not always a sign of pathology but may be an opportunity for positive change and growth.

When the qualities in the same burner tend to be more similar than different, we are witnessing less chaos than when the qualities in all the positions are significantly different. When there is little change in qualities and amplitude and few Empty-type qualities, we have a more stable organism. Further stability is indicated when the pulse and other signs and symptoms are synchronous and not paradoxical. This is also true for the synchronicity of age, sex, height, and weight with the pulse qualities. The relative absence of qualities that indicates excess or deficiency is another positive sign.[2]

17

Interpretation

Jamin Nichols, A.P.

INTRODUCTION

This chapter provides a methodology for pulse interpretation. The case studies in Ch. 18 are excellent tools to help learn this process. This chapter is divided into three main sections:

- **BROAD FOCUS:** This includes the rate, rhythm, wave form, and uniform qualities of the pulse taker's first impressions over the entire pulse. Certain psychological issues such as Heart shock (Rough Vibration) and Heart qi agitation (Change in Rate at Rest) manifest here.

- **CLOSER FOCUS:** Includes the depths, sides, areas, and 'systems', for example, 'digestive system weak' (Deep or Feeble on right side).

- **CLOSEST FOCUS:** Examines the principal and complementary positions and their relationships (general considerations, specific considerations, acute vs. chronic conditions). Qualities also have their psychological implications (see Table 15-1).

Each of these sections is analyzed with regard to stability, substances, and activity.

Other diagnostic tools must be used to confirm the pulse diagnosis. In order to become proficient in identifying the qualities, it is important to train with a qualified instructor.

ORGANIZING PRINCIPLES

Symptoms vs. conditions

One concept guiding the thought process inherent in what follows is the endless interplay in people's lives, and in our assessment of their strengths and vulnerabilities, between the stress in their lives and their underlying terrain. Chinese medicine is one of the few extant medicines that can alter the basic terrain so that people can become less vulnerable to the stress.

Those whose focus is on the stress are more likely to also focus their therapeutic endeavors on relieving the stress rather than on the Chinese medical conditions that they imply. Again, the thrust is either in the direction of the stress (symptom) or the terrain (condition). In the context of this book, our concern with stress is axiomatic, but our primary concern is with the terrain.[1]

THE PROCESS OF DISEASE AND PREVENTION

The pulse is a tool to recognize the disease process from its beginning. This recognition provides us with an exquisite preventive medicine.

THE PULSE AS A LIFE RECORD

Above all, remember this: an accurate pulse record provides us with detailed information about a patient's past, present, and potential future. Not only is it the key to early diagnosis and prevention, it also provides information for productive management and treatment.

METHODOLOGY FOR PULSE INTERPRETATION

DATA

We begin by collecting all the data from the patient's pulse regarding the substances, stability, activity, body areas, and systems. Refer to Ch. 4 to review the method of taking the pulse.

The ultimate goal of pulse diagnosis interpretation is to facilitate management and treatment. We consider and record the age, gender, weight, and occupation of the person in terms of what is appropriate or paradoxical.

Qualities vary according to whether they are accessed at the height or depth of their amplitude. We choose the quality at the height of its amplitude as the one that is correct for interpretation. Furthermore, we access the pulse at the strongest impulse. Qualities on the sides of that impulse vary from those on the principal pulsation. These two principles are essential for a methodology that can be communicated from practitioner to practitioner so that each will know exactly what they felt and another has felt, where to look for it, and what it means.

It is important to note the degree of the presence, on a scale of 1-5, of each quality. A quality rated five [5] is a far more serious sign than the same quality rated one [1]. In our clinical case histories, when describing Chinese medical conditions we describe a reading of [1-2] as mild, [3-4] as moderate, and [4-5] as severe. Therefore, Thin [2] represents only a mild degree of blood deficiency, Thin [3-4] a moderate degree, and Thin [4-5] a severe degree.

The severity or seriousness of a quality can also depend upon its location. A Choppy quality is much more serious if found at the left distal position, signifying Heart or coronary artery issues, than in the Large Intestine position where it might indicate some microbleeding and inflammation.

We should consider the relation of a quality in one position with the same quality when it appears simultaneously over the entire pulse. We rely on the relative strength of that quality in the two places. For example, if there is a Change in Amplitude [3] on first impression, we would record and consider significant a Change in Amplitude in a principal or complementary position only if it differed significantly from the first impression. When a pulse quality is found in only one position, it assumes a more special significance.

Integration of the pulse data compares the initial impression with the individual principal and complementary positions that inform us of general and specific deficiencies and excesses, stagnation, and circulation.

As previously noted, we integrate and organize this diagnostic information with other information obtained from 'looking' (tongue diagnosis, etc.), 'asking', and 'listening'. We then incorporate all of this into a diagnostic catalogue from which we derive a management formulation and management implementation. This is organized into current prevailing issues (immediate interventions), root issues (basic etiologies, including constitution), secondary and derivative issues, and possible prognosis. From this we can offer suggestions for lifestyle changes and referrals to allopathic and other practitioners, if necessary.

PROCEDURE

Table 17-1 provides the simplest outline to approach interpretation. Fig. 17-1 is a form showing the most common qualities that one might expect to find in each position and Fig. 17-2 is a list that is helpful for interpreting the pulse record.

Beginner: List substances and activity

The beginner should first list the status of substances (qi, blood, yin and yang) and activity (heat and cold) of the body, as well as the rate and rhythm. This information alone will provide useful information in formulating a treatment plan, especially with herbs, and avoid many serious mistakes in prescribing. For example, supplementing the qi in someone who has stagnant qi, or yang in someone with excess heat, or removing dampness in someone who is already yin deficient, will only exacerbate these disorders.

Please note that the following lists do not attempt to be all-inclusive. Some qualities have multiple interpretations depending on the depth and position at

Table 17-1 Methodology for Interpretation

I. **Quick Overview of the Entire Pulse**

Sex and age in terms of what is appropriate or paradoxical

Unusual qualities

Paradoxical findings

II. **Broad Focus and Closer Focus**

In-depth evaluation

A. Observations

1. Rhythm and rate: outstanding abnormalities

2. Uniform qualities

3. Unusual wave form

4. Above qi, qi, blood, and organ depths

5. Areas

Neuro-psychological

Burners: similar qualities bilaterally at upper, middle, and lower

Diaphragm

Pelvis/lower body

6. Sides

7. Systems

'Nervous system'

'Circulatory system'

'Digestive system'

'Organ system'

8. Stability

Separation of yin and yang

'Qi wild'

Blood out of control (hemorrhage)

B. Diagnostic impressions

III. **Closest Focus**

A. Substances

1. Qi

2. Yin

3. Yang

4. Blood

5. Dampness

6. Wind

7. Food

8. Essence

9. Parenchyma

B. Activity

1. Heat

Excess

Deficiency

2. Cold

Excess: internal, external

Deficiency

C. Organs (principal and complementary positions)
   1. Heart-circulation
   2. Lungs
   3. Liver
   4. Spleen-Stomach
   5. Kidneys
D. Diagnostic impressions

IV. **Psychology**: Mind, emotion, and spirit

V. **Interpretation**: Initial formulations are not set in stone and serve primarily as a starting point for a flexible process that increases with precision in the course of the success and failure of treatment strategies. Consider multiple etiologies.

A. Summary of specific diagnostic categories
B. Formulation
   1. Current prevailing issues
   2. Root issues and etiology of disharmonies
   3. Derivative issues
      a. Primary derivative issues
      b. Secondary derivative issues
   4. Analysis and synthesis of significant patterns and overall diagnostic concept

VI. **Management**
A. Lifestyle strategies
B. Referrals
C. Acupuncture, herbs, and other healing strategies

For the sake of discussion these strategies are separated into stages that in reality must be flexible and generously blended as the clinical situation unfolds into a clearer diagnostic picture:

   1. Immediate interventions
      – If these interventions succeed, proceed to the next step:
   2. Intermediate interventions
      – If these interventions succeed, proceed to the next step:
   3. Long-range minor and major interventions

VII. **Client History and Integration with Pulse Interpretation**
A. Client history—age, gender, occupation
   1. Chief complaints
   2. Medical history
      a. Review of systems
      b. Habits
      c. Childhood
      d. Family
B. Symptoms and the pulse
   1. Analysis of symptoms with pulse diagnosis
   2. Amendments to analysis and synthesis of significant patterns and diagnostic concepts

Fig. 17-1   Most Common, Less Common, and Uncommon Qualities at Each Position

Rhythm Normal, *Rate Change @ Rest, Interrupted, Intermittent*	**Rate/Min:** Begin: End: w/Exertion: Chng: **Other Rates During Exam:**
First Impressions of Uniform Qualities Tense, Tight, Robust Pounding, Amplitude Change, Smooth Vibration, Rough Vibration, Choppy, Thin, Reduced Substance, Muffled, Diffuse, *Slippery, Leather-Hard, Ropy*	**DEPTHS** **Floating:** Smooth Vibration, *Tense & Slow, Yielding & Rapid, Tight* **Cotton:** Common

Left Side:	**Right Side:**
Amplitude Change from Left-Right	

Qi: Diminished-Absent, Thin & Tight, Tense, Smooth Vibration, *Robust Pounding, Leather-Hard*
Blood: Heat, Thick, Reduced Substance, *Slippery, Rough Vibration, Choppy*
Organ: Robust Pounding, Tense, *Tight, Slippery, Choppy*
O-B/O-S: Robust Pounding, Tense, Choppy, Slippery, *Tight*
Wave: Hesitant, Flooding Deficient, Full-Overflowing, *Flooding Excess, Normal, Suppressed*

PRINCIPAL POSITIONS	**COMPLEMENTARY POSITIONS**

L: DISTAL POSITION R:	**L: NEURO-PSYCHOLOGICAL R:**

| Thin, Tight, Tense, Smooth Vibration, Rough Vibration, Muffled, Feeble-Absent, Slippery, Quality Change, *Robust Pounding, Choppy, Amplitude Change, Flat, Inflated* | Tense, Tight, Thin, Feeble-Absent, Quality Change, Rough Vibration, Muffled, *Choppy, Slippery, Robust Pounding, Inflated* | Doughy, Smooth Vibration, Muffled, *Tight, Rough Vibration* |

L: SPECIAL LUNG POSITION   R:

Tense, Tight, Slippery, Muffled, Narrow, Choppy, Rough Vibration, Qualities Changing to Feeble-Absent, Robust Pounding, Amplitude Change, *Restricted*
Pleura: *(Inflated, Rough, Tight)*

Pericardium:
(Tight)

HEART
Mitral Valve: Smooth Vibration, Rough Vibration, Slippery, *Amplitude Change, Muffled*
Enlarged: *(Inflated, Rough, Tight)*
Large Vessel: *(Tense Inflated)*

L: MIDDLE POSITION R:	**L: DIAPHRAGM R:**

| Tense, Tight, Thin, Robust Pounding, Reduced Substance, Diffuse, Muffled, Separating @ Organ Depth, Quality Change, Rough Vibration, Choppy, Full-Overflowing, *Leather-Hard, Slippery, Diminished/Absent @ Qi Depth, Flooding Excess, Amplitude Change* | Tense, Robust Pounding, Reduced Substance, Diffuse, Muffled, Tight, Thin, Separating @ Organ Depth, Quality Change, *Rough Vibration, Choppy, Diminished/Absent @ Qi Depth, Flooding Excess, Full-Overflowing, Amplitude Change, Leather-Hard* | Inflated | Inflated |

LIVER
ENGORGED
Distal: Inflated, *(Rough, Tight)*   **Ulnar:** *(Inflated)*
Gallbladder: Tense, Tight, Robust Pounding, Choppy, Slippery, Muffled, *Rough Vibration, Inflated*

SPLEEN-STOMACH
Esoph: Rough, Inflated, *(Tight)*   **Spleen:** *(Inflated)*
Stom-Pyl. Exten: Tense, Tight, Robust Pounding, Muffled, Choppy, Slippery, Rough Vibration, *Qualities Changing to Feeble-Absent, Amplitude Change*
Peritoneal Cavity/Pancreas: *(Inflated)*
Duodenum: *(SI & SPEP are identical)*

L: PROXIMAL POSITION R:	**Large: INTESTINES Small:**

| Diminished/Absent @ Qi Depth, Tight, Thin, Tense, Muffled, Qualities Changing to Feeble-Absent, Choppy, Robust Pounding, Deep, *Rough Vibration, Separating @ Organ Depth, Wiry, Flooding Excess, Full-Overflowing Reduced Pounding* | Tense, Tight, Muffled, Robust Pounding, Choppy, Rough Vibration, Qualities Changing to Feeble-Absent, Slippery, Biting, *Amplitude Change* |

FORMATTING LEGEND
More Common   *Less Common*   *(Uncommon)**
*likely when associated quality is present at position

L: PELVIS/LOWER BODY   R:
Tight, Tense, Thin, Choppy, Slippery, Robust Pounding, Muffled, Qualities Changing to Feeble-Absent, Rough Vibration, *Amplitude Change*

Note 1 The More Common and *Less Common* qualities are listed in order from most to least common according to Dr. Hammer's experience.
Note 2 While these qualities are, as indicated, More Common or *Less Common,* it is important to access the position with an open mind and only record what one feels with their fingers.

COMMENTS
Fǎn Quán Mài, *Sān Yīn Mài*

Fig. 17-2 Interpretation of Qualities in the Complementary Positions

<small>LEGEND:</small> Question mark (?) = unsubstantiated
Asterisk (*) = Reduced Substance, Diffuse, Deep, Feeble-Absent, etc.

Neuro-Psychological

Doughy	Kidney yang-essence deficiency?
Rough Vibration	Intractable headaches?
Choppy	Head trauma?
Change of Intensity	Dizziness?
Slippery	Allergies/pollutants?
Robust Pounding	Head trauma, seizures?
Smooth Vibration	Worry, Heart qi agitation?
Inflated	Qi Stagnation?
Flat	Qi Stagnation?
Very Tight	Parenchymal damage to CNS?
Muffled	Use of psychedelics?
Change of Qualities	Severe impaired function?
Reduced Qualities*	Impaired function?

Special Lung Position

Tense	Mild-moderate qi stagnation with excess heat
Tight	Inflammation
Wiry	Extreme inflammation
Rough Vibration	Parenchymal damage
Slippery	Dampness or phlegm
Narrow	Stagnation and functional impairment
Restricted	Severe stagnation and functional impairment
Inflated	Trapped qi
Empty	Recent grief
Choppy	Inhaled toxins
Muffled	Neoplastic process
Change of Amplitude	Impaired function
Change of Qualities	Severe impaired function
Floating	Exterior condition
Reduced Qualities*	Impaired function

Large Vessel ....

    Inflated   Aneurysm

    Tense Hollow Full-
       Overflowing   Hypertension

Pericardium ....

    Tight   Excess heat

    Slippery   Phlegm-heat

    Concentration of qualities   Defensiveness

Mitral Valve Position ....

    Smooth Vibration   Mild Heart qi deficiency

    Slippery   Greater Heart qi deficiency,
                               mitral valve prolapse

Heart Enlarged ....

    Inflated
    Rough   Energetic enlargement,
    Tight   Heart qi-yang deficiency

Diaphragm ....

    Inflated, more on left side   Suppressed tender feelings replaced by anger

    Inflated, more on right side   Heavy lifting, overuse of upper body

    Little or no Inflation   No relationship or perfect relationship

    Inflated, unilateral or   Trapped qi in diaphragm,
       bilateral   possibility of hiatal hernia

Distal Engorgement ....

    Tight
    Rough   Liver blood stagnation
    Inflated

Ulnar Engorgement ....

    Inflated   Liver blood stagnation

Pleura ....

    Tight
    Rough   Past or current inflammatory
    Inflated   Lung illness

Esophagus ....

Inflated

Tight   Parenchymal damage, impaired

Rough   function (Barrett's syndrome)

Slippery

Spleen ....

Inflated   Spleen qi deficiency from
                              Kidney qi-yang deficiency

Gallbladder ....

Tight and Wiry	Inflammation and tissue irritation (from chronic heat)
Rough Vibration	Parenchymal damage
Choppy	Stones, microbleeding, and necrosis
Slippery	Dampness
Tense	Mild-moderate qi stagnation with excess heat
Robust Pounding	Excess heat
Flooding Excess	Infection (excess heat)
Inflated	Trapped gas (associated with infection)
Muffled	Neoplastic process; stones
Change in Amplitude	Impaired function
Change in Qualities	Greater impaired function

Stomach Pylorus Extension ....

Inflated (whole position)	Trapped qi
Inflated (proximal part)	Prolapse from Spleen qi deficiency
Tense	Mild-moderate qi stagnation with excess heat
Robust Pounding	Excess heat
Tight and Wiry	Inflammation and/or pain (from chronic excess heat)
Rough Vibration	Parenchymal damage
Choppy	Microbleeding
Change in Amplitude	Impaired function
Change in Qualities	Greater impaired function
Muffled	Stagnation of all substances, neoplasm
Reduced Qualities*	Impaired function

Large Intestine ···

Inflated	Gas, qi stagnation
Slippery	Dampness
Robust Pounding	Excess heat
Tense	Mild-moderate qi stagnation with excess heat
Tight and Wiry	Inflammation (chronic excess heat); pain
Biting	Abdominal Pain
Choppy	Microbleeding
Muffled	Neoplastic process; fecal impaction
Change in Amplitude	Impaired function
Change in Qualities	Greater impaired function
Reduced Qualities*	Impaired function

Small Intestine ···

Tense	Mild-moderate qi stagnation with excess heat
Robust Pounding	Excess heat
Tight and Wiry	Inflammation (chronic excess heat), loose stools
Rough Vibration	Parenchymal damage
Choppy	Microbleeding
Inflated	Gas, qi stagnation
Slippery	Dampness
Muffled	Stagnation of all substances, neoplasm
Biting	Pain
Change in Amplitude	Impaired function
Change in Qualities	Greater impaired function
Reduced Qualities*	Impaired function

Pelvis Lower Body ···

Choppy	Blood stagnation
Tight and Wiry	Pain, inflammation
Rough Vibration	Parenchymal damage
Muffled	Stagnation of all substances, neoplasm
Flooding Excess	Infection, severe excess heat
Robust Pounding	Excess heat
Change in Amplitude	Impaired function
Change in Qualities	Greater impaired function
Reduced Qualities*	Impaired function

Table 17-2 Substances and Activity

SUBSTANCES			
Qi	Excess (stagnation)	External	Cotton
		Internal	Taut, Tense, Muffled, Inflated, Flat, Short Excess (residual: Tight, Wiry, Leather-Hard)
	Deficiency	Qi depth	Yielding, Diminished, or Absent
		Blood depth	Spreading, Absent
		Wave	Flooding Deficient
		Other depths	Reduced Pounding, Diffuse, Reduced Substance, Deep, Feeble-Absent, Flat, Short Deficient
Blood	Excess	Tissues	Choppy, Muffled, Liver Engorgement, very Tense Inflated
		Vessels	Blood Heat, Blood Thick, Tense-Tight Hollow Full-Overflowing, Slippery at blood depth, Tense Ropy
	Deficiency		Thin, Yielding partially Hollow, Spreading, Leather-Hard, Leather-Empty
	Hemorrhage	Imminent	Leather-like Hollow, Rapid
		Recent	Leather-like Hollow, Slow
Yin	Excess (stagnation)	Damp-Phlegm	Slippery, Muffled
	Deficiency		Tight, Wiry, Leather-Hard, Hesitant Wave (Heart)
Yang	Deficiency		Deep, Feeble-Absent, Hidden Deficient
		Qi-yang deficiency leading to chaos	Empty qualities (Yielding Empty Thread-like, Minute, Scattered), Change in Qualities, Yielding Hollow Full-Overflowing, Yielding Hollow Full-Overflowing Interrupted-Intermittent
Essence	Excess (stagnation)		Very Taut-Tense in proximal positions
	Deficiency	Yang-essence	Deep, Feeble-Absent in proximal positions, Doughy at Neuro-psychological positions
		Yin-essence	Wiry, Leather-Hard at first impression, especially in proximal positions
Wind	External		Floating Tense & Slow, Floating Yielding & Rapid, Floating Slippery
	Internal		Floating Tight
Food	Stagnation	Any signs of qi and/or fluid stagnation in the GI tract would imply some concomitant food stagnation as well	Right middle, Stomach-Pylorus, Small Intestine and Large Intestine positions
Parenchyma	Damage		Rough Vibration in individual positions

Table 17-2 Substances and Activity, cont.

ACTIVITY			
Heat	Excess		Tense, Robust Pounding, Flooding Excess, Long, moderately Tense Inflated
		Blood heat	'Blood Heat', 'Blood Thick,' Tense Ropy, Tense-Tight Hollow Full-Overflowing
		External	Floating Yielding & Slightly Rapid
	Deficiency		Tight, Wiry, Leather-Hard
Cold	Excess	External	Floating Tense and Slow
		Internal	Tense or Tight (rare and usually in one position), Hidden Excess
	Deficiency	Yang deficiency	Deep, Feeble-Absent, Hidden Deficient, Empty, Yielding Hollow Full-Overflowing, Empty Thread-like, Minute, Scattered

Table 17-3 Signs of Chaos

Qi	Separation of yin and yang (in principal positions)	Empty qualities (separating at organ depth, Leather, Tense, Yielding Empty & Thread-like, Minute, Scattered), Change in Qualities, Change in Amplitude, Yielding Hollow Full-Overflowing, Unstable, Nonhomogeneous, Dead, Muffled*
	'Qi wild' (separation of yin and yang in entire organism)	Majority of principal positions indicate separation of yin and yang; qualities at first impression: Change in Qualities, Empty Qualities (see above), Collapsing, Yielding Hollow Full-Overflowing (*Interrupted-Intermittent* most severe 'Qi wild,' *Rapid* due to stopping long-term cardiovascular exercise suddenly, *Slow* due to physical overwork or exercise since early childhood); qualities change from side to side; sides/burners vary greatly
Blood ('blood out of control')		Leather-like Hollow, Very Tense-Tight Hollow Full-Overflowing, Yielding partially Hollow Full-Overflowing
Circulation ('instability of circulation')		Interrupted-Intermittent, one cannot get the rate, Change in Amplitude over the entire pulse, rate differs from side to side
Other qualities implying potentially serious conditions		Wiry, Choppy, Leather-Hard, Restricted, Bean (Spinning), Ropy, Floating Tight, Nonhomogeneous, Unstable, Rate Decrease with Exertion, Heart Enlarged and Large Vessel positions present, Robust Pounding (4-5 degree), Flooding Excess (4-5 degree), Suppressed, Hollow Full-Overflowing, Amorphous (vessel anomalies), high temperature with slow pulse rate and low temperature with fast pulse rate
Common and less common qualities and prevention	Qualities prognostic of impending disease or that appear simultaneously with the earlier stages of disease	Flooding Deficient Wave, Deep, Feeble-Absent (qi deficient); Tight (yin deficient); Thin (blood deficient)
	Qualities associated with stagnation and that can lead to cancer over a long period of time	Flat, Inflated, Muffled, and Cotton

*Although Muffled mostly appears wherever coherent active qi function is impaired at the cellular-molecular level by extraordinary stagnation or physiological chaos equivalent to separation of yin and yang, it should be noted that we often find it at lesser degrees [1-2]. In this case it should certainly be monitored for further progression, but we don't usually consider it a separation of yin and yang.

which they are found, the other qualities with which they are combined, and so forth. Refer to the previous chapters for greater detail regarding their specific description and interpretation.

Advanced: quick overview

We scan the pulse record for qualities suggestive of serious conditions.

Substances (includes broad, closer, and closest focus) and activity
Refer to Table 5-3, Table 17-2, and the appropriate chapters.

Stability (activity and change)
We are concerned here with signs of physiological chaos, which is the most serious pathological threat that can be presented to a living organism and which may signify life-threatening conditions including cancer and autoimmune diseases. Refer to Tables 5-3 and 17-3, Ch. 6, and other appropriate chapters.

Burners: preliminary examination
We scan the burners (see Ch. 14) to get a sense of the person's root/groundedness (proximal positions), centeredness (middle positions), and how well they can interact with the outside world (distal positions; see Ch. 15).

Paradoxical qualities
When certain pulse qualities that ordinarily take many years to develop are found in a younger person it is a paradoxical finding and considered more serious and possibly representative of a constitutional or congenital deficit. The following are some examples:

- Any quality that indicates severe deficiency (Deep, Feeble-Absent) or chaos (various Empty qualities, Changing Qualities, Yielding Hollow Full-Overflowing, severe arrhythmias).

- Any quality that indicates severe excess heat (Robust Pounding [4-5], Flooding Excess [3-5], Tense-Tight Hollow Full-Overflowing, Ropy) or extreme yin-essence deficiency (Tight, Wiry, Leather-Hard).

- Increase in Rate on Exertion > 35 beats/minute indicates severe Heart Blood deficiency.

- If the rate remains constant or decreases on exertion or frequently misses beats, this indicates a severely impaired cardiovascular function (Heart qi-yang deficiency).

- A Ropy quality in a young person (under 40 years) and any of the qualities listed above as signs of instability, severe depletion of qi, blood, or yin and yang and severe excess heat (Tense-Tight Hollow Full-Overflowing, Flooding Excess) are of serious concern.

- The typical gender difference reflected on the pulse is that a woman's pulse is generally Thinner and a man's pulse is generally Wider. If these are reversed, they are signs of illness. The Thin quality in a man has been found to be potentially serious clinically.

- A very high temperature with a very low pulse rate, or vice versa, is a sign of physiological chaos ('qi wild') of the most serious kind, frequently found in the terminal yin stage of illness.
- In an acute disease the pulse should be Robust and Pounding and in a chronic condition it should be Reduced.
- The depth of the pulse is somewhat determined by the amount of connective tissue between the body surface and the vessels. Thus an obese person's pulse tends to be Deeper (depending on degree of obesity) and a thin person's pulse tends to be slightly more Superficial.

List preliminary diagnostic impressions

Include Robust (excess), Reduced (deficient), and Instability (chaos).

Systematic approach: all levels of experience

The following is the most thorough method for interpreting a pulse record. Beginning with the preliminary scan discussed above, it moves from a broad focus ('first impressions' of the entire pulse qualities, and 'wave forms') to a closer focus (qualities of the depths and sides), and then to the closest focus (examination of the individual principal and complementary positions).

• BROAD FOCUS: initial impressions

The broad focus of the pulse consists of the uniform qualities found over the entire pulse, the wave form, and most importantly, the rate and rhythm. We must first attend to the information from the broad focus when developing a treatment strategy or the treatments will not hold.

The abnormalities in rhythm (see Ch. 6) include Change in Rate at Rest, Interrupted, and Intermittent.

Rate abnormalities (see Ch. 7) include Slow, Fast, the rarely-seen varying rate between the sides, burners and positions, different rates over the course of the exam, and small or large Changing Rates on Exertion (see Ch. 6).

If there are disharmonies of rate and rhythm, we should look first to the other qualities and positions associated with Heart disharmony, especially the left distal and Heart complementary positions (see Ch. 12.)

Wave forms

We are concerned with the wave-form (see the appropriate chapters) as part of the larger picture. We may find Normal, Flooding Deficient, Flooding Excess, Hollow Full-Overflowing, Hesitant, or Suppressed waves.

Uniform qualities

Uniform qualities (see Chs. 13 and 14) found frequently over the entire pulse include the Tense, Tight, Thin, Smooth Vibration, Robust Pounding, Reduced Substance or Diffuse, Change in Rate at Rest, Floating, Cotton, Flooding Deficient Wave, Hesitant Wave, and Change in Amplitude.

Uniform qualities found over the entire pulse that suggest more serious conditions are the Choppy (now more common), Wiry, Leather-Hard (now more common), Muffled, Rough Vibration, alterations in rate and rhythm (see above), Empty, Yielding Hollow Full-Overflowing, or Change in Qualities, Blood Unclear, Blood Heat-Thick, Tense very Tight Hollow Full-Overflowing, Ropy, Wiry, Slippery, Flooding Excess, as well as most of the paradoxical qualities listed above.

The uniform qualities at the organ depths (organ qi, blood, and substance), especially the latter two, inform us about the presence and the nature of retained pathogens. These are substances that the body considers a threat to the integrity of vital organs and diverts through the divergent and *luo* channels to places that are less immediately threatening to essential function like the solid organs. Joints, skin, and the sinuses are familiar areas of the body for retained pathogens where, over time, they do great damage. They also deprive the organism of energy to keep them there that would otherwise have been available for growth, development, healing, and function. Qualities commonly found at these positions are Tense, Robust Pounding, Choppy, and Slippery. (See discussion of organ depth in Ch. 13.)

• **CLOSER FOCUS:** depths, sides, wave forms, areas, systems and psychology

Please refer to the appropriate chapters for a more complete discussion of the individual qualities.

Depths

Refer to Ch. 13 for more detail on the depths of the pulse.

Above the qi depth there may be qualities associated with an external etiology (Floating Tense and Slow or Floating Yielding and slightly Rapid) or an internal etiology (Floating Tight, Cotton, Hollow Full-Overflowing, Flooding Excess).

Qualities found at the qi depth are Yielding, Diminished, or Absent, Thin Tight, Thin Yielding, Taut, Tense, Tight, Wiry, Leather-Hard, Robust Pounding, Slippery, and Smooth Vibration. Qualities found consistently at the qi depth and separating or absent at the blood and organ depths are the Empty qualities.

The blood depth has these qualities: starting with pressure from the surface we have Spreading, Yielding Partially Hollow, Leather-like Hollow; beginning at the organ depth and gradually releasing pressure we have Blood Unclear, Blood Heat, and Blood Thick, sometimes with Slippery, Rough Vibration, and Choppy.

The organ depth is subdivided into the organ qi, blood, and substance depths.

Qualities found at the organ qi depth include the Taut, Tense, Tight, Thin, Wiry, Slippery, Robust Pounding, Reduced Pounding, Suppressed Pounding, Vibration, Choppy, Slippery, Leather-Hard, Muffled (if qi and blood depth are Absent), and Separating, Reduced Substance, Diffuse, Deep, and Feeble-Absent,

All qualities found at the organ blood and substance depths imply a retained pathogen. Some of the more common qualities associated with a retained pathogen include Slippery, Robust Pounding, Tense, Tight, Choppy, Rough Vibration, and Leather-Hard.

Uniform qualities found only on one side (see Ch. 14 for more detail) usually involve one of Dr. Shen's 'systems' (see below and Glossary).

Dr. Shen's systems model

Dr. Shen developed the 'systems' model (see Chs. 14 and 15)[2] to explain the relatively mild and shifting complaints of patients who showed no signs of illness by Chinese or biomedical diagnostic methods. His four systems are the 'nervous system', 'digestive system', 'circulatory system', and 'organ system', each of which is defined in the Glossary.

The digestive and organ 'systems' are discussed below in the sections on the right and left sides, respectively.

The 'nervous system' may be tense due to lifelong or constitutional hypervigilance (Slow rate) or current stress-related hypervigilance (rate more Rapid). It may be weak due to a constitutional vulnerability with lifelong and endless physical and emotional problems for which no allopathic etiology can be elicited.

The 'circulatory system' is characterized by occasional migrating joint pain (especially when fatigued), being quick to anger, and a Slow pulse with no other signs.

On the entire left side ('organ system') we may find the Reduced Substance, Diffuse, Deep, Feeble-Absent, or Empty qualities, signifying that the 'organ system' is deficient. In the elderly, this may be due to aging. If the person is under 50, the etiology is likely constitutional and is associated with a 'nervous system weak', essence-deficient condition or major lifestyle abuse, including severe childhood nutritional deprivation and extended physical or sexual exploitation.

If the entire left side has a Thin Tight line at the surface, this shows that the 'nervous system' is affecting the 'organ system'.

If the entire right side ('digestive system') has Reduced Substance, Diffuse Deep, Feeble-Absent, or Empty, it indicates that the 'digestive system' is deficient, which is often the result of eating irregularly, in excessive amounts, or difficult to digest foods.

If the entire right side has a Thin Tight line at the surface it indicates that the 'nervous system' is affecting the 'digestive system'—usually due to eating too rapidly.

The psychological category (see Table 15-1 and Ch. 15) includes all mental, emotional, and spiritual issues associated with each quality as deduced from the pulse exam.

Sides

When the Changes in Amplitude shift from side to side—first one side alone showing this change, then the other side alone—this is usually due to the presence of a current, strong interpersonal conflict. Less frequently it can follow exertion far beyond a person's capacity and lasts for a limited time (weeks).

If the qualities shift from side to side, it is a rare but serious 'qi wild' sign.

When one side is Amorphous, being present without any identifiable shape resembling a quality, we must make sure no anomalous qualities (i.e., the Transposed or Three Yin pulses) are involved, as this may interfere with the diagnostic value of the associated side.

The qualities found in the Neuro-psychological positions, the Special Lung positions, and possibly the Pelvis/Lower Body positions inform us of conditions on the opposite side of the body.

Neuro-psychological positions

The interpretation of Neuro-psychological positions' qualities are open to investigation without concrete data at this point.

Areas and burners

By 'areas' we mean positions that might represent a larger body space; for example, the Special Lung or Diaphragm positions might include the breasts. Areas of the pulse are the three burners, the Diaphragm positions, the Peritoneal, and the Pelvis/Lower Body positions.

Qualities that appear bilaterally in one burner often have a special significance. For example, a Wiry quality appearing simultaneously in both middle positions might indicate pancreatitis rather than a specific disharmony in either the Liver or Spleen-Stomach.

• CLOSEST FOCUS

General considerations were discussed above in the quick overview section.

Specific considerations encompass the interpretation of individual and complementary positions and their relationships. The presence of pathology in the complementary positions associated with an organ informs us that the disease process in that organ is more advanced and serious than otherwise.

See Ch. 12 for more detail on the principal and complementary positions of the organs. Many pulse-takers have observed a trend that the more serious qualities that were once uncommon are now becoming more common, especially those indicating the separation of yin and yang (Empty, Changing Qualities), parenchymal damage (Rough Vibration), and toxicity (Choppy, Leather-Hard).

We also consider the relationships between individual positions (see Ch. 12) that are intimately related to familiar associations in the medicine, such as the findings in the left distal and right distal and Special Lung positions informing us about cardio-pulmonary disease, or between the left distal and left proximal positions about Kidney-Heart disharmony.

The qualities representing qi and yang deficiencies are usually the ones that offer least resistance to our fingers, such as Reduced Substance, Diffuse, Feeble-Absent, and Empty. Those qualities representing yin and essence deficiencies, such as Tight, Wiry, Leather-Hard, that offer more resistance may override those that offer less resistance, and when both exist simultaneously, we may miss the qi-yang aspect of the condition.

Revisiting broad/closer/closest focus

Finally, one returns to the broader initial impressions and searches again for connections between those qualities and the findings in the individual positions. For example, a Deep right side and clear signs on the right middle position would indicate that the condition affecting digestion goes beyond the Spleen to include the Kidneys and Lungs.

INTERPRETATION

To best understand this section, the reader is strongly encouraged to refer to the case histories in Ch. 18.

Summary of findings

Here we present a definitive, coherent statement of the patient's overall and individual conditions and the factors that led to them. We integrate the patient's history, symptoms, and signs (pulse) and make an argument for those that are most central to the individual's health and survival.

Based on the summary of our findings, we decide upon a formulation, or analysis and synthesis, of immediate interventions, root issues, secondary issues, and derivative issues as described below.

Current prevailing issues or patterns

These are the diagnostic categories that require more immediate intervention including such emergencies (hot button issues) and urgent matters as imminent hemorrhage, acute diseases, severe acute cardiac dysfunction, 'blocks'[3] such as stability (chaos), trauma and shock, and various forms of intolerable pain, both physical and emotional. Depending on the situation, some of the root, secondary, and derivative disharmonies may be introduced here. We follow the fundamental dictum that we must move as we build.

Root issues, and often the etiology of the disharmonies

These are the fundamental patterns and vulnerabilities that underlie the patient's condition and often involve in utero, birth, and very early life etiologies. They are also often the least obviously perceived without the aid of the pulse. In our time, these are most often the Kidneys and the Heart, the organs that are most affected by intra-uterine and birth insults. Increasingly, with the escalating use of cold substance such as marijuana, the Liver tends to become a root issue.

Secondary issues

These are the conditions that are not as crucial to the patient's short- or long-term function as those requiring immediate intervention, nor as fundamental as the root issues to the ultimate recovery.

Derivative issues

These conditions are the consequence of the effects of the root and secondary issues, such as blood stagnation, blood heat, neoplastic conditions, and toxicities.

Management

The following is an exercise based initially on the pulse, but the final management should integrate the pulse with the patient's history and other signs and symptoms.

Lifestyle strategies

These are recommendations for changes to aspects of the patient's lifestyle that have led to and sustain his current state of disordered mental, emotional, spiritual, and physical health.

Referrals

These are made for diagnostic or treatment purposes in order to enhance those already available to the practitioner within their own scope of practice. So as not to alarm the patient, you may suggest them in such terms as desiring to "rule out" potential complications in order to best treat him.

Acupuncture, herbal, and other healing strategies

Keep in mind that these interventions are guidelines and you may need to revise them when necessary. Treatment is part of our diagnosis.

Immediate interventions are management strategies that place more emphasis on relieving 'blocks' and on treating conditions that are most urgent. Again, depending upon the situation, management of some of the root, secondary, and derivative disharmonies may be introduced here. It is Dr. Hammer's personal preference, if possible, to simultaneously treat the 'digestive' functions (Spleen-Stomach, etc.) to enhance the patient's participation in their healing.

Following attention to the intermediate interventions, the emphasis shifts to the root issues while also continuing to relieve any problems remaining from our immediate interventions and appropriate secondary and derivative issues.

The long-range major interventions move to include some of the secondary issues, while the management strategy remains to also address the enduring root issues and remaining immediate interventions.

Derivative issues are addressed by the long-range minor interventions, along with what remains of the other issues. Although these conditions are not the primary source of the patient's pathology, they are important to resolve so that they don't develop into more serious conditions in the future.

ACUPUNCTURE AND PULSE DIAGNOSIS

Dr. Shen was very clear that in his experience (and in my own), using this system of evaluation of the pulse immediately after a treatment is inaccurate and not useful until several days have passed due to the ongoing changes set in motion by the introduction of needles and herbs.

CONCLUSION

This chapter has been concerned with the methodology of interpreting the data revealed by the pulse. This process is illustrated in the case records in the following chapter.

Teaching and learning this skill through the written word is unavoidably complex and repetitive. The process of learning involves a dynamic interplay between the didactic material found in these chapters and direct, practical, hands-on experience during intensive pulse seminars.

The acquisition of this skill involves a gradual absorption and integration of experience and awareness. During this diligent study, you will encounter many epiphanies that will deepen and refine your understanding. The reward for the dedicated practitioner is a world of exciting and very useful knowledge that goes far beyond our routine diagnostic assessments.

Above all, you should remember that this is an evolving system. A good example of this occurred during an advance pulse intensive seminar taught by Dr. Hammer. There was a pulse volunteer, a veteran of the Gulf War, who was exposed to a significant amount of chemical warfare. Her pulse had one of the most Choppy qualities we had ever encountered, which ultimately expanded our understanding of this quality to include the possibility of toxicity. Another example is the occurrence of the Leather-Hard quality. Not so long ago this was a rather rare quality, but it seems that with the increased use of wifi, cell phones and the like in recent years, it has become a much more common finding.[4]

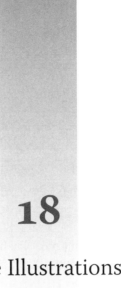

18

Case Illustrations

Leon Hammer, M.D.

INTRODUCTION

Two case histories are presented in this chapter as exercises in pulse interpretation. They follow the procedures used in actual pulse classes that I teach on the pulse to practitioners of Chinese medicine.

I suggest that you begin by reading and analyzing the pulse record (chart) through the section on management, but not the client history, in accordance with the precepts that are set forth in Ch. 17 and in Fig. 17-1. Then compare your analysis and management recommendations with those presented here, and use the comparison to explore aspects that you may have overlooked. (It is of course possible that you may discover issues that I have missed, in which case a message to my website would be appreciated.)

Next, read the client history and its correlation with the pulse. In the context of my classes, the goal here is to explain the patient's problems based on the findings from the pulse so as to provide the referring practitioner with a fresh perspective on a clinical situation that has thus far resisted their efforts to resolve. Again, compare your findings with mine. Additional case illustrations may be posted in the future on my website *www.dragonrises.org* that will reflect more recent developments.

Figs 18-1 and 18-2 have been revised in keeping with our new pulse form, Fig. 4-1. Please note in particular that the organ depth is now subdivided to include organ-qi, organ-blood, and organ-substance. These are important changes in order to account for signs in the latter two positions of retained pathogens, especially retained heat (Robust Pounding), retained toxins (Choppy), retained dampness (Slippery), and retained radiation (Leather-Hard). (See the Closer Focus and Depths sections in Ch. 17.) However, because the pulses reflected in Figs. 18-1 and 18-2 were recorded and analyzed prior to the first edition of the source text, *Chinese Pulse Diagnosis: A Contemporary Approach* in 2001, the organ-blood and organ-substance findings are not recorded here.

These two cases are presented only to illustrate the methodology of pulse interpretation in this pulse system. There have been a few significant changes compared to the original book. We have learned a great deal in the past twenty years since this project began. The client history is included only for the sake of completeness and for comparison with the pulse findings. A discussion of complaints and symptoms as interpreted by the pulse findings is included but is not relevant to the main thrust of this presentation.

The 'management-formulation' format varies slightly from the one normally taught and practiced at Dragon Rises College of Oriental Medicine, with which I am affiliated.[1] Acupuncture or herbal treatments are neither included in the Management-Implementation section here nor in the larger source book due to space considerations. Once diagnosed, there are hundreds of books telling us how to treat a condition, but the trick is to diagnose the correct condition.

While all methods of Chinese medical diagnosis deserve equal attention, remember that this is an exercise illustrating only the potential of Contemporary Chinese Pulse Diagnosis to provide profound practical and in-depth diagnostic information that enhances the management and treatment of patients in the clinic.

Presenting this in a step-by-step fashion inevitably leads to some repetition that may, in final appraisal, become woven into an integrated impression. While this is necessarily a laborious process for teaching purposes, with experience, the total time for the pulse examination done without elaborate note taking can be as little as fifteen minutes, and a quick determination of the significant findings can be assessed as one goes along.

Caveat: The pulse records, Figs. 18-1 and 18-2, and case illustrations in this chapter were recorded almost twenty years ago. At the very end of this chapter I have therefore added a third record, Fig. 18-3, made recently to demonstrate how much more material we are now capable of accessing than we did at the earlier time.

---

1. Dragon Rises College of Oriental Medicine (DRCOM) is the only school of Chinese medicine where Contemporary Chinese Pulse Diagnosis is a major part of the program (165 hours) and has been taught for over ten years. For additional information, visit *www.dragonrises.edu.*

Fig. 18-1   **Contemporary Chinese Pulse Record**

Date:					
Name: Client 1	**Gender:** F	**Age:** 27	**Hgt:** 5' 10"	**Wgt:** 160	**Occup:** Housewife

Rhythm: Interrupted [about 5x/min.]	**Rate/min:** Begin: End: W/exertion: Chg: **Other Rates During Exam:**

First Impressions Of Uniform Qualities
 	
 Thin; Tense-Tight; Robust Pounding [2];
 Rough Vibration at all depths; Change in Amplitude [2]
	DEPTHS
	 Floating: ————————
	 Cotton: [3-4]
	 Qi: Tense-Tight
	 Blood: Thick
	 Organ: Tense
	   O-B: Not Accessed
	   O-S: Not Accessed
	 Wave: Normal → Flooding Deficient

Left Side: ————————	**Right Side:** ————————	

PRINCIPAL POSITIONS		COMPLEMENTARY POSITIONS	

L: DISTAL POSITION **R:**		**L:** NEURO-PSYCHOLOGICAL **R:**	
Tense	Tight	Smooth Vibration Doughy	Smooth Vibration Doughy

L: SPECIAL LUNG POSITION   **R:**

L distal (cont.)	R distal (cont.)	L Lung	R Lung
Slippery [4-5]	Rough Vibration Slippery	Tight Rough Vibration Slippery	Tight Slippery Rough Vibration **Pleura:** ————————

HEART
Mitral Valve: Slippery
Enlarged: Present
Large Vessel: ————————

Pericardium: ————————

L: MIDDLE POSITION **R:**		**L:** DIAPHRAGM **R:**	

Reduced Substance → Thin
 	
 Qi Depth: Tense-Tight
 	
 Blood Depth: Thick
   Slippery
     Rough Vibration [2]
 	
 Organ Depth: Tense-Tight
	Tense
	
	 Robust Pounding [4]
		Inflated [1-2]	Inflated [1-2]

LIVER
ENGORGED
Distal: ————————   **Ulnar:** Present
Gallbladder: Tight; Slippery

SPLEEN-STOMACH
Esophagus: ————————   **Spleen:** ————————
Stom-pyl. Exten: ————————
Peritoneal Cavity/pancreas: ————————
Duodenum: ————————

L: PROXIMAL POSITION **R:**		**Large:** INTESTINES **Small:**	
Qi Depth: Diminished Tight ↕ Absent	Qi Depth: Diminished Tight Change in Amplitude [2]	Tense Slippery	Tight-Biting Slippery

L: PELVIS/LOWER BODY   **R:**

Pelvis L	Pelvis R
Muffled Change in Amplitude [5]	Choppy Change in Amplitude [5]

THREE BURNERS **Upper:** Slippery **Middle:** ———————— **Lower:** Tight	**COMMENTS** △ = Change [1] → [5] = low → high degree

CLIENT 1 Female, Age 27

BROAD FOCUS: INITIAL IMPRESSION OF LARGE SEGMENTS AND UNIFORM QUALITIES

Rhythm

The rhythm is Interrupted, irregularly skipping beats approximately five times per minute. This is ordinarily a sign of severe Heart qi deficiency, its seriousness mitigated because its rate can still be measured. This is also a sign of severe Heart qi agitation.

Rate

The initial rate is only 60 beats/min and 66 at the end. On exertion, the rate increases six points to 72. The Slow rate in a 27-year-old woman is a sign of Heart qi deficiency, and the increase of only six beats with vigorous exertion is a sign of moderate to severe Heart qi-yang deficiency.

Wave

The Flooding Deficient Wave by itself is a sign of mild to moderate general qi deficiency. With regard to patient number one, the wave was Normal at times and the Flooding Deficient Wave not consistently present; this militates toward a milder qi deficiency. Searching the rest of the pulse for confirmation of this impression one finds significant though also inconsistent qi deficiency only in the left proximal position.

Uniform qualities over the entire pulse

Common qualities

The Tense-Tight combination is a sign of qi stagnation and mild excess Heat (Tense) and developing yin-deficiency (Tight).

Robust Pounding (2) is a sign of mild excess heat that the body has been unable to eliminate completely through normal processes of defecation and urination or perspiration.

The Thin quality is a sign of blood deficiency.

Tight is a common quality. While appearing in only four principal positions, it is still unusual in a 27-year-old woman. One must also consider pain as the cause, perhaps from arthritis. (Excess invasive cold is another, but less likely, cause since it is rare in our era of indoor heating.)

Less common qualities

Rough Vibration over the entire pulse at all depths is a sign of Heart shock and possibly consequent Heart qi deficiency. Fear and guilt might be implicated.

Change in Amplitude over the entire pulse is another mild (2) sign of Heart qi deficiency.

Unusual qualities

See Rhythm above.

Paradoxical qualities

'Blood thick' is a form of blood heat and blood vessel congestion rarely found in a young woman.

A rate rising only 6 beats/min on exertion is an unusual finding in a 27-year-old woman.

The developing Flooding Deficient wave is a sign of a growing true qi deficiency, again an unusual sign in a 27-year-old woman.

The Interrupted rhythm is evidence of considerable Heart/circulatory system instability rarely found in such a young person and indicating a profound etiology and serious outcome.

CLOSER FOCUS

Depths

Cotton quality

The Cotton quality is a sign of qi stagnation associated with an acknowledged sense of resignation to a less than satisfactory life situation, and about which she feels stuck. A major physical trauma is the other etiological possibility.

Qi depth

The Tense-Tight combination is, again, a sign of qi stagnation and slight excess Heat (Tense) and developing yin-deficiency (Tight).

Blood depth

Blood Thick is a sign of inflammation of the vessels and turbidity in the blood that could be exacerbated in part by the Slow circulation.

Organ depth

Tense quality is a sign of mild to moderate qi stagnation and mild excess heat.

Sides

Nothing significant.

Three burners

Slippery (4-5 at the left distal position) with a Slow rate bilaterally in the upper burner indicates phlegm disturbing the orifices of the Heart and present in the Lung (bilaterally Slippery in the Special Lung positions) and perhaps chest.

SUMMARY OF INITIAL IMPRESSIONS OF BROAD AND CLOSER FOCUS

The principal findings here are the signs of considerable Heart qi deficiency, Heart shock, and Heart qi agitation, including the Interrupted rhythm, Slow rate, Rough Vibration at all depths, and the Change in Amplitude over the entire pulse.

Phlegm misting the Heart orifices and a damp condition in the upper burner is another significant finding. An excess heat condition (Robust Pounding) is moving at an early age to a yin deficient condition (Tense to Tight). Blood deficiency is evidenced by the Thin quality.

There is considerable qi stagnation (Cotton) indicating a feeling of being stuck in life, general moderate qi deficiency (Flooding Deficient Wave), and 'blood thick' (Blood Thick quality), which is a sign of inflammation and turbidity in the blood circulation.

CLOSEST FOCUS (INDIVIDUAL POSITIONS AND ORGANS)

Quick Overview

All of the principal positions were either Tense (qi stagnation and excess heat), Tight (yin deficiency), or somewhere between these two qualities (Tense-Tight or Tight-Tense), indicating the simultaneous presence of both excess heat and yin deficiency.

Unusual qualities

The presence of the Heart Enlarged position is probably the most unusual and potentially serious sign, especially with the other signs of Heart qi-yang deficiency already mentioned and the Slippery quality at the Mitral Valve position. The Muffled quality at the Pelvis/Lower Body position is relatively unusual in a 27-year-old woman and is a sign of a neoplastic process that should be carefully followed, especially with the extreme Change of Amplitude and Choppy qualities (blood stagnation) at the same position.

Instability: where there is the most activity and change

The Change in Amplitude is extreme [5] at the Pelvis/Lower Body positions, indicating possible serious physiological disturbance with the organs of the lower burner. The greatest change is found at the left proximal position where there is a Change in Qualities (Tight ← → Absent) indicating a Kidney separation of yin and yang—the result of both Kidney yin and qi-yang deficiency. This suggests in such a young woman that the root of her problem began at an early stage of life, in utero or at birth. Changes in Qualities at the left middle position indicates a developing less serious separation of yin and yang condition of the Liver.

Other more serious qualities

Slippery [4-5] at the left distal position indicates phlegm disturbing the orifices of the Heart. Slippery in the right distal position and bilaterally at the Special Lung positions are signs of a serious damp condition in the Lungs and perhaps chest, possibly related to the Slippery quality at the left distal position. Rough Vibration at the right distal position may be pulmonary alveolar damage and qi deficiency.

Rough Vibration and a Slippery quality at the blood depth of the left middle positions indicates damage to the intima of the vessels and are serious signs commensurate with the Thick quality at the general blood depth.

Paradoxical qualities

All of the above are paradoxical in a 27-year-old woman, especially an enlarged Heart position, which may indicate an enlarged Heart, energetically or otherwise.

Individual Positions (Principal & Complementary)

Heart/circulation

The Slippery quality at the left distal position is a sign of phlegm misting/disturbing the Heart orifices, a signal of possible severe emotional instability. The presence of the Heart Enlarged position, and the Slippery quality at the Mitral Valve position, are signs of Heart qi deficiency. The Smooth Vibration quality at the Neuro-psychological is a sign of Heart qi agitation.

Lungs

The Tight quality at the right distal position is a sign of Lung yin deficiency; at the Special Lung positions it is a sign of some inflammation. The Slippery quality at both of these positions is a sign of Lung damp stagnation, and the Rough Vibration quality at both positions is a sign of parenchymal damage and, by implication, of Lung qi deficiency.

Liver-Gallbladder

This position has Reduced Substance and is becoming Thin, which indicates developing Liver qi and blood deficiency. The instability is a sign of a developing separation of yin and yang of the Liver. One engorged position is present, indicating some slight blood stagnation in the Liver. The Gallbladder shows signs of damp-heat and inflammation (Slippery, Tight). In this position, the Tight quality is usually a sign of moderate inflammation.

Spleen/Stomach/Intestines

The Robust Pounding quality [4] at this position, and the Biting and Slippery qualities at the Intestine positions, are indications of considerable excess heat (irritation or inflammation) and compensatory dampness in the gastrointestinal tract as well as some abdominal discomfort (Biting at the Small Intestine position).

Kidneys/Bladder

There are signs of both Kidney yin (Tight quality) and qi-yang deficiency (Absent quality). The Change in Qualities at the left proximal position, from Tight to Absent, is a sign that Kidney yin and yang are separating.

SUMMARY OF CONDITIONS AT INDIVIDUAL POSITIONS (CLOSEST FOCUS)

The Interrupted quality, Change in Amplitude, Rough Vibration over the entire pulse, Slow rate, Enlarged Heart, failure of the rate to increase more than 12 beats/min (6 on exertion), and Slippery quality at the left distal and Mitral Valve positions are all signs of Heart qi-yang deficiency. To find this degree of disharmony in a 27-year-old woman suggests either a constitutional or congenital insult or rheumatic heart disease. A Kidney-Heart disharmony is therefore an important consideration.

Other considerations are damp-heat in the Lungs, damp-heat and damage to the intima of the blood vessels, excess heat and inflammation of the gastrointestinal system, Liver qi and blood deficiency, chaotic Kidney and Liver qi, and possible tumor development in the pelvic area.

SUBSTANCES (INCLUDES BROAD, CLOSER, AND CLOSEST FOCUS)

Qi stagnation

COTTON   The Cotton quality [3-4] is a sign of qi stagnation, discussed above and below.

TENSE   The Tense quality that pervades the entire pulse is a sign of moderate qi stagnation and mild excess heat.

MUFFLED   Present only at the Pelvis-Lower Body position, it is a sign of a developing neoplastic process.

Qi deficiency

The Flooding Deficient Wave is a sign of general qi deficiency. The Change in Amplitude over the entire pulse, the Slow rate, the Slippery quality at the Mitral Valve position, the Interrupted rhythm, the rise on exertion of the rate of between 6 and 11 beats/min, and the presence of the Enlarged Heart position are signs of Heart qi-yang deficiency. Other signs of qi deficiency are found in the Lung (Rough Vibration), Liver (Reduced Substance), and Kidneys (Absent).

Blood stagnation

The Choppy quality at the Pelvis/Lower Body position is a sign of blood stagnation in the pelvis, and the presence of the distal Engorged position indicates mild blood stagnation in the Liver. The Blood Thick quality is a sign of considerable blood stagnation in the general circulation and turbulence (Slippery at the blood depth).

Blood deficiency

The Thin quality mentioned under first impressions and at the left middle position is a sign of blood deficiency.

Yin excess (dampness)

The Slippery quality is a sign of considerable damp stagnation in the Heart, Lungs, Gallbladder, and Intestines. The Slippery quality at the blood depth is a sign of turbulence in the blood.

Yin deficiency

The Tight quality found especially in the Lungs and the Kidneys is a sign of yin deficiency. The appearance of the Tense-Tight qualities generally, and in several positions, indicates a trend toward yin deficiency.

Yang excess

None.

Yang deficiency

The presence of the Interrupted quality, and the increase of less that 6 beats/min on exertion, together with the Enlarged Heart position is convincing evidence of a developing Heart yang deficiency. The Absent quality and Change in Qualities at the left proximal position is an indication of a trend toward Kidney yang deficiency and the previously mentioned Kidney-Heart yang disharmony.

Essence deficiency

The Change in Qualities at the left proximal position from Tight to Absent is a sign of Kidney yang-essence deficiency.

Parenchyma

The Rough Vibration at the right distal and Special Lung positions is a sign of parenchymal damage to the pulmonary alveoli.

ACTIVITY

Excess heat

The Tense quality throughout the pulse, Robust Pounding, and Blood Thick qualities are signs of excess heat.

Combined excess heat and yin deficiency

Excess heat is metabolic heat that has accumulated in a failed attempt to overcome stagnation. In the service of balance, the body brings fluid (yin) to balance the heat that over time is gradually depleted.

Cold excess

The literature cites the Tight quality to be a sign of invasive excess cold. However, in the modern context of central heating, this is now a rare etiology.

Deficient cold (yang deficiency)

Deficient cold is equivalent to yang deficiency, one piece of evidence for which is the occasionally Absent quality and Change in Qualities at the left proximal position. The presence of the Enlarged Heart position, the Interrupted quality and increase of less than 6 beats/min on exertion are signs of developing Heart yang deficiency.

AREAS

Burners: similar qualities bilaterally at same burner

Upper burner

The Slippery quality bilaterally at both distal positions is a sign of dampness in the chest. Emotionally, this could also indicate some inhibition of the normal impulse to open one's heart and arms to the world.

Middle burner

None.

Lower burner

The presence of both the Tight quality and Diminished quality at the qi depth reflects the simultaneous presence of Kidney yin and qi deficiency in the lower burner.

Diaphragm

The bilateral minimal Inflation [1-2] at the Diaphragm position is a sign that there is no currently ongoing stress associated with separation and the acrimonious suppression of tender feelings associated with it. It may also mean that there are no significant relationships.

Pelvis/Lower Body

The extreme Change in Amplitude [5], bilaterally, and the Muffled and Choppy qualities, are signs of extreme stagnation of qi and blood and physiological disorganization in the female pelvic organs.

SIDES

Nothing.

SYSTEMS

'Circulatory system'

The Slow pulse rate is a sign of impairment of the 'circulatory system,' probably due to Heart shock (seen in the Rough Vibration quality at all depths on first impression over the entire pulse).

INTERPRETATION

Summary of specific conditions

The degree of severity of the condition is indicated in parentheses.

- Heart qi/yang deficiency with mitral valve prolapse and enlargement (severe)
- Heart qi agitation (severe)
- Phlegm obstructing orifices of the Heart and dampness in the chest (severe)
- 'Circulatory system' deficient (severe)
- 'Blood thick', turbulence in the blood, and vessel wall damage (moderate to severe)
- Blood and qi stagnation in the lower burner (Pelvis/Lower Body position) (severe)
- Blood deficiency (mild to moderate)
- General qi stagnation (mild) and deficiency (moderate)
- Lung yin and qi deficiency and damp stagnation (moderate)
- Liver blood and qi deficiency and blood congestion (moderate)
- Gallbladder dampness and inflammation (moderate)
- Inflammation and excess heat and dampness (irritation and inflammation) in the gastrointestinal tract (moderate)
- Kidney yin, essence, and qi/yang deficiency; separation of Kidney yin and yang (moderate)

Pulse diagnostic formulation

It must be clear at the beginning of this discussion of diagnosis that one's initial formulations are not set in stone. They serve primarily as a starting point for a flexible process that becomes increasingly precise over the course of treatment, which is also part of the diagnostic process.

Pulse analysis and synthesis

The primary vulnerability for this woman is her Heart qi and yang deficiency, Heart shock (Rough Vibration), Heart qi agitation, and phlegm misting the orifices.

The damp-phlegm condition in the Heart, Lungs, and chest is associated with the Heart and Lung qi deficiency. The bilateral Slippery quality in the upper burner is a signal that her Heart feelings, which should normally reach out through one's arms to the world, are somewhat withdrawn.

Gallbladder damp and inflammation in the Gallbladder and Intestines and Stomach heat have caused the 'blood thick' condition, a drain on Heart qi. The 'blood thick' and Heart/circulation deficient conditions have contributed to the blood stagnation in the lower burner and Liver. Kidney yin has been depleted by compensating for this excess heat. Liver qi and blood are depleted.

Separately, Liver yin and yang are separating (Change in Qualities), suggesting a history of drugs and/or infection (no evidence on the pulse), since she is otherwise too young for such advanced pathology.

The early age of this seemingly significant Heart qi deficiency, and the Change in Qualities to Absent at the left proximal position, suggest the early onset of this problem with concomitant Kidney qi deficiency. With the mitral valve prolapse in conjunction with the Heart instability and deficiencies, we must also consider rheumatic fever as an etiology.

In deciding on the immediate intervention, we take into account the most serious current issues threatening the health and survival of the patient. We must also deal with blocks that diminish the effectiveness of our intervention including severe pain, instability, retained pathogens and trauma as well as structure. I usually also enhance the earth element in the beginning and throughout treatment if possible, attempting to make our main source of qi and blood during life as effective and efficient as possible.

With this client one can see that we must deal with the root issues in the immediate intervention, as these problems are immediate threats to the individual's viability. The seriousness of the situation in such a young person implies an etiology either in utero or very early in life.

MANAGEMENT FORMULATION

A. Immediate interventions

1. Heart-Kidney Disharmony
   a. Heart
      Qi-yang deficiency
      Heart shock
      Severe circulatory instability
      Phlegm misting the orifices as well as phlegm in the Lungs and chest
      Mitral valve prolapse
   b. Kidney
      Qi-yang-essence deficiency
      Separation of Kidney yin-yang-essence

2. Lower burner

    Blood and qi stagnation

    Impaired function

3. Liver-Gallbladder

    Gallbladder damp-heat

    Liver separation of yin and yang

    Stomach heat with damp-heat in the Intestines

B. Root issues and etiology

1. Heart

    As above

2. Kidney

    Qi-yang deficiency

    Yin-essence deficiency

    Separation of Kidney yin and yang-essence

C. Secondary issues

1. Liver-Gallbladder

    Blood deficiencies; qi deficiencies

    Gallbladder damp-heat, inflammation

2. Speen-Stomach-Intestines

    Stomach-Intestine damp-heat

3. Lung

    Yin and qi deficiency

    Damp stagnation

    Parenchymal damage

D. Derivative issues

1. Qi deficiency (Heart-Kidneys)
2. Blood deficiency
3. Blood and qi stagnation in the lower burner
4. Excess heat in the tissues and blood
5. Damp condition

MANAGEMENT IMPLEMENTATION

Lifestyle strategies

Overwork, pregnancy, and birth control

The significant deficiencies of qi and blood in several organs, especially the Heart, and the degree of blood stagnation in the lower burner, make it imperative that she rest and avoid the stresses of pregnancy and the blood-stagnating side effects of birth control medications.

Habits

Avoiding alcohol, tobacco, and recreational drugs and getting her to eat a moderate fat, low sugar, and no spice diet is also imperative because of the damp-heat in the blood, the damp-heat in the Gallbladder and Intestines, the heat in the Stomach, and both Lung yin deficiency and Lung damp-heat.

Emotional stress

See Referrals below (counseling).

Referrals

- The considerable stagnation of qi and blood in the lower burner warrants regular gynecological examination.
- The moderate to severe Cotton [3-4] quality and severe Heart qi agitation both suggest the advisability of counseling.
- The excess damp-heat in the Gallbladder suggests inflammation and stones, which should be investigated with ultrasound.

Acupuncture, herbs, and other strategies

Immediate interventions

1. Heart-circulation and Kidney qi-yang essence deficiency
   Heart shock
   Qi-yang deficiency
   Severe circulatory instability
   Phlegm misting the orifices as well as phlegm in the Lungs and chest
   Mitral valve prolapse

2. Kidney qi-yang deficiency

3. Spleen-Stomach-Intestine-Liver-Gallbladder
   Stomach heat and damp-heat in the Gallbladder and Intestines simultaneously to enhance digestive function and nourish the body-mind with assistance from other interventions. Especially if there are problems digesting the herbs, this strategy might need to precede all else.

Intermediate (root) interventions

Assuming the immediate interventions succeed, the following must be considered: Heart qi-yang deficiency (including phlegm in the Heart, mitral valve and Lungs, and Heart qi agitation) and circulation; blood stagnation in the lower burner (and Liver); and the 'blood thick' conditions are the basic issues to deal with at this stage. Combining treatment of the Heart, Liver, and Kidney deficiencies (qi, blood, yin, essence) is desirable.

Long-range interventions

Assuming the immediate and intermediate interventions are successful, treatment of selective conditions related to the Heart, Lungs, Kidneys, circulation, 'blood thick,' blood stagnation, dampness, and Liver blood deficiency must continue.

The Cotton quality and the 'stuckness' it represents is often benefited by improving Kidney yang-essence, which provides the will and courage to move on in life.

HISTORY AND PREVIOUS TREATMENT

Complaints

■ *Tiredness*

SYMPTOMS:

• 50 percent of time: trouble getting up even after a good sleep

• Could sleep all day but doesn't because then she would not sleep at night

• On 'empty' all of the time for no reason in terms of activities, including sex

• Body is in slow motion, as if carrying a heavy weight

• Hard to concentrate, organize, feels discombobulated and frazzled

• Cannot finish a project

• Hands have lost strength

• Patience is greatly diminished at these times

• Good times (50%): on good days she is tired only after activity or at end of day, and goes to sleep at 10 P.M.

• Somewhat worse before menstrual period when her husband reports increased irritability

• Feels that tiredness is due to stress, too much on her mind, so that she wants to "close my eyes, sleep and hide." In the past she dealt with stress through activity, not talk.

HISTORY:

• Began three years ago before pregnant with latest child, now two years old.

• Routine physical revealed very low platelets, under 100,000.

• Her adolescence was rebellious; she dropped out of school and partied, which involved heavy drug use (cocaine, marijuana, alcohol, cigarettes). Once slept five days. Went to live with father who remarried and had new family.

• Birth control methods: Ortho-Nova from age 16-20. Nausea, headaches, weight gain and sluggish; Depo-Prevara at age 22 for one year with same symptoms, some worse, some less; IUD used from age 23-25 and presently.

- Stress: Pregnant and delivered at age 20 with 60 pound weight gain, restricted activity due to back injury. Left father of child when baby was eight months old due to verbal and physical abuse, followed by a vicious custody battle. Shortly afterwards, her father died.

INTERPRETATION

Fatigue, especially even after a good night's sleep, is associated with Heart qi deficiency for which there is abundant evidence on the pulse. Difficulty organizing and concentrating, and feeling discombobulated, are signs of Heart qi and blood deficiency and Heart phlegm misting the orifices, and the decrease in patience is due in part to Heart qi agitation. In part the latter is due to the inability of Liver qi to contain her emotions.

The history of birth trauma (see discussion of pregnancies and birth histories below) reveals prolonged delivery under anesthesia with the cord wrapped around her neck several times. The multiple pregnancies in the presence of significant Heart qi deficiency is extremely draining. The heaviness and 'body in slow motion' is related to the damp condition that we see in the Gallbladder, Intestines, Heart, and Lungs, and to diminished circulation, in part due to Heart qi deficiency and in part to the 'blood thick' condition.

The excessive use of marijuana probably is a significant contribution to the Liver qi and blood deficiency and stagnation and to her fatigue and inability to recover her energy.

The fifty percent of the time when she feels at her worst and is most irritable is when she is premenstrual or under great stress, again a function of deficient Liver qi to contain her emotions. These symptoms began in the context of a custody battle for her first child, a time of great stress for which she self medicated with 'substances', exacerbating her already deficient terrain, especially the Liver's ability to contain.

Kidney essence deficiency, with its effect on the bone marrow (drop in platelets), and Lung qi deficiency, are contributory factors, as is the superficial qi stagnation.

■ *Easily bruises*

SYMPTOMS:

- Spontaneous and unrelated to trauma
- Sometimes painful and sometimes not
- Platelets normal recently, with less bruising

HISTORY:

- Always bruised easily and just assumed that she was clumsy

- Current increase began three years ago when platelet levels dropped
- Bone marrow biopsy normal, no spider varicose veins or phlebitis

INTERPRETATION

Spontaneous bruising is classically due either to Spleen qi deficiency, for which there is no significant evidence on the pulse, or blood stagnation, for which there is much pulse and historical evidence (IUD, birth control pills). My experience closely ties the low platelets to Kidney essence deficiency since the Kidneys control the bone marrow where platelets are made.

■ *Body aches*

SYMPTOMS:

- Several joints at once
- Almost constant
- Dull ache in knees, hip, elbows, shoulders, and hands
- With activity the dull ache becomes a deeper soreness, pain
- Stiffness without activity
- Worsens with cold, stress, and fatigue
- Constant with cold
- Relieved by warm bath, which relaxes her

HISTORY:

- Hands have always hurt with cold.
- Symptoms began one year ago and have become progressively worse.

INTERPRETATION

Slow circulation due to severe Heart qi-yang deficiency is the foundation for these symptoms (stiffness without activity) that has become fixed because her Kidney qi-yang deficiency has created an internal cold condition that makes her more susceptible to external cold (hands always hurt with cold). This internal cold condition has been with her all her life (see birth history). The fixed aspect is also enhanced by the damp condition in her Heart, Gallbladder, Intestines, and Lungs. Heat improves circulation and warms the extremities.

Exacerbation with activity may be attributed to her qi deficiency condition. Qi moves the blood. Body activities drain the qi, which in turn will worsen the circulation of blood. The obstruction due to internal cold and damp stagnation will create pain in addition on movement.

The stress aspect of the occurrence of these joint pains may also involve Liver qi deficiency and the concomitant inability to move qi and blood. Another factor is the location of joints as a recipient of retained pathogens, in her case emotions and drugs, demonstrating the multiplicity of factors that can contribute to one symptom.

■ *Dizziness*

SYMPTOMS:

- Like a hot wave that washes over her; head tingles, feels flushed from chest up
- Has to hold on to something, then fuzzy-headed and unsteady

HISTORY:

- Began three months ago
- Experienced on three occasions: sitting in kitchen, sitting at dinner table, talking to husband

INTERPRETATION

These episodes of a "hot wave washing over me" are consistent with blood stagnation in the lower burner that enhances a separation of qi and blood since the qi wants to move and the blood cannot. The qi is light and rises rapidly to her chest and head, and is experienced as a wave of heat.

Review of systems

Head

- Frontal headaches, which are persistent and interfere with functioning; pressure and sitting up helps so that they become less intense
- Frontal headaches are associated with damp-heat in the gastrointestinal system *(Gallbladder and Intestinal damp-heat)*

Eyes

- Sensitive to bright light *(Liver blood deficiency)*; difficulty reading, needs glasses

Ears

- Clog easily *(Lung and Gallbladder damp-heat stagnation)*

Nose and inhalant allergies

- Allergic to cats, animal hair, dust, and feathers *(Kidney and Lung qi and protective [wei] qi deficiency)*

Mouth

- Canker sores on gums occasionally *(damp-heat in the gastrointestinal system; Gallbladder and Intestinal damp-heat)*
- Canker sores on tongue after dental surgery
- Lump inside back of jaw, painful, and lasts for a few days; occurred four times last month (TMJ)

Upper respiratory

- Head cold once or twice a year (not throat) that progresses to the chest and tends to last a long time. *(Kidney and Lung qi and protective [wei] qi deficiency. Kidneys make protective qi, Liver stores it, and Lung distributes it.)*

Lungs

- Shortness of breath twice in past few months, once with dizziness, again when doing nothing at the time *(Heart, Lung qi, and Kidney yang deficiency)*

Digestion

- No complaints

Urinary

- Two bladder infections; candida with antibiotics led to painful urination *(damp-heat pouring down from impaired digestion; Robust Pounding at right middle position; Gallbladder and Intestines positions Slippery)*

Skin

- Excema in the winter; upper arms (rarely face) is dry, itches, and occasional circular patch; helped by moisturizer. Acne now on face and shoulders; more now than as adolescent *(blood stagnation and deficiency, Gallbladder damp-heat, and excess heat in the Stomach-Intestines)*

Trauma

- Accident at age 15, went through the windshield *(Cotton quality, Rough Vibration, and diminished circulation, Heart shock)*
- Surgeries included:
  Tonsils, age 5
  Carpal tunnel, age 14
  Back, age 23 (related to car accident)
  Wisdom teeth, age 27

Liver

No history of mononucleosis or hepatitis; drug abuse (see below)

Temperature

All symptoms below due primarily to Kidney qi-yang deficiency and diminished Heart/circulatory qi, and secondarily to cold hands and feet due to Liver qi deficiency and resulting stagnation:

- Deeply chilled when others are warm
- Hands, fingers, feet, and toes are generally cold
- Especially cold in winter when she feels stiff

- Prefers warm climate
- Never overexposed to the cold

Perspiration

- Sweats easily (normally)

Thirst

- Frequently drinks a great deal, depending on activity *(probably due to excess heat, especially in the Stomach-Intestines-Gallbladder)*

Exercise

- Past: gym machine and walking
- Now: crunches 100 several times/week *(further depleting her general extreme deficient qi and blood, especially of the Heart)*; plays with children and takes walks

Diet

- Eats a lot of dairy, cheese, yogurt, and red meat because of husband *(damp-heat in Gallbladder and Intestines)*

Habits

- Currently does not use drugs, cigarettes, or alcohol
- Past: marijuana use several times/week (23 joints); sniffed cocaine 4 to 5 times/week; cigarettes from age 14 to 25, from a few to a pack/day; used all forms of alcohol from age 14 to 20, paralyzed briefly from bourbon, gave up alcohol when she became pregnant at age 20. *(This explains the Liver qi deficiency.)*

Obstetrical and gynecological

MENSTRUAL:

- Menarche at age 12, lasted days with no problems.
- Cycle: 31-33 days, heavy flow for two days (Kidney qi deficiency), lasts at least one week, deep red first three days, then brownish.
- Blood stagnation in pelvis/lower burner from birth control: IUD ages 23-25 and now: cramping increasing, with clots ranging from small to large, and very dark with heavy bleeding. OrthoNova from age 16-20: nausea, headaches, weight gain, and sluggish; Depo-Prevara from age 22 for one year with same symptoms, some worse, some less *(blood and qi stagnation [Choppy, Muffled] and pelvis/lower burner dysfunction [Change of Amplitude: 5]).*

PREGNANCIES:

Two full term pregnancies:

- Female, age 6 years, overdue 3 weeks; induced delivery; gained 60 pounds, greatly stressed
- Male, age 2 years, didn't breathe, cord around neck and incubated.

INFECTION:

- Candida infection once with antibiotics; no venereal disease

SEXUAL ENERGY:

- Sexual energy is low (*Kidney, Heart, and Liver qi deficiency*)

Own gestational and birth history

- Mother had morning sickness, bronchitis, and tonsillitis
- Medication for morning sickness, no drugs or alcohol
- Birth took 12 hours after water broke, with anesthesia
- Umbilical cord wrapped several times around neck (*Heart shock-Rough Vibration at all depths, Kidney qi-yang deficiency*)

Childhood

- Breastfed; tonsillitis

Family history

- Mother: migrating joint pains, sinusitis, chronic fatigue
- Father: alcoholic, died at age 37 from liver failure due to hepatitis
- Maternal grandfather: agranulocytosis, brain tumor, died of heart disease at age 77
- Maternal grandmother: breast cancer, died at age 44

Biomedical medications and treatments

- Surgeries and birth control as listed above

Alternative treatments

- None

Synthesis of Symptoms and Pulse

The original pulse impression of an early shock to the cardiovascular system is borne out in the history of a cord wrapped around the neck during a prolonged birth performed under anesthesia. This early insult is commensurate with Kidney qi-yang deficiency.

The Blood Thick quality and damp-heat in the Gallbladder and Intestines found on the pulse is partially explained by the diet high in milk products, animal protein, and fat; and the Liver qi deficiency by the history of extensive use of recreational drugs.

The pulse findings of Kidney qi-yang deficiency is compatible with the history of feeling a deep chill and cold since childhood and the birth trauma. The blood stagnation in the lower burner on the pulse is partially explained by the presence of an IUD, a history of birth control medication, and severe trauma, including the accident and low back surgery, as well as the other causes (Heart, Kidney, and Liver qi deficiency, and 'blood thick') listed earlier.

CLIENT 2 Female, Age 42

BROAD FOCUS: INITIAL IMPRESSION OF LARGE SEGMENTS AND UNIFORM QUALITIES

Rhythm

Normal

Rate

75 beats/min in beginning and 60 at rest at end indicates possible instability of Heart qi, a sign of Heart qi deficiency. One must consider that at the beginning of the examination, the client's pulse rate might be elevated due to anxiety engaging with an unfamiliar process with a stranger.

Change in Rate on exertion from 60 to 68, and increase of 8 beats/min, is slightly less than the normal increase of rate on exertion, 12-20 beats/min, that are within normal limits. This suggests a mild Heart qi deficiency.

Wave

The Hesitant Wave indicates Heart yin deficiency and obsessive preoccupation.

The Hollow Full-Overflowing quality is restricted at first to the left middle position, indicating excess heat in the blood that appears here because the Liver stores the blood.

Uniform qualities over the entire pulse

Common qualities

Robust Pounding is a sign of excess heat that the body is having difficulty eliminating.

The Tense-Tight quality is a sign of qi stagnation and excess heat (Tense) and the onset of yin deficiency (Tight).

The Hollow Full-Overflowing quality is another sign of excess heat, this time in the blood, which the body is having difficulty eliminating.

Fig. 18-2　　　　　　　**Contemporary Chinese Pulse Record**

Date:					
Name: Client 2		**Gender:** F	**Age:** 42	**Hgt:**	**Wgt:**	**Occup:**

Rhythm:	**Rate/min:** Begin: End: W/exertion: Chg:
Normal	**Other Rates During Exam:**

First Impressions Of Uniform Qualities	**DEPTHS**

Tense-Tight; Robust Pounding; Hollow Full-Overflowing [2]; Empty [more on left]; Change in Amplitude [3]	**Floating:** – – – – – – – –
	Cotton: [1]
	Qi: Tense-Tight
	Blood: Empty; Thick
	Organ: Tense → Empty
	  O-B: – – – – – – – –
	  O-S: – – – – – – – –
	Wave: Hesitant → Hollow Full-Overflowing

Left Side:	**Right Side:**
More Empty	Reduced

PRINCIPAL POSITIONS	**COMPLEMENTARY POSITIONS**

L: DISTAL POSITION **R:**	

L	R
Tense Change in Amplitude [3]	Feeble

L: NEURO-PSYCHOLOGICAL **R:**	
Smooth Vibration [ephemeral]	– – – – – – – –

L: SPECIAL LUNG POSITION **R:**	
Tense Robust Pounding	Tense Robust Pounding

HEART
Mitral Valve: Smooth Vibration [ephemeral]
Enlarged: – – – – – – – –
Large Vessel: – – – – – – – –

Pericardium:

L: MIDDLE POSITION **R:**		**L:** DIAPHRAGM **R:**	

Change in Qualities
 	
Change in Amplitude [3]
  Tense-Tight
  ↕
  Hollow F/O
  ↕
  Empty
	Change in Amplitude [3]
	
	Change in Qualities
	  Thin, Tight-Wiry
	  ↕
	  Tense
	  ↕
	  Empty
		Inflated [2]	Inflated [2]

LIVER
ENGORGED
Distal: – – – – – – – –   **Ulnar:** – – – – – – – –
Gallbladder: Tense

SPLEEN-STOMACH
Esophagus: **Spleen:** Inflated
Stom-pyl. Exten: – – – – – – – –
Peritoneal Cavity/pancreas: Present
Duodenum:

L: PROXIMAL POSITION **R:**	
Deep Thin Tight	Deep Thin Feeble

Large: INTESTINES **Small:**	
Tight	Tense

L: PELVIS/LOWER BODY **R:**	
Tense [5]	Tense [5]

THREE BURNERS	**COMMENTS**
Upper: **Middle:** Tight → Empty **Lower:** Deep; Thin	Δ = Change [1] → [5] = low → high degree

Unusual qualities

The relatively Empty quality on the left side is at most a sign of an 'organ system' deficiency and in this instance, on closer examination, was found only at the middle burner. The significance of this is discussed later.

If the Empty quality were more widespread on the pulse we would consider either a 'qi wild' condition if enduring, or severe emotional shock if temporary.

The presence of a Peritoneal/Pancreas finding is of concern due to its association with pancreatic failure, cancer, lymphomas, and peritoneal abscess.

Paradoxical findings

The following are unusual findings in a relatively young woman: the Tense Hollow Full-Overflowing quality; the relatively Empty quality on the left side (compared to the right side); signs of Kidney yang deficiency (proximal positions Deep, Feeble), Kidney yin deficiency (proximal positions Tight), and blood deficiency (proximal positions Thin) are usually found in older people.

Stability

Change in Amplitude [3] over the entire pulse is a sign of Heart qi deficiency if consistent, and Liver qi stagnation if inconsistent.

Unusual wave form

When the amplitude was robust, the wave was Hollow Full-Overflowing, and when the amplitude was diminished, the wave was Hesitant.

CLOSER FOCUS

Depths

Cotton [2] is usually a sign of mild external qi stagnation associated with resignation and suppression of self about which the person is usually aware. Physical trauma is another less likely etiology.

Qi depth

Tense-Tight indicates qi stagnation and excess heat changing to yin deficiency. Again, excess heat is metabolic heat that has accumulated in a failed attempt to overcome stagnation. In the service of balance, the body brings fluids (yin) to balance the heat that over time is gradually depleted.

Blood depth

Blood Thick when the amplitude is high is a sign of inflammation in the vessels and the accumulation of solid materials in the inflamed, damaged areas of the vessels.

Organ depth

Absent. The absence of the organ depth is one type of the Empty quality on the pulse that suggests a 'qi wild' quality (not borne out here on later examination, which limits it to the middle burner).

Sides and systems

The left side is more Empty than the right side. The Empty quality on the left, if borne out on further examination, would be a sign of separation of yin and yang of the 'organ system' if persistent, or the possibility of an ongoing severe emotional shock if lasting only a few weeks. (Further examination of the individual positions indicated that the Emptiness is found only at the middle burner.)

The Reduced right side would indicate a deficient 'digestive system'. (Given the Empty qualities in the middle burner, this diagnosis is validated.)

SUMMARY OF INITIAL IMPRESSIONS AT BROAD AND CLOSER FOCUS

Heart and circulation

Qi deficiency

The rate decreases during the four-hour examination from 75 to 60. A Slow rate is a sign of Heart qi deficiency in a 42-year-old woman.

Change in Amplitude on first impression and at the left distal position indicates Heart qi deficiency.

On exertion the rate increases only 8 beats/min—borderline for Heart qi deficiency.

Mild Heart yin deficiency with obsessive activity

Hesitant Wave

Blood vessels

Blood Heat and Blood Thick and Hollow Full-Overflowing wave with a Tight left proximal position could be signs of early hypertension.

Kidney yang and yin deficiency

The Deep quality at both proximal positions, and the Feeble one at the right proximal position, are strong signs of Kidney qi-yang deficiency.

The Tight quality at the left proximal position is a sign of Kidney yin deficiency and/or pain due to kidney stones. The Thin quality is a sign of Kidney blood-essence deficiency (bone marrow).

Closest Focus (Individual Positions and Organs)

Overview

Unusual qualities

The Wiry quality in the right middle position may be a sign of abdominal pain or, much less likely, a very early sign of diabetes.

Instability (where there is the most activity and change)

Change in Qualities at both middle positions is a sign of a separation of yin and yang and severe qi deficiency in the middle burner, the one associated with centering.

Other more serious qualities

Empty at both middle positions is another sign of the separation of yin and yang and severe qi deficiency of the middle burner. Its presence bilterally in the middle burner is also a potential sign of the presence of a Peritoneal/Pancreas finding. This is of concern due to its association with pancreatic failure, cancer, lymphomas, and peritoneal abscess.

Paradoxical qualities

Hollow Full-Overflowing changing to Empty at the left middle position is a combined sign of heat in the blood occurring simultaneously with separation of yin and yang and severe qi-yang deficiency in the Liver (and in the middle burner, since the right middle position is sometimes also Empty). The message here is that the pulse (the organism) is informing us that there is more than one serious condition in the Liver.

Individual positions (principal and complementary)

Left distal, Large Vessel, Enlarged, Neuro-psychological, Mitral Valve (Heart circulation) positions

A rate of 75/min in the beginning and a significantly different rate of 60/min at the end is a possible sign of mild Heart qi deficiency. Change in Amplitude over the entire pulse, if constant, and especially at the left distal position, and Slow circulation (60/min), are also signs of Heart qi deficiency. The Hesitant quality indicates mild Heart yin deficiency with obsessive mental activity. There is mild qi stagnation and excess heat in the Heart, as evidenced by the Tense quality at the left distal position. The ephemeral Smooth Vibration at the Neuro-psychological and Mitral Valve positions suggests mild Heart qi agitation.

Right distal and Special Lung positions (Lungs)

Lung qi deficiency is signified by a Feeble quality at the right distal position. Lung excess heat is signified by the Tense Robust Pounding quality at the Special Lung position.

Left middle, Gallbladder, and Liver Engorgement positions (Liver-Gallbladder)

The Change in Amplitude [3] and Qualities, and especially the Emptiness, at the left middle position signify a separation of Liver yin and yang, probably due to Liver qi-yang deficiency. The simultaneous Emptiness at the right middle position indicates qi-yang deficiency of Liver and Spleen. The Tense quality at the left middle position indicates simultaneous mild Liver qi stagnation and excess Liver heat.

Liver excess heat and mild blood stagnation is seen in the Hollow Full-Overflowing quality at the left middle position. This suggests 'blood heat' or 'blood thick' in at least the Liver, and a consideration of very early hypertension.

Right middle, Intestines, Esophagus, Spleen, Stomach Pylorus Extension, Peritoneum (Spleen-Stomach positions)

The Empty quality in the right middle position and the Inflated Spleen position suggests Spleen qi deficiency and separation of Spleen yin and yang. The simultaneous Emptiness at the left middle position indicates qi deficiency and separation of yin and yang over the entire middle burner, as well as a specific sign of Spleen and Liver qi deficiency. It is also a sign that she has a problem with 'centering', the ability to focus on goals and to do the work necessary to realize them by eliminating the extraneous. It is also associated with a sense of self.

The Thin Tight-Wiry quality at the right middle position, along with Tightness and Tension in the Intestine positions, suggests irritation/inflammation that will contribute to the heat in the blood, and pain along the alimentary canal, possibly gastritis, and, with the Wiry quality, possibly associated with a stomach ulcer. This can be due to poor eating habits and incomplete digestion, as indicated by the deficient 'digestive system' and Spleen qi.

The presence of a Peritoneal/Pancreas finding based on simultaneous Emptiness in the middle burner is of concern due to its association with pancreatic failure, cancer, lymphomas, and peritoneal abscess.

Proximal positions (Kidneys)

With the left proximal position Deep, and the right proximal Feeble, we have significant Kidney qi-yang deficiency. The Thin Tight quality on the left is a sign of Kidney yin deficiency.

Summary of Conditions at Individual Positions (Closest Focus)

'Digestive system' deficiency and separation of yin and yang in the middle burner

Spleen and Liver qi-yang deficiency

Heart qi and yin deficiency and Heart qi agitation

Kidney qi-yang and Kidney yin deficiency

Possible pre-diabetic condition

Gastritis (possible stomach ulcer) and irritability in the intestines

Lung qi deficiency and Lung excess heat

Heat in the blood and possible hypertension

SUBSTANCES (INCLUDES BROAD, CLOSER, AND CLOSEST FOCUS)

Qi deficiency

As noted above, there are signs of Heart qi, Lung, Liver, Spleen, and Kidney qi deficiency.

Searching for the root of these deficiencies, Kidney qi-yang and yin deficiency are evidenced by the Deep and Tight qualities at the proximal positions. The Deep quality here in a 42-year-old woman suggests a constitutional or congenital qi-yang deficit, or it may be attributable to very early insults due to illness or trauma. The stresses and shocks of daily life that drain the other organs will not be supported sufficiently by the Kidneys to avoid their deficiencies.

Qi stagnation

COTTON   The slight Cotton quality [1] indicates minimal qi stagnation associated with a mild emotional state of resignation due possibility to compromises she is making in her current life situation.

TENSE-TIGHT   The Tense quality in general and at the left distal, left middle, and Gallbladder positions, and the very Tense quality at the Pelvis/Lower Body position indicate qi stagnation in those organs and areas.

INFLATED [2] AT THE DIAPHRAGM AREA   The very slight qi stagnation here is associated with the mild repression of tender feelings and the exaggeration of angry ones, usually associated with interpersonal separation.

Blood excess heat and stagnation

Hollow Full-Overflowing and Robust Pounding (only on initial impression) suggest a 'blood heat-thick' condition.

Blood deficiency

The Thin quality at the proximal positions is a sign of Kidney blood deficiency (marrow) not recognized by TCM.

Yin excess

There is no evidence of yin excess (no Slippery quality), which in itself is somewhat unusual in a 42-year-old woman, unless she is taking diuretic medication.

Yin deficiency

Tightness at the proximal positions, and the Tense-Tight qualities at the middle positions, suggest yin deficiency. This is probably the result of overworking the mind (Hesitant Wave-OCD) and the 'nervous system' (alcoholic father), both of which deplete yin, which is supplied by the Kidneys that especially nourishes the Heart and Liver yin.

Yang excess

There is no evidence on the pulse of yang excess.

Yang deficiency

The Deep quality at the proximal positions, the Empty quality at the middle burner, the presence of the Spleen position, and Feeble quality at the right distal position are signs of qi-yang deficiency of the Kidney, Liver, Spleen, and Lung respectively. A complaint of coldness would be one deciding factor in determining whether this is a sign of qi or yang deficiency.

There is Heart qi deficiency evidenced by an increase of only 8 beats/min on exertion (borderline for Heart qi deficiency), the Slow rate (60 beats/min) during the four hour seminar at which the pulse was taken, and a Change in Amplitude [3] over the entire pulse (if it is constant).

Essence deficiency

The Wiry quality at the right middle position is probably due to abdominal pain but is a quality associated with essence deficiency

Wind

There is no evidence of internal or external wind.

Food

There is no evidence of food stagnation.

ACTIVITY

Excess heat

The Tense quality at many positions is a sign of mild excess heat and the consequence of qi stagnation (due to excess or deficiency of which there is more of the latter here). The Hollow Full-Overflowing Wave and Blood Thick are signs of heat in the blood, and Robust Pounding is a sign of excess heat in the tissues.

Tightness at three positions, especially the Kidneys, indicates yin deficiency and a diminishment of the Kidneys ability to supply the fluid necessary to balance the excess heat. This excess heat may have been one important original drain on the Kidneys.

Rising yang

The separation of yin and yang in the middle burner allows the yang to leave the area and interfere with function in the most vulnerable area or organ. From the record this would seem to be the Lungs, the digestion, and/or the lower burner.

Cold excess

None. The Tight quality at the left proximal position might once have indicated possible excess cold prior to central heating, but is now only a rare finding and with this etiology, the Tight quality is usually bilateral.

Deficient cold

See 'Yang Deficiency' above.

Agitation

The ephemeral Smooth Vibration at the Neuro-psychological and Mitral Valve positions suggests mild Heart qi agitation.

AREAS

Middle burner

The simultaneous Emptiness at the right and left middle positions indicates qi deficiency and separation of yin and yang over the entire middle burner as well as the problem with 'centering' described above.

Diaphragm

The slight Inflated quality at the Diaphragm position [2] is a sign of minimal trapped qi in the diaphragm area, the implications of which were discussed above.

Peritoneal/Pancreas position

The presence of a Peritoneal/Pancreas finding is of concern due to its association with pancreatic failure, cancer, lymphomas, and peritoneal abscess.

Pelvis/lower body

The very Tense quality [5] at the Pelvis/Lower Body positions is a sign of severe qi stagnation in the reproductive organs.

SYSTEMS

'Digestive system'

The qualities on the right side of the pulse, identified as the 'digestive system', are all signs of deficiency (Feeble and Empty).

'Organ system'

Most of the qualities on the left side of the pulse, identified as the 'organ system', are signs of deficiency (Rate on Exertion rises only 8 beats/min; Feeble and Empty).

INTERPRETATION

Summary of specific conditions

- 'Digestive system' deficiency and separation of yin and yang in the middle burner (severe)
- Blood heat, blood thick (moderate)
- Mild blood congestion in the Liver
- Heart qi deficiency (moderate)
- Heart yin deficiency with obsessive activity (and slight Heart qi agitation)
- Lung qi deficiency (severe)
- Lung excess heat (moderate)
- Liver qi stagnation (mild)
- Liver yang deficiency (severe)
- Spleen qi/yang deficiency (severe)
- Gastritis (or stomach ulcer) and irritability in the intestines with abdominal pain (moderate)
- Stomach yin deficiency
- Kidney yin deficiency (moderate)
- Kidney qi-yang deficiency (severe)
- Kidney-Heart disharmony, both yin and yang type
- Qi stagnation at the Pelvis/Lower Body position (very severe)
- Possible very early signs of diabetes, hypertension (moderate)
- Possible pancreatic or peritoneal pathology
- Excess heat (moderate)
- Trapped qi in diaphragm area (mild)
- Qi stagnation and excess heat in the Gallbladder (mild)
- Peritoneal/Pancreatic pathology

MANAGEMENT FORMULATION

A. Immediate interventions

1. Middle burner qi collapse and pain
      Separation of Spleen and Liver

> Abdominal pain
>
> Stomach yin deficiency

2. Blood

> Severe excess heat

3. Heart and circulation

> Qi deficiency
>
> Qi agitation
>
> Yin deficiency

B. Root issues and etiology

1. Kidney

> Qi-yang deficiency
>
> Yin deficiency

2. Liver

> Separation of yin and yang

3. Heart

> As above

C. Secondary issues

1. Lung

> Qi deficiency
>
> Excess heat

2. Spleen-Stomach-Intestines

> Spleen qi-yang deficiency
>
> Stomach yin deficiency

D. Derivative issues

1. Blood excess heat

2. Lower burner qi stagnation

3. Trapped qi in the Diaphragm area

Management Implementation

Lifestyle strategies

Food diary

Investigate energy drains, including eating habits, that have led to the 'digestive system' deficiency, the separation of yin and yang in the middle burner, and the irritability-inflammation and possible pain in the alimentary canal (Wiry quality in the left middle position, indicating possible gastritis and/or stomach ulcer with abdominal discomfort). Provide nutritional counseling and intervene immediately if there is danger of hemorrhage.

Exercise and work

Investigate lifestyle causes of slow circulation (over-exercise, overwork, medications) and or trauma.

Substance abuse

Do a complete drug history and a history of liver disease to explain the Empty and Change in Qualities at the left middle position.

Referrals

- Blood chemistry tests to explore the status of liver, kidney, and lipid functions, and glucose tolerance (diabetes), including a complete blood count and thyroid profile, would be useful. Ruling out hepatitis and other sources of Liver separation of yin and yang (drugs, toxins) is essential.
- Rule out hypertension with a complete biomedical physical examination.
- Gynecological examination to explore the stagnation in the lower burner and other menstrual implications of the Kidney, Spleen, Liver, and Heart/ circulation deficiencies.
- Chest x-ray and tests of lung capacity and function to explain the Feeble left distal position and Robust Pounding at the Special Lung positions.
- Gastrointestinal examination for gastritis, ulcer, and intestinal polyps.
- Psychotherapy for obsessive thinking (Hesitant Wave)

Acupuncture, herbs, and other strategies

Immediate interventions

1. Middle burner qi collapse and pain

   a. To address the Spleen qi and 'digestive system' deficiency, Intestinal heat, and Liver qi-yang deficiency, we need to treat gastritis and the irritable alimentary canal first so that she will better digest food and contribute qi and blood to her terrain and secondly tolerate the other herbal treatments that follow.

   b. Building Spleen-Stomach qi is ongoing as it is the source of energy upon which all other physiological functions and healing depend.

   c. We build Liver qi-yang because of the Liver's key function of moving the qi in the gastrointestinal system and to mitigate the destructive aspects of the Liver qi-yang that is interfering with the function of vulnerable areas (chest) and organs (Lungs).

2. Blood (severe excess heat)

   Heat in the blood, 'blood thick' and Hollow-Full-Overflowing Wave conditions are signs of blood stagnation that can lead to serious consequences (i.e., hypertension). They must be treated with some urgency, and this treatment, in the service of prevention, must be ongoing, more in the short term than long.

Explained in terms of the Liver's function of moving Stomach-Intestine qi downward, the excess heat is also a consequence of the effort by the deficient Liver to perform this task, like any engine that is asked to work beyond its capacity to overcome the stagnation. The Liver stores the blood and the left middle position will be the first and most evident pulse position to reveal problems in the blood such as toxicity, heat, and increasing turbidity and denseness ('blood thick'), evidenced in this instance by the Hollow Full-Overflowing quality at the left middle position

Qi stagnation in the Gallbladder is mild (Tense) and probably associated with its function of removing heat from the Liver that is excessive. The absence of Slipperiness and Robust Pounding or Choppy qualities with the Tense quality mitigates the possible seriousness of the qi stagnation in the Gallbladder.

3. Heart (qi and yin deficiency; agitation)

   a. The Slow circulation should be evaluated in terms of etiology. If it is due partly to trauma, herbs to overcome the effects of trauma should be used immediately.

   b. For the Heart qi and yin deficiency and Heart qi agitation, we must simultaneously build Heart qi and mitigate the process of obsessive thinking that is affecting the Heart and Kidney and creating agitation, when her recovery may depend on inner quiet.

   c. Kidney and Lung nourishing herbs can be included.

Intermediate (root) interventions

1. Kidney qi-yang deficiency is the single most important intervention for the long term and is a primary constitutional issue for this patient, giving rise to and affecting all other pathological processes. Kidney yin should be included in the plan to offset the depletion of yin by her overworking mind, which affects all function, especially the Heart.

2. It is important to continue to treat the Heart qi deficiency, slow circulation, Heart yin deficiency, and Heart qi agitation conditions as part of correcting the Kidney-Heart imbalance, and because the Heart is the 'emperor' whose well-being affects all other 'subjects' (organ function).

Secondary interventions

1. 'Digestive system' middle burner chaos including the Spleen and Liver qi-yang and irritable alimentary canal (ongoing).

   a. The Empty quality at the left middle position has been associated with lymphomas, and the Peritoneal/Pancreas finding with pancreatic failure and cancer and peritoneal abscess. In our time, substance abuse must be considered as an etiology. Other factors commonly encountered with an Empty quality bilaterally at the middle burner are hepatitis, mononucleosis, sitting in a bent-over position at work (e.g., a secretary), resuming physical labor too soon after eating, parasites, and trauma. Pancreatic involvement must be considered when we have a similar quality in both middle positions

b. Since the signs of heat in the blood, blood congestion in the Liver, and 'blood thick' conditions can lead to serious consequences (i.e., hypertension, coronary occlusion) they must be treated as ongoing issues, in the service of prevention.

c. The Reduced qualities on the right side, Feeble at the right distal (Lungs), Deep at the right proximal position, and the Empty quality at the right middle and left middle positions, as well as the Inflated Spleen position, suggest deficiency of the 'digestive system' and Spleen qi deficiency.

d. The patient's relatively young age suggests Spleen deficiency due to constitutional Kidney qi-yang deficiency.

e. With Client 2's inadequate review of systems we are left to speculate if there could also be a substantial contribution from harmful eating habits: irregularity, eating rapidly, excessive dieting, perhaps reaching the extremes in anorexia and bulimia, and excessive rumination while eating.

2. Lung qi deficiency should likewise already be a focus of the treatment for the 'digestive system' deficiency (Lung, Spleen, and Kidney). The Feeble quality at the right distal position indicates considerable Lung qi deficiency. Robust Pounding at the Special Lung position suggests either excess heat in the Lungs or a compensatory attempt to function.

Derivative issues

While these will ultimately be addressed automatically by attending to the above causes of these conditions, management reducing excess blood heat, moving qi in the lower burner and trapped qi in the chest are addressed along with the management of the Spleen, Liver, Heart, Kidney and Lungs.

COMPLAINTS AND REVIEW OF SYSTEMS

Gynecolgical

- Amenorrhea for several months (with normal period after treatment with herbs and acupuncture). Hot flashes and sweats.

Obstetrics

- Infertility, irregular periods, hot flashes and sweats
- Eight years ago a fluid cyst was found on one ovary and she had two blocked fallopian tubes, one of which was cleared. Irregular periods.

Gastrointestinal

- Abdominal distention

Psychosomatic

She has often had intense emotional crises, resulting in sinus infections with chest tightening that simulated asthma, the symptoms of which are relieved after the emotional crisis passes.

Relationships

A conflict with an authority at school, where she was supported by her fellow students, resulted in her expulsion. For years she fought unsuccessfully to be reinstated, and is finally, after considerable difficulty, trying to put this behind her. This is being helped by a new satisfying relationship.

Oncology and operations

Ten years ago a melanoma was removed from her side.

Family history

Father alcoholic and parents divorced when she was young

Prior treatments

Treatment by the referring practitioner focused on Liver qi stagnation, blood and yin deficiency, and rising Liver yang. The lower burner was treated for blood stagnation, now not in evidence except for the extraordinary qi stagnation in the Pelvis/Lower Body. The Slow pulse rate and sluggish circulation would also contribute to stagnation in that dependent area.

Synthesis of symptoms and the pulse

Amenorrhea and infertility

Short-term amenorrhea, easily reversed, is usually a malfunction of the Liver's function to deliver blood to the uterus due to some passing stress. This stress is usually emotional, calling upon the Liver to contain it and reducing the Liver qi available for moving blood. The Liver pulse picture is one of the 'separation of yin and yang' at the left middle position and a severe deficiency of Liver qi-yang.

More persistent amenorrhea is usually associated with Kidney essence deficiency, a frequent cause as well of infertility, that is evidenced here by the Deep proximal positions.

The cause of irregular periods depends upon the pattern, which is not mentioned here. Skipping periods is associated with Liver dysfunction that we find here at the left middle position. Periods that start and stop in the middle are more related to lower burner blood stagnation, for which the only pulse sign is the extreme qi stagnation in the Pelvis/Lower Body. The latter is probably associated with the history of the obstructed fallopian tubes and possibly the fluid cysts. If the periods are short, yin-essence deficiency is usually involved, for which there is ample substantiation with the Tight quality at the left proximal position. Prolonged periods are usually caused by Kidney yang-essence deficiency, as evidenced by the Deep and Feeble qualities at the proximal positions.

Hot flashes and sweats is a function of the 'separation of yin and yang' that is more often in our time to be rarely due to yin deficiency and more likely to be due to yang deficiency. The formula Two Immortals recommended for this condition has more herbs for yang than yin. If the yin cannot hold onto the yang, the yang leaves with a sensation of heat (hot flash), and later the yin will follow (sweats) since yin does not like to be separated from yang. Furthermore, nature wants the cooler yin to balance the warmer yang.

Abdominal distention

The Liver qi is responsible for the movement of qi in the entire body, and especially the process of peristalsis assisting Stomach qi to move food downward. The separation of yin and yang in the middle burner, 'digestive system' deficiency, and deficiency of Spleen and Liver qi-yang are all contributing to stagnation and irritation in the alimentary canal, with resultant qi stagnation and abdominal bloating. The presence of the positive Spleen position suggests that her Spleen-Stomach dysfunction began with early vulnerability due to the obvious Kidney qi-yang deficiency in utero.

Intense emotional crises (see Relationships above)

The Liver is the yin organ most affected by frustration, tension, and inner emotional conflict. Client 2 has severe Liver dysfunction ('separation of yin and yang') so that containing and 'detoxifying' stressful emotions would be inadequate. A hypervigilant state engendered by an alcoholic father and her parents' divorce would be expected to drain the Liver qi and make emotional containment difficult.

Part of the Liver's detoxifying function is to detoxify emotions that are contained when the wisdom of the organism decides that expressing these emotions (Heart function) is not in its best interests. The alternative is to send these potentially destructive emotions through the divergent and *luo* vessels to become retained pathogens where they cannot impair vital organs.

The sinus is one of these places, especially for Client 2, since her qi-deficient Lungs and Lung excess heat render the upper burner vulnerable. Another is the chest (tightness) and the lower burner/uterus where she has had serious problems in the past. Chest tightening is also often a sign of Liver yang that is separated from the yin, as it is here, moving upward to the vulnerable chest and Lungs (right distal position Feeble).

The inability to let go of the incident at school when she was fired may be a metal issue, defined in *Dragon Rises, Red Bird Flies* as a failure of metal yang deficiency (Large Intestine).

Melanoma

Melanoma is one of the most virulent forms of cancer, one that I have increasingly found in young people. Cancer is traditionally thought of as a condition involving stagnation of substances, a concept with which I only partially agree.

I have found it more often in situations in which the yin and yang have separated, either in one organ or area, or as a 'qi wild' condition affecting the entire organism. Despite six years of treatment, this patient continues to show signs of separation of yin and yang in the middle burner. There was also one initial impression of Emptiness over the entire left side, possibly a sign of a separation of yin and yang in the 'organ system' of the fundamental Heart, Kidney, and Liver organs.

Another important aspect is that of cancer as the result of a pathogen, in this case emotional (and/or drugs), retained in the skin. My experience with this form of cancer in young people is that it includes a history of heavy abuse of recreational drugs contributing to the middle burner chaos ('separation of yin and yang'), not mentioned in this brief history.

Comment

Due to the extreme deficiencies and instability on this pulse, the conditions exist now for some other form of chaos—such as cancer, autoimmune disease, or degenerative neurological disease—to occur within the next five to ten years unless therapeutic attention is given to these findings.

Fig. 18-3   **Contemporary Chinese Pulse Record**

Date:							
Name: Client 3		**Gender:** M	**Age:** 27	**Hgt:** 6' 0"	**Wgt:** 160	**Occup:** Former student	

Rhythm:
Occasional Change in Rate at Rest

Rate/min: Begin: 68   End: 82   W/exertion: 90   Chg: +8
Other Rates During Exam: 78

First Impressions Of Uniform Qualities	**DEPTHS**
Tense; Robust Pounding; Amplitude Change [3]; Rough Vibration [2+]; Muffled [1]	**Floating:** ——————— **Cotton:** [4] **Qi:** Diminished; Reduced Pounding; Occasionally Slippery

Blood: Heat; Robust Pounding [2+]; Rough Vibration [2+]
Organ: Tense; Robust Pounding [3]; Occasionally Slippery
  O-B: Tense; Robust Pounding [3+]
  O-S: Tense; Robust Pounding [3]
Wave: Hesitant

Left Side:	**Right Side:**
Robust Pounding ↑ Ropy Leather-Hard ↑	Robust Pounding ↓ Leather-Hard ↓

PRINCIPAL POSITIONS	**COMPLEMENTARY POSITIONS**

L: DISTAL POSITION **R:**		**L:** NEURO-PSYCHOLOGICAL **R:**	
Muffled Tense-Tight ↕ Amorphous Nonhomogeneous ↕ Absent	Muffled Reduced Pounding ↓ Absent	Doughy Smooth → Rough Vibration Slippery Robust Pounding	Doughy

L: SPECIAL LUNG POSITION **R:**	
Muffled [1]; Narrow [2] Tense-Tight Robust Pounding [3] Choppy [2] Occasionally Slippery	Reduced Pounding Suppressed Wave Rough Vibration [3] Choppy [3+] **Pleura:**

Pericardium:	

HEART	
Mitral Valve: Smooth Vibration	
Enlarged: ? Qualities Changing	
Large Vessel: ———————	

L: MIDDLE POSITION **R:**		**L:** DIAPHRAGM **R:**	
Muffled [3] Tense → Tight Robust Pounding [2+] ↕ Tense Hollow Full-Overflowing	Muffled [2] Thin [3] Leather-Hard → Wiry Robust Pounding [2+]	Inflated [3]	Inflated [3]

ENGORGED   LIVER
Distal: ———————   **Ulnar:** ———————
Gallbladder: Thin; Tight-Wiry; Robust Pounding [2+]; Choppy [3]

SPLEEN-STOMACH	
Esophagus: ——————— **Spleen:** ———————	
Stom-pyl. Exten: Tight-Wiry; Choppy [2+]; Robust Pounding [2]	
Peritoneal Cavity/pancreas: Present	
Duodenum:	

L: PROXIMAL POSITION **R:**		**Large:** INTESTINES **Small:**	
Muffled [3] Tense Robust Pounding [2] ↕ Thin Tight-Wiry	Wiry Robust Pounding [3]	Muffled [3] Tense-Tight Robust Pounding [2] Amplitude Change [4]	Muffled Robust Pounding [2-3] Tight-Biting → Feeble

L: PELVIS/LOWER BODY **R:**	
Tense-Tight Amplitude Change [5] Robust Pounding [2] Choppy [3]	Choppy [4]; Wiry Rough Vibration [3] Robust Pounding [3+] → Feeble/Absent

THREE BURNERS	**COMMENTS** *Qualities, Amplitude, Pounding --- Changing Fequently
Upper: Absent **Middle:** ——————— **Lower:** Wiry	Δ = Change [1] → [5] = low → high degree

Epilogue

Soulié De Morant stated the case concisely when he wrote:

> The knowledge of pulses is absolutely indispensable for the practice of true acupuncture, which is based on treating the root condition. Using only memorized formulae and treating only visible problems does not constitute true acupuncture.[1]

One of my missions in life is to reawaken an awareness of the importance of pulse diagnosis, which was recognized since antiquity and in all cultures as necessary to gaining a profound knowledge of a person. Yet it is also necessary for traditions to evolve and remain relevant to the times in which they are practiced.

Knowledge of Chinese pulse diagnosis has steadily diminished in recent times. In part, the problem has been that it relies on ideas that are expressed in an archaic language that is often incomprehensible to a practitioner of the twenty-first century. Moreover, the ideas themselves are based on texts and traditional lore that were passed down from an agrarian civilization whose daily life was so different from our own that the information is often no longer relevant in the modern clinic. To that extent, Chinese medicine has increasingly lost its ability to predict and thereby prevent illness.

During the modern era, the industrial, information, nuclear, and 'space' revo-

---

1. George Soulié de Morant, *Chinese Acupuncture*, trans. Lawrence Grinnell et al. (Brookline, MA: Paradigm Publications, 1994) 56.

lutions have made new demands on every aspect of our physiology, particularly our nervous and immune systems, demands which are historically sudden and cataclysmic. This has happened to a creature, homo sapiens, who has otherwise evolved in a remarkably stable and slowly-changing cultural environment for at least the last ten thousand years. While the human organism seems to have remained more or less constant, the stresses to which it is subject have changed radically in recent times. And now there is evidence that even man has changed. There are said to be between 50 and 150 chemicals in our blood that were not there fifty years ago. In the book *Nature through Nurture*,[2] the author points out that genes turn on and off and even change with experience.

The only thing that never changes is change itself. Pulse diagnosis must be brought up to date to reflect our current situation. The human organism has a limited reservoir of symbols with which to express its internal anguish. We call these symptoms. The causes of each symptom are legion, and a patient can rarely tell you that they have an ulcer or a tumor, to say nothing of its cause. This limitation is the genesis of the art and science of diagnosis.

The pulse qualities themselves, likewise, limited in the variety of sensations, have not changed. What has changed in many cases are the causes for these qualities, our ability to distinguish them from one another, and the language we use to communicate them. Many of the images, metaphors, and interpretations of the past no longer resonate with modern man.

Even the best of traditions must evolve to remain relevant. And while the contents of this book mark a significant departure from the past, its goal is to return Chinese medicine to its diagnostic roots. It draws upon the written classics, but even more from the clan-based, oral tradition with its emphasis on learning from actual practice. It is based on the work of a teacher from the Ding clan, Dr. John H.F. Shen, and the work of his students. The goal is to bring pulse diagnosis into the twenty-first century in terms of sensation, expressed in modern, easily identified terminology, and interpretation, which is in accord with the enormous changes in all aspects of our existence since ancient times.

Students in my classes tell me that their otherwise competent teachers discourage them from pursuing the study of pulse diagnosis because "it is really not that important." For those who do not know pulse diagnosis, it cannot be very important. Furthermore, the time and patience necessary to master Chinese pulse diagnosis are not synchronous with a culture such as ours, which encourages short-term vision and short-term investment in all positive human attributes. Yet, within the traditional Chinese diagnostic system of asking, looking, listening, and touching, pulse diagnosis is the most informative and profound diagnostic modality concerned with the physical, emotional, and mental status of an individual.

The Normal pulse is the most sensitive indicator of the state of our health.

---

2. Matt Ridely, *Nature through Nurture* (London: Fourth Estate, 2003).

Of all diagnostic modalities, it provides the most reliable basis of a preventive medicine by giving us the most precise picture of every subtle and complex deviation from this standard. In addition, the pulse provides information about the root cause of any deviation, allowing our patients the opportunity to change their lives and their habits, or adapt to constitutional deficits, in the direction of health. And the more precise the diagnosis, the more precisely we can design a therapeutic regime for the patient. The pulse record is an instant picture of the current status of a person's voyage from birth to death. It permits us to diagnose and treat people as individuals, rather than diseases.

When practiced with dedication, quiet patience, and consistency, becoming attuned to pulse qualities is an ongoing meditation, a training ground for the development of awareness and mindfulness. Finally, pulse diagnosis is an opportunity for practitioners to obtain the ultimate satisfaction of being one with their patients, one with themselves, one with the diagnostic process, and perhaps with the universal forces which are expressed through the pulse.

Dr. Shen once asked the question, "Why did God put eyes in front of our head instead of behind?" The answer, he said, is that "We were meant to always look ahead, not behind." In a similar vein, Martin Prechtel, who lived and studied in Guatemala for many years with a Mayan shaman, recorded these words from his teacher:

> If God gives us life and we continue as we have, some day when I'm a pile of ashes and the smell of smoke in your memory is all you have left of these days, then you will see situations and sicknesses never seen before. I've no idea what they may be; I have no way of recognizing them with our very old ways and traditional roots. But you're the new one who's going to have to find special medicines to deal with them, instead of just using the old things because they're old. You must find new ways to do old things, and new medicines with old roots to cure the bad times made by new things.[3]

---

3. Martin Prechtel, *Secrets of the Talking Jaguar: Unmasking the Mysterious World of the Living Maya* (New York: Penguin-Putnam, 1998).

Notes

CHAPTER 1: Preliminary Reflections

1. Wang Shu-He, *The Pulse Classic*, trans. Yang Shou-Zhong (Boulder, CO: Blue Poppy Press)

2. Li Shi-Zhen, *Pulse Diagnosis*, trans. Hoe Ku Huynh (Brookline, MA: Paradigm Publications, 1981) 70; Ted Kaptchuk, *The Web That Has No Weaver* (New York: Congdon and Weed, 1983) 309; Wu Shui-Wan, *The Chinese Pulse Diagnosis* (San Francisco: Writers Guild of America, 1973) 20; Deng Tietao, *Practical Diagnosis in Traditional Chinese Medicine*, trans. Marnae Ergil (Edinburgh: Churchill Livingstone, 1999) 119–21.

3. Lu Yubin, *Pulse Diagnosis* (Jinan: Shandong Science and Technology Press, 1996) 70–71.

4. Wu, 34.

5. R.B. Amber, *The Pulse in Occident and Orient: Its Philosophy and Practice in India, China, Iran, and the West* (New York: Santa Barbara Press, 1966) v–vi.

6. Leon Hammer, "Science East and West" *Medical Acupuncture* 2010;22(2).

7. Ilza Veith, trans., *Huang Ti Nei Ching Su Wen* (Berkeley: The University of California Press, 1972) 151.

CHAPTER 2: Pulse Positions through History

1. Wang Shu-He, *The Pulse Classic*, trans. Yang Shou-Zhong (Boulder, CO: Blue Poppy Press, 1997).

2. Ding Gan-Ren, *Maixue jiyao* 脈學輯要 *(Summary of Pulse Study)*. (Shanghai: Shanghai zhongyi zhuanmen xuexiao 上海中醫專門學校, 1917).

3. See Volker Scheid, *Currents of Tradition in Chinese Medicine 1626-2006* (Seattle: Eastland Press, 2007) 393-95, and 466, n. 16.

4. John Shen, *Chinese Medicine* (New York: Educational Solutions, 1980) 43, 45.

5. George Soulié de Morant, *Chinese Acupuncture*, trans. Lawrence Grinnell et al. (Brookline, MA: Paradigm Publications, 1994) 61–63.

5. Paul Unschuld, trans., *Nan-Ching* (Berkeley: University of California Press, 1986) 258.

7. Wang, 23.

8. Deng Tietao, *Practical Diagnosis in Traditional Chinese Medicine*, trans. Marnae Ergil (Edinburgh: Churchill Livingstone, 1999) 90.

CHAPTER 3: Basic Axioms and Other Considerations

1. Deng Tietao, *Practical Diagnosis in Traditional Chinese Medicine*, trans. Marnae Ergil (Edinburgh: Churchill Livingstone, 1999) 85.

2. Leon Hammer, "The Pulse and the Individual" *The American Acupuncturist* Spring 2008;43.

3. Leon Hammer, "Science East and West" *Medical Acupuncture* 2010;22(2).

4. Jiang Jing, "A Brief Survey of the Korean Dong Han System of Pulse Diagnosis" *Oriental Medicine* 1993;2(1):19, 21.

5. Leon Hammer, Ross Rosen, "The Pulse, The Electronic Age and Radiation: Early Detection" *The American Acupuncturist* Spring 2009:47.

6. This section is based on Leon Hammer, "The Paradox of the Unity and Duality of the Kidneys According to Chinese Medicine" *American Journal of Acupuncture* 1999;27(3&4):179.

7. Leon Hammer, *Dragon Rises Red Bird Flies*, Rev. Ed. (Seattle: Eastland Press, 2005) Ch. 14.

8. Leon Hammer, "Ecology in Chinese Medicine, Part One" *Chinese Medicine Times*, Vol. 5, Issue 2, Summer 2010.

——"Ecology in Chinese Medicine, Part Two" *Chinese Medicine Times*, Vol. 5, Issue 3, Winter 2010.

CHAPTER 4: Taking the Pulse: Methodology

1. Deng Tietao's recommendation of an average of three minutes does not provide the practitioner of this exquisite art-science the time it requires and deserves. *Practical Diagnosis in Traditional Chinese Medicine*, trans. Marnae Ergil (Edinburgh: Churchill Livingstone, 1999) 89.

2. Leon Hammer, "Towards a Unified Theory of Chronic Disease: with Regard to the Separation of Yin and Yang and 'The Qi is Wild'" *Oriental Medicine*, 1998: 6[2&3]:15.

3. Ibid.

4. The finding of Heart Enlarged at this position, or for that matter a positive finding in almost any position, is often concurrent with a biomedically-defined 'organic' problem. When such qualities are found on the pulse they are assessed in terms of the total pulse picture, in conjunction with other signs and symptoms. However, Dr. Hammer always recommends that a thorough physical examination, with all appropriate testing, be performed to determine which of these findings are energetic and which are 'organic'.

CHAPTER 6: Rhythm and Stability

1. R.B. Amber, *The Pulse in Occident and Orient: Its Philosophy and Practice in India, China, Iran,*

and the West (New York: Santa Barbara Press, 1966) 115.

2. Leon Hammer, *Dragon Rises, Red Bird Flies* (Barrytown, NY: Station Hill, 1990) 347.

3. This occurs especially in individuals whose eyebrows are continuous from one side to the other; such eyebrows are a sign of a constitutional propensity to constantly change one's mind. Both Dr. Shen and Dr. Hammer confirmed this correlation time and again in their practices.

4. John Shen, *Chinese Medicine* (New York: Educational Solutions, 1980) 64.

5. Leon Hammer, "The Unified Field Theory of Chronic Disease with Regard to the Separation of Yin and Yang and 'The Qi is Wild'" *Oriental Medicine* 1998;6(2&3):15.

6. Leon Hammer, "The Pulse and the Individual" *American Acupuncturist*, Spring 2008, Vol 43.

7. *Pulse Diagnosis*, trans. Hoe Ku Huynh (Brookline, MA: Paradigm Publications, 1981) 88.

8. Russell Jaffe, in a personal communication to Dr. Hammer, claimed that if on inhalation the pulse increases in intensity and/or amplitude, the direction of transition is positive, and if the pulse decreases in strength, the direction is negative.

9. In the early 1990s Dr. Hammer began to do seminars in Berkeley, California. There he found for the first time the ubiquity of these 'qi wild' qualities in a way that he had never encountered elsewhere during the nearly twenty years that he had used this system. It was not so prevalent elsewhere in California, although more so than in the eastern United States, Europe, China, Japan, or Australia.

10. Dr. Hammer has not come across a descriptive quality for this phenomenon in any of the literature. The closest is the description of Tung by Amber (164): "a tremulous pulse, quick and jerky; its pulsation covering a space no longer than a pea." It is interesting that this description is extraordinarily similar to his own, particularly considering that he wrote his description of the Unstable quality before reading Amber. A personal communication from five element practitioners informed him that in their tradition, the Unstable quality is associated with an Akabane disharmony, an imbalance within a phase (element) between one side of the body and the other. Thus this quality seems to have been subsumed unofficially under the categories of Hurried and Knotted, which only confuses the clear interpretation of all three. But because the Unstable pulse is relatively common and sufficiently significant, it deserves its own place in the spectrum of qualities.

11. Amber (164) says that the Tung pulse "is indicative of pain caused by internal heat or excessive sweating and hemorrhage."

CHAPTER 7: **Rate**

1. Deng Tietao, *Practical Diagnosis in Traditional Chinese Medicine*, trans. Marnae Ergil (Edinburgh: Churchill Livingstone, 1999) 84.

2. Deng (112) mentions the heart only once in connection with a rapid rate, and then only as a sequela of diphtheria, rheumatic heart disease, or myocarditis.

3. John Shen, *Chinese Medicine* (New York: Educational Solutions, 1980) 50, 57.

4. Li Shi-Zhen states that the Rapid pulse "results when excessive or yin fluid is damaged. Clinically, there are symptoms of restlessness, mental confusion and delirium." He also associates a Rapid pulse with excessive "yang qi" as with "heart or kidney fire," which can be a "deficient or excessive condition." He attributes a Rapid quality during autumn to "excess internal fire burning the lung yin," which he says is difficult to treat. *Pulse Diagnosis*, trans. Hoe Ku Huynh

(Brookline, MA: Paradigm Publications, 1981) 66, 67. Elsewhere (22), he notes that a rapid pulse accompanies hot diseases of the yin organs, especially when the pulse is also strong. A Rapid pulse without strength is felt when a small amount of heat in the blood remains, as after pus is discharged from an abscess. In addition, Li alludes to a Rapid rate in individual positions and bilaterally at the same burner, which are outside of Dr. Hammer's experience. Therefore, we have not included it here, but refer readers to the source.

Ted Kaptchuk says that the Rapid pulse reflects the presence of "Heat accelerating the movement of Blood." "A rapid pulse with strength signifies Excess Heat; a rapid but weak pulse points to Deficient Heat or Empty Fire." The exception is when it accompanies a pattern of cold from deficiency, "in which it is a serious sign of extreme Deficient Yang floating to the outside of the body." *The Web That Has No Weaver* (New York: Congdon and Weed, 1983) 162, 304.

CHAPTER 8: Volume

1. Though not immediately relevant to this discussion of volume, for those who are interested, R.B. Amber has commented on volume from a Western perspective. *The Pulse in Occident and Orient: Its Philosophy and Practice in India, China, Iran, and the West* (New York: Santa Barbara Press, 1966) 114.

2. Leon Hammer, *Dragon Rises, Red Bird Flies* (Barrytown, NY: Station Hill Press, 1990) 313.

3. Li Shi-Zhen considers this pulse to be normal in the summer, and otherwise a sign of fire or heat from excess. This heat may be accompanied by fever during a febrile illness, which gradually depletes yin, or "when blood deficiency produces heart fire blazing upwards." Li Shi–Zhen, *Pulse Diagnosis*, trans. Hoe Ku Huynh (Brookline, MA: Paradigm Publications, 1981), 77. It is Dr. Hammer's impression that with heat from deficiency, the pulse may show a tendency to recede more quickly.

   Ted Kaptchuk's principal assertion is that "heat has injured the Fluids and Yin of the body." Ted Kaptchuk, *The Web That Has No Weaver* (New York: Congdon and Weed, 1983), 168. Although it can accompany the heat from excess which we normally associate with this quality, it has not been our experience to identify a condition of yin deficiency as the principal pathology associated with the Flooding quality.

   According to Kaptchuk (314), with a febrile illness the Flooding pulse is accompanied by symptoms of "thirst, irritability" and "red swollen skin ulceration" and signs of "vomiting of blood." He states that "Heart disharmonies" and "Heat in the Interior being restrained or bottled up by Cold on the Exterior" are other etiologies of this quality. He also describes a Flooding pulse "whose surging forward movement is big but lacks strength and which recedes like a regular flooding pulse. If this pulse is accompanied by such signs as diarrhea, the interpretation is that the bigness signifies deficiency [as does an empty pulse], and the pulse is then considered a sign of deficiency." This is possibly the deficient Flooding 'push pulse' observed by Dr. Shen, characteristic of a person who is literally pushing himself in work or exercise beyond his energy. (This quality is discussed with the reduced volume qualities.)

   Manfred Porkert, who otherwise associates this quality with "profuse heat", also describes it as a sign of deficiency and "grave danger" if the quality "persists for some time" during the convalescence of a seriously ill person. Here he fears the "dissociation of active and structive energies", which is essentially what Dr. Shen describes as 'qi wild'. Manfred Porkert, *The Essentials of Chinese Diagnostics* (Zurich: Chinese Medicine Publications, 1983), 214.

   J.R. Worsley calls this the "Large" pulse characterized by constipation, mania, anxiety, headache, thirst, and dry throat. *Acupuncturists' Therapeutic Pocket Book: The Little Black Book*

(Columbia, MD: Center for Traditional Acupunture, 1975), D-8.

4. According to Kaptchuk (315), a Flooding and Big pulse is a sign of ascending heat while a Flooding and Floating pulse signifies exterior heat from yin deficiency. A Flooding and Tight pulse can be felt when heat from excess has persisted for a long time, depleting the fluids and giving rise to heat from yin stasis and deficiency. A Flooding and Sinking pulse indicates "Internal Heat or Cold Restraining Heat" and a Flooding and Slippery pulse indicates "Heat/Mucus."

CHAPTER 9: Depth

1. Ted Kaptchuk classifies the Floating quality under the aegis of depth as "yang" because of its "exteriorness." (Ted Kaptchuk, *The Web That Has No Weaver* [New York: Congdon and Weed, 1983], 161.) Other descriptions of the Floating quality are "floating like a log or piece of dry wood on water" (Paul Unschuld, trans., *Nan-Ching* [Berkeley: University of California Press, 1986] 245); "like a piece of dry stick floating on the surface of the water" (C.S. Cheung and Jenny Belluomini, "An Overview of Pulse Types Used In Traditional Chinese Medical Diagnosis" *Journal of the American College of Traditional Chinese Medicine* 1982;1:14); and "like bird's feathers being ruffled by wind" (Li, 61). In addition to these characterizations, Li observes that it is "steady and moves gently like a slight breeze blowing over a feather on the back of a bird.

2. With regard to the Empty pulse and qi deficiency, Li Shi-Zhen observes: "The Empty pulse appears when the upright qi is damaged—after perspiration caused by unconsolidated Wei [protective] qi, after palpitations caused by heart blood deficiency, or after fear or fright caused by heart shen [spirit] deficiency." Li Shi–Zhen, *Pulse Diagnosis*, trans. Hoe Ku Huynh (Brookline, MA: Paradigm Publications, 1981), 72.

   Some sources also allude to blood deficiency as a cause of the Empty quality, as in the following passage from Ted Kaptchuk:

   > In general, if the Empty pulse is especially superficial, it is said to signify Deficient blood (that is, to have a Deficient yin aspect); if it is less superficial, then it signifies Deficient qi (that is, it has a Deficient yang aspect). Compared with a thin pulse, an Empty pulse is more indicative of Deficient qi; compared with a frail pulse, it is more indicative of Deficient blood.

   Ted Kaptchuk, *The Web That Has No Weaver* (New York: Congdon and Weed, 1983), 306.

   Wu Shui-Wan speaks of two kinds of Empty pulse: "The Soft Empty pulse denotes that the blood is deficient while the Real Empty Pulse indicates that the patient is very weak or weakness due to long illness." *The Chinese Pulse Diagnosis* (San Francisco: Writers Guild of America, 1973), 22. Manfred Porkert, who refers to this as the Dispersed pulse, believes that "the structive part of the qi nativum (the resources of energy acquired at birth and stored in the renal orb) has dispersed, has become diffuse." Manfred Porkert, *The Essentials of Chinese Diagnostics* (Zurich: Chinese Medicine Publications, 1983), 220. In addition, Wu, Li, and Kaptchuk all mention this pulse in connection with attack of summerheat.

3. Kaptchuk (169) calls this quality Soggy, and categorizes it as one of the ten less important pulses. Li Shi-Zhen (188) refers to it as the Soft pulse. Cheung and Belluomini use the term synonymously with "Soft–floating." Chinese Medical Diagnosis" *Journal of the American College of Traditional Chinese Medicine* 1982;1:21. Wu Shui-Wan (32) and Mann refer to the pulse as "Weak–Floating," Felix Mann, *Acupuncture: The Ancient Art of Chinese Healing and How It Works Scientifically* (New York: Vintage Books, 1971), 169. And Wu says further that it can also be called "Soft." She categorizes this with the "Empty Kind." Although not mentioned by its English name, R. B. Amber spells it in the Wade-Giles transliteration as *ju*, which is the same as

ru in pinyin. R.B. Amber, *The Pulse in Occident and Orient: Its Philosophy and Practice in India, China, Iran, and the West* (New York: Santa Barbara Press, 1966), 164.

4. Amber (164) describes this quality as "a soft pulse, superficial and fine—like a thread floating on water." The "thread floating on water" is the description that comes closest to Dr. Hammer's own experience. Kaptchuk (169) describes the Soggy pulse as a combination of the Thin, Empty, and Floating pulses. It is extremely soft, is less clear than a Thin pulse and is perceptible only in the superficial position. The slightest pressure makes it disappear. A Soggy pulse feels like a bubble floating on water. Li Shi-Zhen (88) and Wu Shui-Wan (32) are consistent with both of the above descriptions. Li (61) adds that this quality "is like a bubble, which bursts when pressure is lightly increased." Under the Floating quality he says that the "floating pulse which is spongy, weak and thin is called a soft pulse." Worsley (D–12) calls this the Soft pulse and notes that it is "insufficient, weak and soft; it is without power like a lump of cotton wool dipped in water." Although he does not allude directly to the Empty quality of this pulse, his expression "without power" can be interpreted to have this meaning. For beginners, this pulse quality is relatively obscure. The following comparisons of this quality with other similar superficial and deficient pulse qualities may be helpful. They are drawn from Li Shi-Zhen and Wu Shui-Wan. The Empty pulse is "bigger" (Wu, 32), the Minute pulse is "intermittently indistinct" (Li, 89), the "Weak" (Feeble-Absent) pulse is deep (Li, 89), and the Thin pulse "can be clearly felt at a sinking position" (Li, 89).

5. Kaptchuk (317, 169) asserts that this pulse is a sign of extreme deficiency of blood, essence, and, to a lesser extent, yang. This is due primarily to a loss of fluids and blood after a serious illness, childbirth or miscarriage (including abortion), or after surgery, when the patient has not received rest and nourishing therapy. Li Shi-Zhen (89) attributes the deficiency to "damage to the ying–blood and severe deficiency of yin jing," and "with deficiency in the sea of marrow and deficiency of dan–tian." Even in the absence of disease, the pulse "is said to be without root, due to failure of the kidney and spleen", which should be treated promptly. Li (89) has also found this pulse with "Spleen deficiency with inability to control dampness." Kaptchuk (317) adds that the Soggy quality can accompany a "damp pattern, because the dampness 'spreads everywhere' and obstructs qi and blood movement.... In this case, the Soggy pulse is likely to have a tight, hindered quality." With this pattern, the dampness is interfering with the free flow of qi and blood, and there may be water stagnation at the surface in the form of non-pitting edema in the connective tissue. Thus, the patient is not as wasted as when the pulse is due to depletion of fluids and blood. Finally, Worsley (D–12) describes a Soft pulse to which he ascribes "anemia, bleeding, internal wounds caused by damp and moisture," and Wu Shui-Wan (32) always regards this quality as "a sign of danger," independent of the duration of the illness.

6. Li Shi-Zhen (12) classifies this pulse among the Floating pulses. Kaptchuk (172) includes it among the "other pulses" which he considers to be less important refinements of the first eighteen pulses. Porkert (220) calls it the Dispersed pulse.

7. Ilza Veith, trans., *Huang Ti Nei Ching Su Wen* (Berkeley: The University of California, 1972) 164.

8. Kaptchuk (315) points out that this quality can appear either at the final stage of the depletion of qi and yang, or at the end stage of "Vanquished Yin" and "Vanquished Yang," as an example of the principle that at their extremes, conditions transform into their opposites. The reason for this is the interdependence of yin and yang, such that a severe depletion of one will force the other into almost complete dysfunction. It is at this point that the yin and yang separate and can no longer interact to preserve and enhance life. This condition is signaled by cold symptoms

such as extreme weakness, oily perspiration, loose stools, intolerance of cold, shallow respiration, or what Kaptchuk calls "Vanquished Yang."

For this pulse quality Li Shi-Zhen (24, 79) refers to "the five types of fatigue and the six types of extreme fatigue in men." Wu Shui-Wan (27) mentions "that the body has very weak metabolism ... [that] may lead to death." She also states that if this quality appears suddenly in the course of an acute illness, the prognosis is better than if the quality appears when "the patient has been ill for a long time." Cheung and Belluomini (23) include "shock or pre–shock due to decreased blood volume" as the source of this quality. According to Dr. Shen, who concurs with Li Shi-Zhen, one etiology is excessive menstrual flow at a very early age, which depletes the blood and qi at a vulnerable time in energetic development. Li (24, 79) says that "both blood and qi are Empty." Thus, the patient has less resistance to disease and more difficulty recovering, thereby draining the system continuously throughout life, which may itself be shortened by this vicious cycle of devitalization.

9. Porkert (218) agrees with my picture of the Hollow quality as being completely or partially missing at the blood depth. As he says, "This is a long superficial pulse which readily collapses under the exploring finger and disappears, only to reappear in depth upon increased pressure of palpation." Mann (175) describes "the sensation [as] being shaped like an onion stem; either floating or deep with a hollow area in the middle." In their diagrams and written material, neither Li Shi-Zhen (83) nor Kaptchuk (172) says that the pulse has a bottom. This is a clear departure from Porkert, Mann, and Dr. Hammer's own experience. Cheung and Belluomini (28) refer to this quality as "Leakstalk" and say that it is an "Empty-centered quality," but in their diagram, they show no organ depth. This is somewhat puzzling since Li, Kaptchuk, and Cheung and Belluomini all use the terms "spring onion," "green onion," "onion stem," and "green leakstalk" in describing this quality; these terms imply a hollowness in the center only.

10. Kaptchuk's (319) interpretations of Hollow combinations include the following:

    • Hollow, Empty and Soft: deficient essence, loss of blood
    • Hollow and Rapid: deficient yin
    • Hollow and Knotted: stagnant blood

    Jiang Jing (21) indicates that the Hollow and Stringy quality "means there is an imbalance between qi and blood, and usually extreme deficiency of blood."

11. Wu, 31.

12. Wu (ibid.) writes of "an internal chill which causes poor blood circulation and poor functioning of the organs, forming accumulation internally." She and others who refer to cold are not clear on the pathogenesis of the "internal chill" or internal cold. Li Shi- Zhen (88), for example, regards this pulse as a sign of excess, and alludes to an undefined "excessive perverse qi" causing "excessive internal cold with symptoms like cold pain in the heart region and abdomen," in addition to symptoms "like hernia and lumps in the abdomen." The latter could be interpreted as a neoplastic process, but the translation is not clear. He states that this pulse can exist with excess, as above, which is not serious because the pulse is going "with the current" (meaning with the etiology of internal cold from excess), or with diseases of deficiency, in which case the problem is more serious because the pulse is going "against the current."

    Kaptchuk (171) believes that the Firm quality is a sign of obstruction due to cold, characterized as yang within yin. Porkert (219) mentions "painful blocks in the abdomen," and indicates that when found in a pattern of deficiency "as part of a general 'exhaustion' diagnosis, there is immediate danger of death."

    Whether this quality can be associated with deficiency is unclear. None of the sources seems to refer explicitly to cold from deficiency, such as chronic Spleen or Kidney yang deficiency, although it is suggested. Li (88) and Kaptchuk (318) mention the possible association of this quality with deficiency, including "running piglet disease."

13. Worsley (D–11) is the only source who mentions individual positions and the associated symptoms as follows:

   - Left distal: "thirst, baked tongue, bifid tongue"
   - Right distal: "suffocation, diabetes"
   - Left middle: "abdominal pain"
   - Right middle: "poor appetite, palpitations"
   - Left proximal: "rupture (e.g., of the appendix), tumor"
   - Right proximal: "sore loin and knee, constipation, and dysuria"

CHAPTER 10 Size: **Width & Length**

1. Li Shi-Zhen does not list the terms 'wide' or 'big' among his categories of twenty-seven pulse qualities, but he often does use the word 'big' in his book on the pulse. *Pulse Diagnosis*, trans. Hoe Ku Huynh (Brookline, MA: Paradigm Publications, 1981)

2. Ted Kaptchuk notes, "A Big pulse is usually strong, which makes it similar to a Full pulse, or weak, which makes it similar to the Empty pulse." However, he also says that "clinically, it is possible for a Full pulse to be part of a Deficiency pattern if all the other elements of a configuration indicate Deficiency. Such a pulse is illusionary and is thought to be a sign that the prognosis is poor." Ted Kaptchuk, *The Web That Has No Weaver* (New York: Congdon and Weed, 1983), 305, 307. I believe that Kaptchuk's deficient Full pulse and deficient Big pulse are compatible with the Wide (Big) Yielding Hollow (Deficient) and the Full-Overflowing (Full) qualities described in our text.

3. **Combinations**

   LONG HOLLOW FULL-OVERFLOWING

   This combination denotes heat from excess in the blood, which can be found with such disorders as hypertension. It can also be a sign of diabetes, especially if found on the left side, and especially if it is more Wiry.

   LONG TENSE

   These qualities may indicate a 'nervous system tense' condition if found over the entire pulse (see Chapter 7 for elaboration).

   LONG TENSE WITH NORMAL RATE

   This is a 'nervous system tense' condition, usually constitutional in origin.

   LONG TENSE AND RAPID

   This is another 'nervous system tense' condition, usually associated with tension from daily stress.

   LONG SLIPPERY

   LONG SLIPPERY AND RAPID

   This combination is a sign of heat from excess associated with subacute infection, such as hepatitis. (Acute infection would be associated with Flooding Excess.)

   LONG SLIPPERY AND SLOW

   This is a sign of a lower grade chronic infection, such as parasites or candida, where there is lingering heat from excess in a deficient person.

LONG TIGHT

This combination usually indicates stagnation of Liver qi with symptoms of heat from both excess and deficiency.

LONG TENSE (WIRY) AND RAPID

Kaptchuk (313) states that with this pulse there may be signs of "Lung Heat with coughing of blood," which Dr. Hammer has not encountered. Bleeding, in his experience, is usually accompanied by a Leather-like Hollow quality. Kaptchuk reports that this pulse also accompanies "Cold/Excess with pain and asthma."

LONG FLOATING

This combination signifies a lingering external pathogenic factor, such as a cold or flu, which has been partially internalized with some heat from excess.

LONG FLOODING

This combination is a sign of yang brightness syndrome with severe heat symptoms in the Stomach and Large Intestine, as with appendicitis, dysentery, and peritonitis. Kaptchuk (314) mentions "Yang insanity or epilepsy." He also notes the following combinations, which are outside Dr. Hammer's experience: Long Soggy, described as indicating "alcohol intoxication or Cold;" Long Sinking Thin, a combination said by Kaptchuk to be a sign of "lumps and tumors;" and Long Slippery, a quality which he associates with "Mucous Heat."

Positions

BILATERALLY AT SAME POSITION

By definition, the Long quality cannot be confined to a single position or burner.

SIDES

When one side is longer than the other, some disease process is indicated. *Left:* If the left is Long and the right side is shorter and the rate and other qualities are Normal, this is an indication of a strong 'organ system' and a deficient 'digestive system.' If the rate is Rapid and the pulse is Tight, then we have heat from both excess and deficiency in the yin organs, usually due to an overworking 'nervous system.' *Right:* The 'digestive system' has good qi if the right side is Long and the rate and other qualities are Normal. If the left side is shorter, we can say that the 'organ system' is deficient and that the 'digestive system' is supporting it. If the rate is Rapid and the right side is Tight, then we have heat from excess and deficiency in the 'digestive system,' usually due to eating too rapidly.

INDIVIDUAL POSITIONS

By definition, the Long pulse would not be limited to one position at a time.

CHAPTER 11 Shape

1. C.S. Cheung and Jenny Belluomini also associate the Slippery quality with blood. They observe, "The Su Wen describes the Slippery pulse as present in cases of overabundance of yin Chi, so it must follow that blood volume necessarily increases. Other sources describe the Slippery pulse as reflecting Excess blood and Congestion of Chi." "An Overview of Pulse Types Used In Traditional Chinese Medical Diagnosis" *Journal of the American College of Traditional Chinese Medicine* 1982;1:20. Wu Shui-Wan notes that "If a normal person has a slippery pulse, it denotes that his blood is abundant" and "If a patient has a slippery pulse, it generally denotes that

he suffers from disease due to phlegm." *The Chinese Pulse Diagnosis* (San Francisco: Writers Guild of America, 1973) 19.

Li Shi-Zhen (69, 22) states that "The Slippery pulse usually results when there is an abundance of yang qi. . . when yuan qi fails and is unable to hold the liver and kidney fire, causing heat at the blood level." It is also from "internal abundance of wind-phlegm blocking upward or food stagnation, counterflowing upward, causing vomiting, or remaining below, causing stasis" and from pregnancy. He also notes that "The slippery pulse occurs with internal excesses of perverse qi. These include accumulation or stagnation of phlegm, qi stagnation due to damaged digestion, accumulation of extravasated blood and qi stagnation due to vomiting."

Kaptchuk (308) also mentions "Damp Heat pouring into the Bladder, and Damp Heat in the Intestines." Giovanni Maciocia observes that "Generally speaking, the slippery pulse is Full by definition, but in some cases it can also be Weak, indicating Phlegm or Dampness with a background of Qi deficiency." *The Foundations of Chinese Medicine* (London: Churchill Livingstone, 1989) 168.

2. Leon Hammer, *Dragon Rises, Red Bird Flies* (Seattle: Eastland Press, 2003) 312.

3. Ibid., 168.

4. These are findings and correlations that we make from our collective experiences with Contemporary Chinese Pulse Diagnosis, Contemporary Oriental Medicine®, and history-taking of lifestyle and other factors. We have written about this previously.

5. Li Shi-Zhen (80) describes a Tight pulse as being "like a tightly stretched rope and feels twisted" and "vibrates to the left and right." In the hierarchy of increasing loss of flexibility, a Tight pulse feels thinner and harder than a "stretched rope," which Dr. Hammer calls Tense, and which does not feel "twisted." It should be noted that in extreme cases of life-threatening cold, such as hypothermia, Dr. Hammer finds that the pulse is Hidden Excess (Tense) near the level of the bone, and does feel as Li described it. The "vibrating left and right" with extreme internal cold is akin to the Rough Vibration quality, which, in our system, is associated with parenchymal damage, or what Dr. Shen calls 'organ dead.' Closely allied would be the Choppy quality associated with blood stagnation, which, at the Hidden position, would represent the congealing of blood in the vessels and impending death.

6. Kaptchuk, 309.

7. These citations include: (1) Berg, David E., Hannan, K. L. et al. "Activation of the coagulation system in Gulf War Illness: a potential pathophyiological link with chronic fatigue syndrome" in *A Laboratory Approach to Diagnosis* (Philadelphia: Lippincott, Williams & Wilkins Inc., 2000) 673-678; (2) Bhatnagagar, A., Environmental Cardiology, Department of Medicine, University of Louisville; (3) Bhakdi, S. et al; "Staphylococcal α toxin promotes blood coagulation via attack on human platelets" *Journal of Experimental Medicine* 1988: 527-542; (4) Yamazaki,Y. and Morita, T., "Snake venom components affecting blood coagulation and the vascular system: structural similarities and marked diversity" *Current Pharmaceutical Design* 2007; 13(8): 2872-86.

8. Li, 88.

9. Ibid., 92.

10. Ibid., 93.

11. Deng Tietao describes this briefly in terms of the "pulse on the back of the wrist *(fan guan mai)*." *Practical Diagnosis in Traditional Chinese Medicine*, trans. Marnae Ergil (Edinburgh: Churchill Livingstone, 1999) 91.

CHAPTER 12 **Individual Positions**

1. Leon Hammer, "The Liver in Chinese Medicine" *Medical Acupuncture* 2009 21(3):173-8. For a more complete discussion, see www.dragonrises.org.

2. Leon Hammer, "The Paradox of the Unity and Duality of the Kidneys according to Chinese Medicine" *The American Journal of Acupuncture* 1999 27(3-4).

3. Manfred Porkert, *The Essentials of Chinese Diagnostics* (Zurich: Chinese Medicine Publications, 1983) 244.

4. Leon Hammer, *Dragon Rises, Red Bird Flies*, Rev. Ed. (Seattle: Eastland Press, 2005), Ch. 14.

CHAPTER 13 **The Three (Eight) Depths and Common Qualities Found Uniformly over the Entire Pulse**

1. Anton Jayasuria, *Textbook of Acupuncture Science* (Dehiwala, Sri Lanka: Chandrakanthi Industrial Press, 1981) 517:

   > The distinction between the deep and superficial pulses requires a discriminating sense of touch and the ability to vary in a controlled manner the pressure exerted by the examining finger. ... Little wonder then that many Western physicians after a few trials, or no experiment at all, have dismissed Chinese pulse diagnosis as an impracticable art, based on highly subjective impressions, derived wholly from the amount of pressure exerted by the examining finger and therefore not worth bothering about.

2. Leon Hammer, Ross Rosen, "The Pulse, the Electronic Age and Radiation: Early Detection" *The American Acupuncturist* Spring 2009.

3. John Shen, *Chinese Medicine* (New York: Educational Solutions, 1980) 115.

4. Leon Hammer, *Dragon Rises, Red Bird Flies* (Barrytown, NY: Station Hill Press, 1990) 324.

5. R.B. Amber, *The Pulse in Occident and Orient: Its Philosophy and Practice in India, China, Iran, and the West* (New York: Santa Barbara Press, 1966) 164.

6. Li Shi-Zhen, *Pulse Diagnosis*, trans Hoe Ku Huynh (Brookline, MA: Paradigm Publications, 1981) 95.

CHAPTER 14 **Uniform Qualities on Other Large Segments of the Pulse**

1 Personal communications, 1973, 1995.

2 Li Shi-Zhen, *Pulse Diagnosis*, trans Hoe Ku Huynh (Brookline, MA: Paradigm Publications, 1981) 4.

3 Jiang Jing offers this view:

   > The more common of the two methods compared RENYING on the left radial artery and CHUNKOU on the right radial artery. In this method, the yin and yang energy balance is analyzed through the comparison of left and right sides: right side being yin and left side being yang. Because there are two positions on each hand when Shenmen is included, four types of energy can be distinguished: yang of yang, yin of yang, yang of yin and yin of yin.

   Jiang Jing, " A Brief Survey of the Korean Dong Han System of Pulse Diagnosis" *Oriental Medicine* 22 (1993):18.

4 R.B. Amber, *The Pulse in Occident and Orient* (New York: Santa Barbara Press, 1966) 102.

5 Leon Hammer, *Dragon Rises, Red Bird Flies* (Barrytown, NY: Station Hill) 311.

6 Leon Hammer, *Dragon Rises, Red Bird Flies*, Rev. Ed. (Seattle: Eastland Press, 2005) Ch. 14.

CHAPTER 15 Uniform Qualities on Other Large Segments of the Pulse

1. Leon Hammer, *Dragon Rises, Red Bird Flies* (Seattle: Eastland Press, 2003) 187-205.

2. Leon Hammer, "The Liver in Chinese Medicine" *Medical Acupuncture* September 2009, Vol. 21, No. 3: 173-178.

3. *Dragon Rises*, 300.

4. Ibid., 302.

5. Leon Hammer, "Case Study—Stopping Long-Term Strenuous Exercise Suddenly: An Epidemic Treated with Chinese Herbal Medicine" *Chinese Medicine Times*, April 2011.

6. *Dragon Rises*, Ch. 8.

7. Ibid., Ch. 14.

8. Ibid., 291-92.

9. Ibid., Ch. 13.

10. Ibid., 326.

11. Ibid., 324.

12. See notes 1, 2, and 3 above; also Leon Hammer, "The Pulse and the Individual" *The American Acupuncturist* Spring 2008, v. 43.

13. Ibid.

CHAPTER 16 Prognosis and Prevention

1. Deng Tietao, *Practical Diagnosis in Traditional Chinese Medicine*, trans. Marnae Ergil (Edinburgh: Churchill Livingstone, 1999) 85.

2. Ibid., 140. Another sign of prognosis is the effect of the breath on the intensity and amplitude of the pulse. According to Russell Jaffe, if, upon taking a deep breath, both of these aspects increase, the prognosis is good; if they decrease, the prognosis is unfavorable. We cannot confirm this.

CHAPTER 17 Interpretation

1. Leon Hammer, "A Discussion of Terrain, Stress, Root and Vulnerability within Chinese Medicine" *Chinese Medicine Times*, Vol. 5, Issue 1, Spring 2010.

2. Leon Hammer, *Dragon Rises, Red Bird Flies* (Seattle: Eastland Press, 2003), Ch. 14.

3. Leon Hammer, "The Concept of 'Blocks'" *The American Acupuncturist* Winter 2006, vol. 38.

4. Leon Hammer and Ross Rosen, "The Pulse, the Electronic Age and Radiation: Early Detection" *The American Acupuncturist* Spring 2009:47.

Glossary

NOTE: This glossary contains special terms that were used by Dr. John H.F. Shen, and which are likely to be unfamiliar to other students of traditional Chinese medicine.

'Blood heat'

This is a condition, called heat in the blood in traditional Chinese medicine, in which the thickness of the blood depth is more readily palpable. As one raises one's finger from the organ depth the pulse expands even more in the blood depth than is the case with 'blood unclear.' This is a sign of heat from excess in the blood. Often the blood depth is also Slippery. (According to Dr. Shen, 'blood heat' without Slipperiness is due to overworking the nervous system, while 'blood heat' with Slipperiness is associated with the metabolism of lipids and digestion.) Dr. Shen likens this pattern to a glass containing hot water, in contrast to one containing dirty water, his metaphor for the 'blood unclear' condition.

Two patterns can give rise to this pulse. The first is heat from excess associated with such foods as spices, wine, shellfish, coffee, chocolate and other heat-inducing items. The organs that are usually affected are the Liver, Stomach, Heart, and the Lungs. The second pattern is one of heat from deficiency, which is usually associated with an extremely tense nervous system; from the Chinese perspective, such a system has been working beyond its capacity. Kidney yin depletion usually ensues.

'Blood thick'

With this pattern and its associated quality (Blood Thick), the pulse at the blood depth has become extremely Wide, Slippery (sometimes Rough Vibration) when it is accessed, as described under 'blood heat' and 'blood unclear' conditions. However, with the 'blood thick' condition the pulse continues to widen even to the qi depth. Later, it often develops into a Tense Hollow Full-Overflowing quality, a sign of the later stages of the 'blood thick' process in which the heat from the blood has overflowed into the qi depth, thereby becoming a very prominent feature of the pulse. According to Dr. Shen, an early sign of this condition can be persistent acne after adolescence. The late signs are usually of a cardiovascular nature, such as hypertension.

'Blood thick' has several etiologies and courses. One develops from heat in the blood and is a damp-heat condition involving heat from the Liver and dampness from the Spleen. The causes for this disorder are primarily excessive intake of fat and sugar, leading to elevated levels of serum glucose, cholesterol, and triglycerides. The pulse shows more Slipperiness, especially where the dampness predominates, and less of the very Tense Hollow quality which is characteristic of advancing hypertension associated with the other causes described below. This process gradually interferes with Heart function due to increasing resistance in both the peripheral as well as coronary circulation, which in turn leads to even higher blood pressure, especially the diastolic.

Another contributing factor is a tense nervous system, which causes Liver qi congestion, interfering with the proper digestion and absorption of fats in the alimentary system (Liver attacking Spleen and Stomach), as well as with efficient metabolism of these substances by the Liver. There is a concomitant increase in Liver fire, and later Liver and Kidney yin deficiency along with the development of 'blood thick.' Both processes lead eventually to a Ropy pulse, a sign of arteriosclerosis and atherosclerosis.

'Blood unclear'

This is Dr. Shen's term for a condition in which the blood depth just barely increases (rather than decreases) in size as one raises the finger from the organ depth toward the qi depth. Often the pulse is also slightly Slippery. There is no equivalent term in traditional Chinese medicine.

The most common cause of this quality is exposure to environmental toxins. I first encountered it with artists using highly toxic solvents, often in poorly ventilated rooms, and with the use of acetylene torches, both in art and industry (welders).

Skin symptoms (eczema, psoriasis) are one obvious way in which the body attempts to discharge that toxicity. Another common symptom is fatigue. Dr. Shen likens this condition to a glass of water in which dirt is suspended: the quality of the blood is not good.

A related origin is a stagnant or deficient Liver that does not properly detoxify. In addition to storing the blood itself, the Liver also stores the blood toxins that are not metabolized by the Liver. These toxins contaminate the blood and ultimately the entire organism which it nourishes.

Another cause of this pattern is a qi-deficient Spleen which does not build the blood well due to poor absorption and digestion of food, especially protein. The protein is only partially digested into small chain polypetides the size of viruses, instead of being completely digested down to amino acids. The small chain polypetides are absorbed and the body reacts to them as if they were viruses by inappropriately mobilizing the immune system. Eventually, autoimmune diseases develop.[1]

'Circulatory system'

While all systems are concerned with qi, the 'circulatory system' especially involves the movement of blood, or heavier energy, throughout the channels. There is no known classical source for this connection between Dr. Shen's 'circulatory system' and the lesser yang, except perhaps for its place between the 'nervous system' involving the tai yang and the rapid movement of the most superficial and lightest qi energies, and the 'digestive system' and its logical connection with yang brightness, the deepest of the yang energies.

If the 'circulatory system' is in fact operating at an energetic level between tai yang and yang brightness, this intermediate energy would coincide with the lesser yang level (half interior, half exterior). It is my understanding that Dr. Shen also identifies this level with the muscles.

Because of its involvement with blood, it is especially connected with the function of the Heart. It is particularly affected by the shock of trauma, which tends to diminish the flow. Both overexercise over an extended period of time, and the sudden cessation of heavy, prolonged exercise, may cause a separation of yin and yang in the vessels, resulting in blood out of control, and in turn chaos in the qi ('qi wild'), since the blood nourishes the qi. Milder manifestations are fluctuating symptoms of being easily fatigued, cold hands and feet, migrating joint problems, and being easily angered. More serious manifestations are severe anxiety and depersonalization.

There is no clear equivalent to the 'circulatory system' in traditional Chinese medicine. The *bi* syndrome due to wind describes the migrating aspect of the disorder associated with this system, and Liver qi stagnation is similar to an aspect of its ephemeral nature, but neither of these accounts for the Heart/circulatory aspect of the syndrome.

'Digestive system'

The 'digestive system' (yang brightness) includes the Lungs, the Stomach-Spleen, and the Bladder-Kidneys. According to Dr. Shen, the Lungs digest mucus, the

---

1. William Philpott and Dwight Kalita, *Brain Allergies: The Psychosomatic Connection* (New Canaan, CT: Keats, 1980) 71–72.

Stomach-Spleen digest food, and the Kidneys digest water. The 'digestive system' can be accessed over the entire right side of the pulse when all of the qualities on that side are approximately the same.

Both Small and Large Intestine are involved. The Small Intestine is reflected at the proximal position on the right side, and the Large Intestine at the proximal position on the left side. Both positions represent the Kidneys, which in conventional traditional Chinese medicine control the lower burner, where each of these organs reside.

Symptoms associated with 'digestive system' disorders include fluctuating appetite and irregular bowel movements (changing from constipation to diarrhea). There is no equivalent term or condition in traditional Chinese medicine.

'Heart closed'

In terms of traditional Chinese medicine, the closest equivalent term to the 'Heart closed' pattern would be Heart qi stagnation. This is a pattern in which a moderately Flat quality is a sign that qi and blood are slightly stagnant in the Pericardium, and cannot freely reach into the Heart. The reason is that circulation of qi, and to a lesser extent blood, to the Heart has been blocked from entering the Heart, usually due to a shock. This ultimately leads to Heart qi deficiency and diminished peripheral blood circulation. While with 'Heart nervous' the shock affects the nervous innervation of the Heart, with 'Heart closed' the substance of the Heart (parenchyma) is slightly affected, though much less so than in the case of either 'Heart small' or 'Heart full.'

The shock is most often an emotional one experienced during childhood while the body's qi is still immature, and usually involves the loss of someone very close, such as a parent. However, it can occur later in life due to a major emotional shock, such as sudden bad news or the sudden breakup of a romance in which the person withdraws their 'heart' feelings. Other causes include Heart qi agitation ('Heart nervous') over a long period of time, or even a physical shock to the chest. The Flat wave associated with a Heart Closed pulse quality usually occurs in a person whose qi is already deficient or undeveloped.

This type of person seems to be in some kind of constant emotional difficulty. By nature the person tends to be vengeful and spiteful. The spirit of the eyes can seem somewhat withdrawn, or angry. The person may experience some chest pain in connection with the closing of qi circulation.

'Heart disease '

By 'Heart disease' Dr. Shen meant, as best I can understand it, Heart yang deficiency. This is the end of the process in the gradual depletion of Heart qi and blood described under the headings of other Heart disorders in this glossary, especially 'Heart weak,' 'Heart full,' 'Heart large,' and 'Heart small.'

Commonly, the entire pulse is very Rapid, arrhythmic (either Interrupted or Intermittent), and sometimes Hollow, with the most serious forms of 'Heart disease.' The left distal position is Deep, shows Changes in Intensity and Qualities, there is constant Deep Rough Vibration and/or an Unstable quality (very serious), and probably Slipperiness. Both proximal positions are almost always Feeble-Absent.

Among the causes are constitutional predisposition, congenital defects, work beyond one's energy as a child, rheumatic fever, extreme abuse of drugs, alcohol and nicotine, prolonged chronic disease, and severe emotional shocks to the Heart and circulation early in life. Repressed anger can always be a contributing factor. All of the etiologies lead to a gradual and ultimately extreme weakening of Heart qi and yang, until the Heart can no longer control the circulation.

The symptoms are the same as those associated with 'Heart large' and 'Heart full,' with the addition of greater chest pain, greater fatigue and shortness of breath on exertion, excessive spontaneous cold or beady perspiration during the day with minimal exertion, coldness in body and especially limbs, dependent pitting edema, and greater need to sleep in a sitting position.

Other symptoms are poor concentration and forgetfulness, palpitation even on mild exertion, numbness of the upper limbs, and a suffocated sensation in the chest. If the etiology is constitutional or congenital, the person will be anxious and vulnerable their entire life.

'Heart full' (trapped qi in the Heart)

This is a condition in which the qi is unable to exit the Heart, which I call trapped qi in the Heart. There is no known equivalent in traditional Chinese medicine, but in quasi-biomedical terms, it would be a very slight energetic enlargement of the heart undetected by x-ray, and might also be accompanied by incipient hypertension.

This condition manifests on the pulse as a Tense Inflated quality at the left distal position. When the condition is less serious, the left distal position can be a little Inflated Yielding, and the rate Normal or a little Rapid. According to Dr. Shen, but outside of my own experience, when the condition is more serious the left distal position is Deep, Thin, and Tight, and the entire pulse rate is Rapid.

A minor cause is sudden and very profound repressed anger at a time when a person is extremely active. A more serious etiology is a prolonged birth with the head inside (breech delivery), because it begins at such an early age. Other causes are trauma to the chest, prolonged grief, or following an episode of sudden extreme lifting beyond one's energy, whose seriousness depends on the events. Uncorrected, 'Heart full' can develop into either an enlarged heart ('Heart large,' see below) or hypertension, or both.

Such individuals will feel tired their entire lives, have little energy, and may be rather depressed. They are frequently very quick to anger. These symptoms are similar to, but more severe than, those associated with Heart blood deficiency ('Heart weak'). The entire body may be uncomfortable. There is more difficulty breathing out than in, and some discomfort when lying down on the left side. In a more advanced stage there may be coughing up of blood, because frequently the Lungs become secondarily stagnant due to cardiopulmonary insufficiency from diminished heart function.

'Heart large'

This is the equivalent of severe Heart qi deficiency in traditional Chinese medicine, or an enlarged heart in conventional medicine, as evidenced by x-ray. Some of the qualities associated with this condition are Change in Intensity or Qualities, and Rough Vibration at the left distal position. There can be a positive response at the Heart Large position in the area between the left distal and left middle positions, which is very Inflated and/or Rough as one moves the finger from distal to proximal, compared to moving from proximal to distal.

Another pulse sign associated with the 'Heart Large' condition is a Deep, Thin, and Feeble quality at the left distal position, with a rate in excess of 100 beats per minute. Dr. Shen associates this sign with prolonged overwork in a person with constitutionally deficient Heart qi. An Interrupted or Intermittent quality may also be present, and the Mitral Valve position will be Slippery. A Tense Hollow Full-Overflowing quality at the left distal position, with a rate exceeding 100 beats per minute, is another combination associated with the 'Heart large' condition. Dr. Shen associates this with suppressed emotion over a long period of time. An Interrupted or Intermittent quality, and a Slippery quality at the Mitral Valve position, can also be found with both of these latter qualities. The rate will increase precipitously with movement and stress, and one will find widely different rates at different times during a pulse examination.

The underlying causes are constitutional Heart qi deficiency, any of the other Heart conditions, especially Trapped qi in the Heart ('Heart full') and Heart blood stagnation ('Heart small') with coronary occlusion over a long period of time, and rheumatic heart disease. All of these factors may be exacerbated by chronic, repressed, and profound anger which occurs especially while active.

Also, more common before the advent of child labor laws, but still prevalent in the underdeveloped world, is child labor with excessive physical work at an early age, together with malnutrition. With this etiology there is usually an Interrupted or Intermittent rhythm, and the pulse is Yielding Hollow.

Symptoms include extreme shortness of breath, especially on exertion, difficulty breathing if lying flat on the back or on the left side, and chronic chest discomfort, as well as extensive fatigue. Hypertension is often present.

Heart Vibration

The Vibration quality over the entire pulse or at individual positions is defined by whether it is transient or consistent, superficial or deep, and rough or smooth. Transient, superficial, and smooth characteristics at the left distal position or even over the entire pulse indicate a relatively innocuous process involving passing worries or a tendency to worry, which I define as mild Heart qi agitation (very mild Heart yin deficiency). This sometimes begins with a very mild emotional shock, and often there is a background of very mild Heart qi deficiency.

Consistent Smooth Vibration over the entire pulse is a sign that one is highly susceptible to worry, and will find something to worry about even when there is no reason to.

Consistent Vibration which is rougher and deeper over the entire pulse is a sign of shock, guilt, or fear, and at individual positions indicates parenchymal damage.

'Heart nervous'

This is a condition, and associated pulse quality (Heart Nervous), in which the Heart yin is deficient and the qi is consequently agitated, erratic, and mildly deficient. I refer to this condition as Heart qi agitation. There is often a predisposition toward constitutional Heart qi deficiency.

There are two types of 'Heart nervous.' Less serious is the one due to prolonged worry, either a 'Heart vibration' or 'Heart tight' condition in which the pulse rate tends to be somewhat rapid, 80-84 beats per minute. With this type of condition, the individual will report feeling nervous.

With the second, more serious type, which is due to emotional shock, physical trauma (often at birth and sometimes in utero), there is Occasional Change in Rate at Rest, with no missed beats. When the change in rate is significant, there will be a propensity to panic. If the cause is trauma, there may be a horizontal line under the lower eyelid, a small purple blister on the tongue, and a bluish-green color at the chin and around the mouth. A large change in rate tends to accompany a propensity to panic. A little Change in Rate at Rest is often associated with an etiology before birth, and one after birth with a larger Change in Rate at Rest.

A 'Heart weak' condition (see below) may also lead to the more serious 'Heart nervous' pattern in which case the pulse will generally be Deep and Thin, and the rate on exertion will increase by more than 8-12 beats per minute. On the other hand, a 'Heart nervous' disorder may lead to 'Heart weak.' Smooth Vibration at the Neuropsychological positions accompanies and is another sign of the 'Heart nervous' condition.

The 'Heart nervous' person will complain of easy fatigue, especially in the morning when awakening. Sleep is restless, marked by frequent wakening, so that one is in and out of an agitated state of sleep throughout the night. Palpitations may occur occasionally. The person will report frequent and disturbing mood swings, changes of mind about others and the chosen course of one's life, and as if they are on a "roller coaster" and mildly out of control. There will also be increased irritability, of a relatively mild nature.

'Heart small'

In terms of traditional Chinese medicine, the closest equivalent term to 'Heart small' would be Heart blood stagnation, and in conventional medicine, the closest equivalent condition would be coronary artery spasm and angina. There are mild and temporary, and serious and enduring, varieties.

With the mild and temporary forms, the pattern is usually the result of a sudden shock during which the heart contracts, thereby constricting the arteries of the heart. The constriction of these vessels due to shock deprives the Heart of qi and blood, leading to transient blood stagnation in the coronary arteries and capillaries, and an insufficient oxygen supply to the coronary muscles. The cardiac muscles are tense, the coronary arteries are in spasm, and breathing is difficult. In Dr. Shen's terms, the Heart is "suffocating." The left distal position can be extremely Flat.

With the more serious form the pulse becomes very Deep, Thin, and Feeble. The rate is Normal, slightly Rapid, or slightly Slow. Less often, a Choppy quality has been observed here in the presence of this condition. 'Heart Small' is permanent unless treated, and is equated by Dr. Shen with what he calls "true heart disease," by which he means coronary artery disease.

The etiology of the more serious 'Heart small' disorder is a profound shock at birth when there is prolonged labor and the head has already reached the outside of the birth canal, but is being held back by something like the cord around the neck of the infant. Prolonged fear and unexpressed anger may also lead to this condition, though these emotions may also be the consequence, since one finds in people with the 'Heart small' condition a lifelong, unexpressed, and unexplained fear, as well as some anger and tension. Night terrors and being easily startled are common complaints. There is shortness of breath, in which it is easy to expel air and difficult to take it in. There may be chest pain, usually of a needle-like or stabbing quality in one spot, in the left shoulder and/or down the left arm. Other symptoms are palpitations and cold extremities.

'Heart tight'

This is both a condition ('Heart tight') and the pulse quality associated with that condition (Heart Tight). It is equivalent to mild to moderate Heart qi agitation, which is initially a condition of heat from excess of the Heart (Heart fire flaring up), and subsequently Heart yin deficiency. With heat from excess the left distal position will at first feel Tight in the Pericardium position, as if a strong, sharp point is sticking the middle of the finger with each beat. If the heat becomes overwhelming, the entire position can feel Tense with Robust Pounding. This heat usually has its origins in the Liver, Gallbladder, and Stomach.

With heat from deficiency, Tightness is felt over the entire left distal position. If the condition has existed for a short period of time owing to an emotional shock, the pulse is usually relatively Rapid, between 84-90 beats per minute. Over a much longer period of time, the pulse rate will be Slower, as this condition weakens Heart qi and affects overall circulation. There may also be some coincidental transient, superficial Vibration at the left distal position from time to time, reflecting episodes of worry.

The Heart Tight quality can also be associated with heat from yin deficiency due to overwork of the Heart as it tries to balance the heat from excess in the Liver, Gallbladder, and Stomach associated with worry, shock, Grave's disease, and the manic phases of bipolar disease, and from stimulating drugs and herbs such as cocaine or Herba Ephedra *(ma huang).*

The 'Heart tight' condition associated with excess is marked by symptoms of irritability, tension, and difficulty getting to sleep. With the yin-deficient variety, one is more restless and complains of constant worry, a "racing mind," and sleep marked by constant awakening throughout the night. With both there is mild to moderate anxiety.

Occasionally, there will be some discomfort in the left side of the chest over a relatively large area. This discomfort is an early form of mild angina, which is due to heat from excess or stagnant qi migrating to the Pericardium from the Liver, Gallbladder, or Stomach, and causing a mild spasm of the coronary arteries. There may also be some shortness of breath during episodes of anxiety.

'Heart weak'

This condition, and associated pulse quality (Heart Weak), is one in which the Heart blood is deficient, with some consequent Heart qi deficiency, both of which cause a deficit in Heart function. The pulse shows a large Change in Rate on Exertion, more than 20 beats per minute if the Heart is very blood deficient, and a lesser change (12-20 beats) if the Heart is only slightly blood deficient. The rate may be a little Rapid, Normal, or Slow, depending upon the chronicity of the condition: the longer the condition has lasted, the Slower the pulse. The left distal position is often Thin when the blood deficiency is more severe, accompanied by Reduced Substance if the Heart qi is also deficient.

While constitutional Heart qi deficiency is sometimes a predisposing factor, Heart blood deficiency is most often due to prolonged and severe Heart qi agitation ('Heart nervous,' see above). If the'Heart nervous' condition continues, the pulse will generally be more Tight and the vessels under the eyes will be normal. However, Heart blood deficiency can be due to one or any combination of the following: Kidney essence deficiency, Spleen qi deficiency, and gradual blood loss over time. When blood deficiency is the cause, the entire pulse is Thin and a little Feeble and the vessels inside the lower eyelid are pale.

The patient may experience palpitations throughout the day, especially with activity, because there is not enough blood in the Heart. There is also a general feeling of weakness, depression, poor concentration, and forgetfulness. The sleep pattern is one of waking up and being unable to return to sleep for a short time after five hours of solid sleep, after which sleep returns, sometimes lightly, and sometimes deeply. One will be tired in the morning, though less so than with Heart qi deficiency. A prolonged 'Heart weak' pattern can lead to serious 'Heart disease,' with manifestations such as congestive heart failure.

'Nervous system'

The 'nervous system' is associated by Dr. Shen with the lightest and quickest energy, which would be closest to the surface of the body and therefore identified with greater yang, and especially the Bladder channel whose outer course is accessed for the treatment of psychological disorders. 'Nervous system' messages are by far the most rapidly conducted compared to the speed of the endocrine or circulatory systems.

The equivalent of the 'nervous system' in traditional Chinese medicine would be one of the singular organs, the sea of marrow, which is engendered and maintained by Kidney essence; this refers to the substance of the brain, the spinal cord, and the central nervous system.

'Nervous system tense'

When Tension is found uniformly over the entire pulse, I refer to it as the 'vigilance' pulse because it appears constitutionally in ethnic groups whose survival through the centuries has required extraordinary vigilance. A similar pulse quality can be found today in almost anyone living in a large city, or living constantly with the need to be vigilant. Therefore, a differential diagnosis is required between a constitutional 'nervous system tense,' and one that is due to ongoing chronic stress. Making this distinction is important since individuals whose tension is related to their current life situation can alter their lifestyle as part of treatment, which is not true for those for whom the etiology is constitutional.

The principal symptom is an ongoing tension that may or may not be related to a particular life stress. The tension can be in the family over several generations. Accompanying symptoms depend on the vulnerability of other organ systems that are affected by the heat from excess, and especially stasis, which can be a consequence of this condition when it persists over a long period of time.

'Nervous system weak'

Another condition in which this quality is found uniformly over the entire pulse is termed 'nervous system weak' by Dr. Shen. Again, this is a constitutional condition in which the pulse goes through a series of stages, ending eventually in a generally Feeble-Absent pulse quality with a Tight quality at the surface of the pulse, especially on the left side, and sometimes with concomitant Smooth Vibration. This type of pulse is often found in a person who has a lifelong history of neurasthenia, one whose symptoms are always changing and who is highly vulnerable, unstable, and easily disturbed or stressed, and subject to constantly fluctuating allergies. The pulse does not represent illness as much as physical and mental instability and vulnerability to illness.

The closest (but imperfect) equivalents in traditional Chinese medicine would be Kidney qi/yang/essence deficiency and Heart qi/yang deficiency.

'Organ system'

The 'organ system' (greater, lesser, and absolute yin) includes the yin solid organs, especially the Heart, Liver, and Kidneys, which are accessed on the left side of the pulse when all of the qualities on the left side are approximately the same.

The condition associated with this system is primarily yang deficiency, but includes yin-deficient symptoms as well. Symptoms include spontaneous sweating, being easily fatigued, frequent pale urination, aversion to cold and preference for warmth, diarrhea with undigested food or infrequent bowel movements, and an extreme vulnerability to chronic illness and infections from which it is difficult to recover. There is no equivalent term or condition in traditional Chinese medicine.

'Push pulse' (Hesitant and Flooding Deficient Wave)

The Hesitant Wave is one of two pulse qualities which Dr. Shen referred to as a 'push pulse,' which he associated with individuals who pushed themselves too hard. The Hesitant quality reflects a person who pushes herself mentally. It occurs over the entire pulse and is found in cases of Heart yin deficiency with agitated qi. Descriptively, the pulse wave has lost its normal sine wave form whereby the flow to and from the wave peak becomes sharp and abrupt, instead of gradually rising and falling. The term Hesitant is used because some practitioners experience this quality as faltering or balking, yet not missing a beat.

By contrast, the Flooding Deficient quality is the form of the 'push pulse' associated with an individual who pushes herself more physically.

In traditional medical terms, the Hesitant quality is closest to mild to moderate Heart yin deficiency. I have found that this quality occurs in one who tends to think incessantly about one subject. In its most extreme form, this would be a monomaniacal obsessive preoccupation with a particular aspect of life, usually work, in which the person's mind never ceases to rest, even when asleep. This is to be distinguished from a tendency to worry about things in general, both real and imaginary, which is expressed over the entire pulse as a superficial Smooth Vibration at all depths.

In the early stages, except for the symptom of worry or difficulty in getting to sleep, there are no other related signs or symptoms. Later, the person will seek help because of a strong sense of malaise and a feeling that one cannot keep up the pace one has set for oneself. Individuals with this pulse quality often collapse suddenly, physically and/or emotionally.

'Qi wild'

This is a condition of extreme functional deficit in which, for one reason or another, the yin and yang have lost operative contact and are unable to support each other.

The yin, which is the material energy of the universe, can be thought of as a gravitational force that holds the more effervescent yang energies in check, and when drained can no longer serve that function. Under these circumstances, the lighter yang energies wander aimlessly to all parts of the organism, unable to function effectively without the organizing force of the yin. The result is physiological disarray, which disrupts the orderly circulation of yang to the channels and organs, impairing their ability to maintain function.

Thus, 'qi wild' is a condition characterized by chaos and represents a very serious physiological disorganization and disruption. A person suffering from this condition is highly vulnerable to serious and fast-spreading, even life-threatening disease within a very short time, including cancer, autoimmune, and degenerative central nervous system disease. Mental illness is another form of this chaos.

The pulse qualities associated with the 'qi wild' condition are Empty Interrupted-Intermittent; Yielding Hollow Interrupted-Intermittent; Empty; Yielding Hollow Full-Overflowing (Rapid or Slow); Leather; Empty and Thread-like; Scattered; Minute; and Change in Qualities. To be pathognomonic of a 'qi wild' condition, the quality must appear over the entire pulse.

'Systems'

Dr. Shen gradually developed the systems model when patients complained of symptoms for which he could find none of the familiar signs on the pulse, tongue, and eye examinations that were associated with disease in the traditional Chinese medical system. Neither were there any biomedical diagnostic findings. The symptoms were somewhat vague and shifting and inconsistent. What Dr. Shen discovered was that, rather than specific organ dysfunction, functional systems in their entirety were disturbed. He reduced these to four major systems— circulatory, digestive, nervous, and organ—drawing upon the layering of energy from superficial to deep, as described by Zhang Zhong-Jing in *Discussion of Cold Damage (Shang han lun)*.

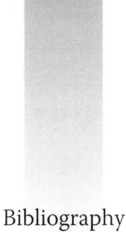

Bibliography

Allport, Gordon. *Becoming*. New Haven, CT: Yale University Press, 1955.

Amber, R.B. *The Pulse in Occident and Orient: Its Philosophy and Practice in India, China, Iran, and the West*. New York: Santa Barbara Press, 1966.

Beijing College of Traditional Chinese Medicine. *Essentials of Chinese Acupuncture*. Beijing: Foreign Languages Press, 1980.

Bilton, Karen. Investigating the reliability of contemporary chinese pulse diagnosis. *Australian Journal of Acupuncture and Chinese Medicine;* 2010;5(1).

Cheung, C.S. and Belluomini, J. An overview of pulse types used in traditional chinese medical differential diagnosis. *Journal of the American College of Traditional Chinese Medicine* 1982;1:1

Dale, Ralph Alan. The demystification of chinese pulse diagnosis. *American Journal of Acupuncture* 1993;21(1):63

de Morant and George Soulié. *Chinese Acupuncture,* trans. Lawrence Grinnell et al. Brookline, MA: Paradigm Publications, 1994.

Deng Tietao. *Practical Diagnosis in Traditional Chinese Medicine,* trans. Marnae Ergil. Edinburgh: Churchill Livingstone, 1999.

Donden, Yeshi. *Healing from the Source: The Science and Lore of Tibetan Medicine,* trans. B. Alan Wallace. Ithaca, NY: Snow Lion Publications, 2000.

Eckman, Peter. Korean acupuncture. *Traditional Acupuncture Society Journal* 1990;7:1

Hammer, Leon. *Dragon Rises, Red Bird Flies.* Barrytown, NY: Station Hill Press, 1990. (Revised edition: Seattle: Eastland Press, 2005.)

—— A discussion of terrain, stress, root and vulnerability within chinese medicine. *Chinese Medicine Times*, Vol. 5, Issue 1, Spring 2010

—— Case study—stopping long-term strenuous exercise suddenly: an epidemic treated with chinese herbal medicine. *Chinese Medicine Times*, April 2011

—— Ecology in chinese medicine. *Chinese Medicine Times,* Vol. 5, Issues 2 & 3, Summer 2010

—— Science east and west. *Medical Acupuncture* 2010;22(2)

—— The concept of 'blocks.' *The American Acupuncturist* Winter 2006, vol. 38

—— The liver in chinese medicine. *Medical Acupuncture* 2009;21(3):173-8

—— The paradox of the unity and duality of the kidneys according to chinese medicine. *American Journal of Acupuncture* 1999;27(3&4):179

—— The pulse and the individual. *The American Acupuncturist* Spring 2008; 43

—— The unified field theory of chronic disease with regard to the separation of yin and yang and 'the qi is wild.' *Oriental Medicine* 1998;6(2&3):15

—— Tradition and revision. *Oriental Medicine* 2001;8(3&4):27

Hammer, Leon and Rosen, Ross. The pulse, the electronic age and radiation: early detection. *The American Acupuncturist* Spring 2009:47

Jayasuria, Anton. *Textbook of Acupuncture Science.* Dehiwala, Sri Lanka: Chandrakanthi Industrial Press, 1981.

Jiang Jing. A brief survey of the korean dong han system of pulse diagnosis. *Oriental Medicine* 1993;2(1):8

Jones, Sandy. *Crying Baby, Sleepless Nights.* New York: Warner Books, 1983.

Kaptchuk, Ted. *The Web That Has No Weaver.* New York: Congdon & Weed, 1983.

Larre, Claude and Rochat de la Vallée, Elisabeth. *The Lung.* Cambridge: Monkey Press, Ricci Institute, 1989.

Larre, Claude, Schatz, Jean and Rochat de la Vallée, Elisabeth. *Survey of Traditional Chinese Medicine.* Paris: Institut Ricci and Columbia, MD: Traditional Acupuncture Foundation, 1986.

Li Shi-Zhen. *Pulse Diagnosis,* trans. Hoe Ku Huynh. Brookline, MA: Paradigm Publications, 1981.

Lowe, Royston. *Secondary Vessels of Acupuncture.* Northamptonshire: Thorsons Publishing Group, 1983.

Lu Yubin. *Pulse Diagnosis.* Jinan: Shandong Science and Technology Press, 1996.

Maciocia, Giovanni. *The Foundations of Chinese Medicine.* Edinburgh: Churchill Livingstone, 1989.

—— *Tongue Diagnosis in Chinese Medicine.* Seattle: Eastland Press, 1987.

Mann, Felix. *Acupuncture: The Ancient Art of Chinese Healing and How It Works Scientifically.* New York: Vintage Books, 1971.

Matsumoto, Kiiko and Birch, Stephen. *Five Elements and Ten Stems.* Brookline, MA: Paradigm Publications, 1983.

Nachman of Breslov. *The Stories of Rabbi Nachman of Breslov,* trans. Aryeh Kaplan. Brooklyn: Breslov Research Institute, 1983.

Needham, Joseph and Lu Gwei-Djen. *Celestial Lancets.* Cambridge: Cambridge University Press, 1980.

Nguyen, Quang Van and Privar, Margie. *Fourth Uncle in the Mountain.* New York, NY: St. Martin's Press, 2004.

Philpott, William and Kalita, Dwight. *Brain Allergies: The Psychosomatic Connection.* New Canaan, CT: Keats, 1980.

Porkert, Manfred. *The Essentials of Chinese Diagnostics.* Zurich: Chinese Medicine Publications, 1983.

Ramholz, James. An introduction to advanced pulse diagnosis. *Oriental Medicine,* 2000;8(1&2):17

Veith, Ilza (trans.) *The Yellow Emperor's Classic of Internal Medicine.* Berkeley: University of California Press, 1966.

Shanghai College of Traditional Medicine. *Acupuncture: A Comprehensive Text,* trans. & ed. John O'Connor and Dan Bensky. Chicago: Eastland Press, 1981.

Shen, John. *Chinese Medicine.* New York: Educational Solutions, 1980.

Townsend, Graham and DeDonna, Ysha. *Pulses and Impulses.* Northampton-shire: Thorsons Publishing Group, 1990.

Unschuld, Paul. *Forgotten Traditions of Chinese Medicine.* Brookline, MA: Paradigm Publications, 1990.

——— (trans.) *Nan-Ching.* Berkeley: University of California Press, 1986.

Wang Shu-He. *The Pulse Classic,* trans. Yang Shou-Zhong. Boulder, CO: Blue Poppy Press, 1997.

Worsley, J.R. *Acupuncturists' Therapeutic Pocket Book: The Little Black Book.* Columbia, MD: Center for Traditional Acupuncture, 1975.

Wu Shui-Wan. *The Chinese Pulse Diagnosis.* San Francisco: Writers Guild of America, 1973.

Index

Bold page numbers refer to principal entries.
Italicized page numbers refer to a table or figure.